STOMA CARE NURSING
a patient-centred approach

STOMA CARE NURSING
a patient-centred approach

Edited by

Celia Myers RGN, ENB216
Clinical Nurse Specialist in Stoma Care, St Mark's Hospital,
Northwick Park NHS Trust, Harrow, Middlesex, UK

Foreword by

James P S Thomson DM, MS, FRCS
Consultant Surgeon and Clinical Director, St Mark's Hospital,
Northwick Park NHS Trust, Harrow, Middlesex, UK

A member of the Hodder Headline Group
LONDON • SYDNEY • AUCKLAND

First published in Great Britain 1996 by
Arnold, a member of the Hodder Headline Group,
338 Euston Road, London NW1 3BH

Second impression 1996

British Library Cataloguing in Publication Data
A catalogue record for this book is available from the British Library

Library of Congress Cataloging-in-Publication Data
A catalog record for this book is available from the Library of Congress

ISBN 0 340 59491 8 (pb)

Typeset in Times 10/11 pt by Anneset, Weston-super-Mare
Printed and bound in Great Britain by J W Arrowsmith Ltd, Bristol

Contents

List of contributors

Marion Allison, BA(Hons), RGN, DipN, DipNEd, RNT
CliniMed Lecturer in Stoma Care Nursing, St Bartholomew's College of
Nursing and Midwifery, City University, London EC1

Carol L. Cox, PhD, MSc, MAEd, PGDipEd, BSc, RN
Head of Department of Nursing and Course Director, Doctor of Nursing
Science Programme, City University – St Bartholomew's School of
Nursing and Midwifery, London

Karen Davis, RGN, ENB216, RN
Formerly Stoma Care Nurse for Croydon Health Authority

Michael J. G. Farthing, MD, FRCP
Professor of Gastroenterology, St Bartholomew's Hospital, London

Gail Fitzpatrick, RGN, RSCN
Clinical Nurse Specialist, Stoma Care, The Birmingham Children's
Hospital NHS Trust, Birmingham

Alastair Forbes, BSc, MD, MRCP
Consultant Physician, St Mark's Hospital, Northwick Park and St. Mark's
NHS Trust, Harrow, Midlesex

Christina Harocopos, RGN, ENB216
Imperial Cancer Research Fund, Clinical Nurse Specialist (Family Cancer
Research) St Mark's Hospital, Northwick Park and St. Mark's NHS Trust,
Harrow, Middlesex

Jacqueline Joels, RGN, ENB216
Clinical Nurse Specialist in Stoma Care, Southend Community Care Trust,
Southend

Rachel Busuttil Leaver, RGN
Clinical Nurse Specialist, Continent Urinary Diversions, St Peter's
Hospital, UCL Hospitals NHS Trust, London

Peter B. Loder, MB, BS, FRACS
Former Robert Luff Research Fellow, St Mark's Hospital, Northwick Park
and St. Mark's NHS Trust, Harrow, Middlesex

Maxine L.V.-T. McVey, RN
Senior Sister, Salmon Ward, St Mark's Hospital, Northwick Park and St.
Mark's NHS Trust, Harrow, Middlesex

Celia Myers, SRN, ENB216
Clinical Nurse Specialist in Stoma Care, St Mark's Hospital, Northwick
Park and St. Mark's NHS Trust, Harrow, Middlesex

Kay F. Neale, MSc, SRN
Registrar, The Polyposis Registry, St Mark's Hospital, Northwick Park and
St. Mark's NHS Trust, Harrow, Middlesex

R. John Nicholls, FRCS
Dean, St Mark's Academic Institute, Northwick Park and St. Mark's NHS
Trust, Harrow, Middlesex

Theresa Porrett, SRN, ENB216
Nurse Practitioner in Coloproctology, Homerton Hospital, London

Mave Salter, RGN, NDN(Cert), CertEdRNT, ENB216 Stoma Care Cert,
CSCT Counselling Cert, BSc(Hons), NursMSc
Clinical Nurse Specialist, The Royal Marsden NHS Trust, Sutton, Surrey

Barbara Stuchfield, RGN, ENB216
Clinical Nurse Specialist, The Royal London Hospital, London

Susanne Wood, RGN, DipN
Nutrition Nurse Specialist, St Mark's Hospital, Northwick Park and St.
Mark's NHS Trust, Harrow, Middlesex

Foreword

Specialist nurses now have an established place in the clinical environment. Their prime role is the provision of excellent patient care, but in addition, and like their medical colleagues, specialist nurses have an important role in teaching, training and research. There is therefore a strong desire to pass on valuable clinical information to others, either by speaking at meetings or writing.

Celia Myers, an outstanding Stoma Care Nurse, has assembled a strong team of nursing and medical staff to share their knowledge with a wider audience. They are all to be congratulated on the excellence of their chapters, all of which will prove of value to the reader.

In addition to chapters dealing with state-of-the-art Stoma Care, including the paediatric aspects, discharge planning, care in the community and the effects of a stoma on sexual function, there are excellent chapters on a wide range of other subjects. These include the two very important types of inherited colorectal cancer (polyposis and hereditary non-polyposis colorectal cancer – HNPCC); physiology, the problems of disordered function and some of the exciting new ways in which they may be corrected; the ways in which both urinary and faecal stoma may be avoided; nutrition support, and the management of p atients with enterocutaneous fistulae and inflammatory bowel disease. Finally current views about the nursing care of patients are discussed. All the chapters are at the forefront of coloproctology and should be the concern of many responsible for stoma care.

St Mark's Hospital for Intestinal and Colorectal Disorders was founded 160 years ago. All the staff realised that the hospital would not be able to provide the high standard of care expected of it on an isolated site and after much negotiation the excellent plan to relocate to the Northwick Park campus took place in July 1995. Celia Myers and her longstanding colleague in Nutritional Care, Susanne Wood, have transferred to the new site and will soon be joined by two more specialist nurses to care for patients after pouch surgery and for those with problems of bowel control. The hospital has a clear vision for the future which will be enhanced considerably by the clinical and academic activity of these specialist nurses.

It is a great privilege to write the foreword to this book which is being published at this exciting time in the history of St Mark's. The text is strongly commended. In wishing this volume well thanks must be expressed to the editor for creating *Stoma care – a patient centred approach* and for all she does at St mark's and wider afield in the teaching and training of staff.

James P S Thomson DM MS FRCS
Consultant Surgeon and Clinical Director, St Mark's Hospital for Intestinal and Colorectal Disorders, Northwick Park and St Mark's NHS Trust.
1996

Acknowledgements

I would like to thank Marion Allison (Tutor College of Nursing and Midwifery, St Bartholomew's Hospital, London) for all her help and support.

Celia Myers

1 Polyposis and the work of the St Mark's Hospital Polyposis Registry*

Kay F. Neale

It would be difficult to find a more promising field for the exercise of cancer control than a polyposis family, because both diagnosis and treatment are possible in the precancerous stage and because the results of surgical treatment are excellent.

C.E. Dukes (1958)

WHAT IS FAMILIAL ADENOMATOUS POLYPOSIS?

Familial adenomatous polyposis (FAP) is a rare, genetically inherited disease affecting about 1 : 10 000 live births (Jarvinen 1992). FAP predominantly affects the large bowel, such that cancer of the colon or rectum will develop from one or more of the polyps. Indeed, 66% of people carrying the gene will already have developed colorectal cancer when they present at the outpatient clinic with symptoms unless they are part of a screening programme that includes prophylactic colectomy. Colorectal malignancy in patients with FAP treated at St Mark's Hospital has been known to occur as young as 17 years of age. The average age at diagnosis of cancer in this group of patients is 40 years, most being in the 25–50 years range. This contrasts with an average age of 65 years for colorectal malignancy in the general population, the majority of cases falling into the 60–80 years range.

In order to 'exercise…control' over cancer as Dr Dukes suggests, it is important to understand how FAP manifests itself and how it is inherited.

Familial adenomatous polyposis is a disease that affects the intestine and other organs, caused by a faulty gene which has been localized to the long arm of chromosome 5 (Bodmer et al. 1987). In 1991 the exact position of the gene was determined. The gene consists of about 8000 base pairs. This compares with 4600 base pairs which make up the gene for retinoblastoma and 6500 base pairs which make up the gene for cystic fibrosis. The genes for Huntington's disease and muscular dystrophy are larger, consisting of 11 000 and 16 000 base pairs respectively. The mutation, or fault, that causes FAP varies from family to family (Miyoshi et al. 1992). In some families 5 base pairs are missing at the same point in the gene: to date, this is the most common mutation to have been found. Many other different mutations have also been detected. In some cases, only a single base pair is found to have been deleted and, in others, there is an extra

*Kay Neale is funded by the Imperial Cancer Research Fund.

base pair. These mutations have been noted to occur at various positions along the gene. It is not yet known how, or indeed if, the variety of manifestations of FAP relates to these genetic changes. It is well known that the clinical manifestations of the disease vary between affected members of the same family, so the relationship cannot be a simple one.

In genetic terms, FAP is an autosomal dominant inherited condition. This means that every person, male or female, with an affected parent has a 50:50 chance of inheriting the gene. The offspring who do not inherit the gene cannot pass it on, so the disease cannot skip a generation. Nevertheless, when reassuring a person that he or she is not at risk, it is essential to confirm that the 'at risk' parent has been thoroughly investigated and not just assumed to be clear of the disease.

The first recorded cases of FAP were characterized by multiple colorectal polyps which, on histological examination, were found to be adenomas (Fig. 1.1). An examination of colectomy specimens prior to 1970 revealed that on average these numbered 1000 in the colon, and ranged from 104 to over 5000 (Bussey 1975). As each adenoma is a premalignant growth, it is easy to see why these patients develop bowel cancer so readily.

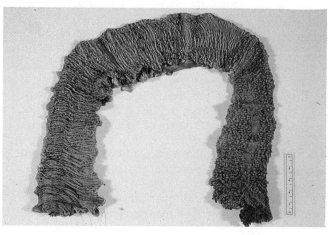

Fig. 1.1 Colon showing the multiple adenomatous polyps found in familial adenomatous polyposis.

Colorectal polyps can often be detected when screening starts in the mid-teens. In some cases, where it has been necessary to examine very young children, polyps have been visible; in other people, who have been examined regularly from the teenage years, the polyps have not developed until the patients were in their mid-thirties (St Mark's Polyposis Registry data).

Extracolonic manifestations of the disease were first recognized in the 1950s when Gardner reported a family with multiple epidermoid cysts and multiple osteomas in addition to FAP (Gardner and Richards 1953), hence the term 'Gardner's syndrome'. Other extracolonic features of FAP have been described subsequently.

ASSOCIATED BENIGN CONDITIONS

The benign conditions associated with FAP are as follows.

Epidermoid cysts

Epidermoid cysts are benign, soft, subcutaneous tumours which may appear anywhere on the body. Removal of these cysts is not necessary unless they are unsightly or inconveniently placed. Epidermoid cysts are rarely found in children outside FAP families.

Osteomas

Osteomas are bony lumps which most commonly develop in the cranium and mandibles of people with FAP. They are benign but the local growth may be unsightly or cause other problems.

Supernumerary teeth

Supernumerary teeth are more common in people with FAP than in the general population.

Congenital hypertrophy of the retinal pigment epithelium

Congenital hypertrophy of the retinal pigment epithelium (CHRPE) has been found to be present in about 80% of people with the gene for FAP. These pigmented patches (freckles), which are thought to be harmless, differ in size, shape and number between individuals. Whilst the presence of the freckles may run in some families, this is not always the case. Their absence cannot therefore be relied on to indicate the absence of the faulty gene (Chapman et al. 1989).

LIFE-THREATENING ASSOCIATED CONDITIONS

The life-threatening conditions associated with FAP are as follows.

Upper gastrointestinal adenomas

Upper gastrointestinal adenomas occur in the majority of patients with FAP and are commonly found in the second and third parts of the duodenum. Gastric polyps are found in just under half of the patients but these are usually hamartomas, a type of polyp not usually considered to be pre-malignant (Domizio et al. 1990). The extent and severity of the adenomas are as diverse in the duodenum as in the colon and rectum. The treatment, however, is not as simple. Individual polyps with a stalk can be snared easily during an endoscopic examination but flat areas of adenomatous tissue are not so easily removed. In those patients in whom a duodenotomy has been performed to facilitate removal, more adenomas have subsequently grown. A few patients have successfully undergone major surgical procedures to remove their duodenum but this type of surgery is not recommended routinely. Trials have been done to test the effectiveness of various drugs (such as the non-steroidal anti-inflammatory drug sulindac) and whilst the results are encouraging it is not thought that significant duodenal disease could be managed by pharmaceutical agents in the long term. A trial using a photosensitizing agent before treatment of the affected areas of the duodenum with a light source (photodynamic therapy) is currently underway and preliminary results are encouraging.

It is difficult to recommend that patients should have regular monitoring of their upper gastrointestinal tract unless a successful treatment can be offered. People working with patients suffering from FAP need, however, to be aware that the duodenum is likely to be affected by this disease and that, although the adenomas do not appear to have the same malignant potential as those in the large bowel, carcinoma of the upper gastrointestinal tract is now one of the most common causes of death in patients with FAP. In fact, the entire hepato-pancreatico-biliary system appears to be at risk (Jagelman, DeCosse and Bussey 1988; Spigelman et al. 1991).

Desmoid tumours

Desmoid tumours are fibrous tissue tumours which may grow on the anterior abdominal wall, in the abdomen (Fig. 1.2) and occasionally outside the abdomen in sites such as the chest wall or shoulder. They occur in about 9% of FAP patients. Whilst they do not metastasize and often remain quite small, they do in some cases cause death. This may be because of their sheer bulk and their location – for example, they may block the ureters or require massive small bowel resection. Surgical intervention is usually avoided (unless these serious side effects occur) for two reasons. The first is that the desmoid tissue will have adhered to other structures, making it impossible to remove the tumour as a whole. This means that early recurrence is likely (Jones et al. 1986), and it is thought that the surgical trauma itself may cause the desmoid tissue to grow even more aggressively than before. Furthermore, it may be impossible to remove the structures to which the tumour has adhered. When a large amount of the small bowel is removed the patient will need total parenteral nutrition. The other reason that surgeons have been reluctant to operate on these patients is that desmoid tumours tend to be very vascular and there is a significant risk of haemorrhage. On the other hand, encapsulated desmoid tumours can usually be successfully removed (Berk et al. 1992).

Statistically sound information about the best way to deal with these tumours is as yet unavailable because these large and aggressive tumours

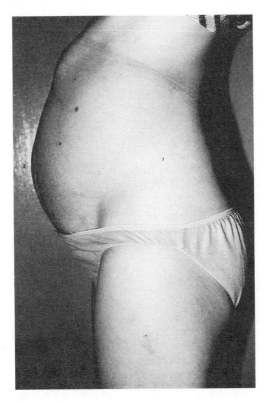

Fig. 1.2 Patient with large intra-abdominal desmoid.

are rare. Furthermore, they will have been treated in a variety of ways, with anti-oestrogens and/or radiotherapy with or without debulking surgery by clinicians trying to find a solution to the individual patient's problems.

Papillary thyroid carcinoma

Papillary thyroid carcinoma occurs more often in women with FAP than in the normal population, the risk being 100–160 times greater (Plail et al. 1987; Bulow, Holm and Mellemgaard 1988).

OTHER MALIGNANCIES

Patients with FAP appear to be at increased risk of developing a malignancy. In addition to those already mentioned, the whole spectrum of malignant conditions has occurred in these patients. Whilst it may be difficult to prove an association with any one malignancy in particular, clinicians need to be alert to the increased risk of serious disease if symptoms occur, thus ensuring early intervention.

When examined carefully, the majority of FAP patients will be found to have one or more extracolonic manifestations of the disease; most authors now agree that the term 'Gardner's syndrome' has lost its clinical significance and should no longer be used (Bulow 1987).

WHAT IS THE TREATMENT FOR FAP?

It was because of the very high average number of adenomas in the large bowel of a person with FAP and because every adenoma has malignant potential that the consultant surgeons at St Mark's Hospital decided that major prophylactic surgery was justified. Indeed, a colectomy with ileo-sigmoid anastomosis was done by J. P. Lockhart-Mummery in 1918 (Lockhart-Mummery and Dukes 1939) and the patient lived for 20 years before dying from a carcinoma of the sigmoid colon. Before World War II, however, major surgery of this kind was rarely attempted. The risk of death was extremely high: anaesthetics, blood transfusions and antibiotics were primitive and the importance of electrolyte balance had yet to be discovered. By the end of the 1940s knowledge about such things had greatly improved, and with the introduction of the National Health Service major surgery was available to everyone.

On 8 December 1948 O. V. Lloyd Davies performed the first colectomy with an ileorectal anastomosis (IRA) at St Mark's Hospital. It was believed that, by taking away the whole of the colon and monitoring the rectum by regular sigmoidoscopy, it would be possible to prevent people dying from colorectal cancer.

By the end of 1992 a total of 252 patients with FAP had undergone an IRA at St Mark's Hospital. The early beliefs proved, on the whole, to be correct. It is of course essential that these patients attend the outpatient clinic at least twice a year for surveillance by sigmoidoscopy of the retained rectum. If rectal polyps are seen to be large or confluent the clinician will recommend that the patient be admitted and the polyps removed under anaesthesia.

Over the years, however, cases of rectal cancer did occur, even in patients who were regularly examined. By 1992 sufficient data were available to show that until the age of 50 years the cumulative risk of rectal cancer following an IRA is 10% but that this risk increases dramatically to 29% at the age of 60 years (Nugent and Phillips 1992). This new information indicated that patients who reach middle age with an IRA must be monitored very carefully and that it would be wise to consider the removal of the rectum and the formation of an ileal reservoir at this time.

Indeed at many centres a restorative proctocolectomy (RPC) is the operation of choice for all patients regardless of age once FAP has been diagnosed. The functional results are very similar to those after IRA and most patients need to open their bowels three to four times in 24 hours. Morbidity, however, is greater following an RPC. The patient will need to stay longer in hospital and the complication rate is higher (Madden et al. 1991). (The advantages and disadvantages of the temporary ileostomy which is sometimes necessary are discussed in Chapter 6 of this book.) It is for these reasons that at St Mark's the IRA remains the operation of choice in most cases. An RPC is normally recommended to patients at higher risk of developing rectal cancer or to those who present with a malignancy high in the rectum.

It is occasionally necessary for a patient with FAP to have a total proctocolectomy with permanent ileostomy. This is usually considered only when there is malignancy in the lower rectum or when the construction of an ileal reservoir is not possible for technical reasons. Even in such cases, lifelong follow-up is recommended. This is because of the risk of other cancers and to ensure that contact is maintained with the family. In this way the next generation will be more likely to be screened at puberty and thus avoid colorectal cancer.

LIFE AFTER SURGERY

The majority of patients who undergo surgery for FAP are young and fit. Following an IRA the patient will, on average, return to normal activities in 14 weeks. Following an RPC this period is, on average, 33 weeks (Madden et al. 1991). There are, however, some patients who find that their work or their social life or both are compromized by the removal of their large bowel.

Patients having an IRA are very likely to have increased frequency of bowel action following surgery, with about half of them unable to delay defaecation for more than 15 minutes. With the need to defaecate occurring about three times a day this can, in certain situations, make life difficult. Following an RPC, patients need to open their bowels an average of five times in 24 hours. The majority, however, can delay until it is convenient. About half of all patients who undergo removal of the large bowel also find it necessary to avoid certain types of food such as fibrous vegetables, spicy foods and beer.

SCREENING ISSUES

In order to 'control cancer' in a polyposis family every person who is 'at risk' must be identified, warned of that risk and, subject to their agreement, screening tests should be arranged. It is important to realize that of those people who carry the FAP gene and wait until they have symptoms before presenting at an outpatient clinic, 60% already have a colorectal carcinoma at the time of presentation. Of those who have been identified as being at risk of inheriting FAP and who attend for a screening examination, only 5% have a colorectal malignancy at that time.

Most commonly a person is identified as 'at risk' if they have a parent with FAP. In some families, however, it is one of the offspring who presents with symptoms and the parents who are subsequently screened. If both parents are found to be free from the disease (and are the true parents) the probability that another of their offspring will be affected is low. Nevertheless many clinicians consider it wise to screen them. When one of the parents is found to have FAP, other offspring have a 50:50 risk of having inherited the faulty gene. It is then important to consider whether the parent has inherited FAP or has the disease as a result of a new mutation. If that parent's own parents are still alive the process can be repeated but they are likely to be elderly and to be unwilling to be screened. It is also possible that one or both of the grandparents have died. In these cases the affected parent's brothers and sisters should be considered to be 'at risk'. If any of them is found to be affected, the children in turn should be screened and so on.

Regardless of the way in which a person is identified, it will be necessary to spend time helping him or her to come to terms with the idea of inheriting and passing on the affected gene. Some people find it difficult to accept that it is better to be screened and, if necessary, treated rather than to wait for symptoms to occur. It can be particularly difficult for a person who has not seen a close relative suffer the consequences of the disease that was left untreated.

The screening tests themselves need to be carefully explained. The method of screening varies from hospital to hospital but should include examination of the bowel to look for polyps. This should be done regularly with a rigid or flexible sigmoidoscope or a colonoscope. If polyps are found, a biopsy must be taken so that the diagnosis can be confirmed histologically. The frequency between examinations will depend on whether DNA analysis is also available. In some establishments barium enema is used but this is not the best screening test for FAP. There is a firm belief in most specialist centres that simple sigmoidoscopy rather than more invasive investigation, such as colonoscopy or barium studies, encourages compliance, especially among teenagers.

In some centres, people who have been identified as 'at risk' will be seen by a geneticist or genetic nurse who will take blood for DNA analysis before the screening of the bowel is arranged. If, however, the patient arrives for bowel examination first, a genetic consultation should be arranged. In a family in which the mutation has already been identified it is a relatively simple matter for the blood from the new patient to be checked to ascertain whether that mutation is present. This is called 'mutation analysis'. In some areas of the UK it will not be possible to arrange for mutation analysis because it is not yet routinely provided by the National Health Service and is carried out only in specialist centres. In addition, there are families in which the mutation responsible for FAP cannot be found. If mutation analysis cannot be done, it may be possible to arrange for 'linkage analysis' to be carried out.

Linkage analysis is not as accurate as mutation analysis and relies on blood or tissue samples being available from several close relatives, both affected and unaffected by FAP. In simple terms the DNA is cut in the laboratory either side of the gene by different enzymes. The resulting lengths vary in size depending upon the enzyme used. These small pieces of DNA are then run on a special gel and a pattern of lines is produced (Fig. 1.3). The pattern produced by the DNA from the affected relatives will often differ from the pattern produced by the unaffected relatives. By comparing the pattern of lines produced from the DNA of the new patient it can be possible to predict with a fair degree of certainty whether the faulty gene has been inherited.

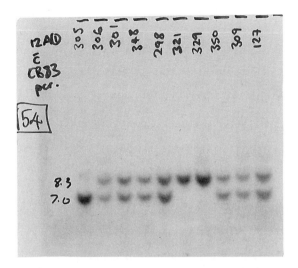

Fig. 1.3 Pattern produced by ten members of the same family when the DNA is run on the special gel.

When DNA analysis is available, it is possible to offer prenatal diagnosis. A consultation with a clinical geneticist should be arranged for those interested. Information about DNA analysis for people living in London can be obtained from the Thames Region's Polyposis Registry, which is based at St Mark's Hospital. For those under the care of clinicians outside London the appropriate Regional Genetic Centre should be able to give advice.

THE ST MARK'S POLYPOSIS REGISTRY

The register of polyposis patients at St Mark's was started in 1924. Initially the aim was to learn more about adenomas, multiple adenomas, the hereditary factor and the link between adenomas and cancer. It was Dr Cuthbert Dukes, the consultant pathologist at St Mark's, and Mr J. P. Lockhart-Mummery, one of the consultant surgeons, who decided that a register should be kept and who, in the early years, interviewed relatives to obtain a detailed history of each family. This work was documented by H. J. R. Bussey who had been employed, at the age of 17 in 1924, to assist Dr Dukes and who, over the years that followed, became more and more involved with FAP and the families attending St Mark's. It was from these records that the mode of inheritance and much of what we know today about FAP was determined.

At that time and right up to World War II there was no point in having a screening programme because there was no treatment to offer. When a person with FAP developed cancer it would, when possible, be surgically removed but the remainder of the bowel and the other polyps would be left. It was inevitable that, given time, another malignancy would develop. By the time many of the patients complained of symptoms, the cancer would be too far advanced to be treated and many died young. But the kindness and understanding that the families received from Dr Dukes, Mr Lockhart-Mummery and H. J. R. Bussey encouraged them to remain in touch with the hospital and they encouraged other relatives to seek help when they too became ill.

By 1948 not only was it possible to remove the colon safely but in addition Dr Dukes had described the adenoma–carcinoma sequence, thus justifying prophylactic surgery. Once a treatment could be offered to prevent bowel cancer, it became sensible to offer screening to all relatives who were identified as being at risk.

From this time onwards, interest in polyposis both at St Mark's and elsewhere increased. Bussey continued to record every detail available to him. Information was sent from doctors practising in other hospitals, both in the UK and beyond. He developed an extensive name index which enabled him to link small family units that did not know of each other's existence and from this he produced family pedigrees for many extended families. By this time he had obtained a BSc in chemistry and in the 1960s worked for a Doctorate of Philosophy on his polyposis studies, which was granted in 1970. In 1974 he retired from his appointment but continued to work four days a week as a Consulting Research Fellow right up to the time of his death in 1991. It is to Dr Bussey that we owe the continuity of the St Mark's Polyposis Registry.

So far, this chapter has concentrated on familial adenomatous polyposis. Two other forms of inherited polyposis – Peutz–Jeghers syndrome and juvenile polyposis – are extremely rare and are associated with an increased risk of cancer. Some of the earliest families recorded by Dr Bussey belong to these categories. For a description of all forms of polyposis the reader is referred to the book by Phillips, Spigelman and Thomson (1994).

When a new case of polyposis (of any type) is diagnosed or referred to St Mark's, the staff in the Polyposis Registry are notified, usually by the sister in the Outpatient Department but sometimes by other members of staff. It is necessary, as soon as possible, to take a detailed history of the family. This can be a time-consuming task. Whilst the aim is to obtain as much information as possible, many people are too upset, nervous or shy at a first meeting to give all the details needed. On the other hand, the process is usually a necessary therapeutic exercise for the patient and any other relatives who are present. It is the Registry's aim to obtain the details of as many relatives as possible and so the names, former names and maiden names, dates of birth and of death, dates of serious illnesses and operations, names of hospitals and addresses are recorded. This information is used in several ways. Names are cross-referenced against those already recorded and, where possible, new small family units are linked into families already registered. Diagnoses are checked by obtaining pathology reports and slides.

The information obtained is entered onto the computer database which is updated as more information, both about an individual's medical status and about additional family members, becomes available. In addition to being an invaluable source for research workers, this database enables a family tree to be generated. If the family is large this pictorial view helps identify those people who are at risk and who have not previously been screened. The majority of relatives who need to be informed that they are at risk are contacted through another member of their family. When this is not possible general practitioners (GPs) and hospital doctors are contacted and warned that one of their patients is considered to be at risk.

From time to time someone will alert the Registry to a baby who has been adopted at birth. People rarely reveal this kind of information readily and it is important to get to know as many members of each family as possible and to get to know them as well as possible. We have learned about adopted babies from grandmothers, uncles, aunts, brothers and sisters as well as from the natural mother or father. Most informants are at pains to make us promise not to reveal to anyone else in the family about what we have been told and, particularly, by whom. Adopted children are traced by contacting the various agencies who may have been involved in placing them. Although it is easier to trace family members while they are young, we have been successful in tracing people of all ages up to the fourth decade.

It is unusual for a person to know or even remember all the details requested by us about their relatives when first seen. It usually takes several meetings to build up a complete picture of the family. We do not ask them to attend formal interview sessions but see them when they are attending the hospital for another appointment. This may be in the outpatient or endoscopy department or when they are admitted to one of the wards. In such a way a family pedigree will grow and become more complete year by year.

Throughout their lives, members of a polyposis family need information, advice, reassurance and support as well as help with the simple practical problems that occur throughout a lifetime of hospital attendances and admissions. The staff in the St Mark's Polyposis Registry are always available, not only for the patients themselves but also for the husbands and wives and anyone else intimately involved with their family. It would be naive to believe that one explanation of all the information needed by a new patient would be sufficient. During any discussion many key facts will be overlooked. For the patient who has just been diagnosed, and perhaps been told that major surgery is needed, details about the genetic nature of the disease may seem unimportant. If that person has children, the details about the surgery may pass them by while their concentration is centred on the details of inheritance.

HOW CAN OTHERS HELP?

Suffice to say that all patients differ and that it is always important to allow time to go over the information that is needed and then to be available to discuss the same thing again or to elaborate other points at other times. A person in a strange environment, such as a hospital, who is being given unpleasant information about an unfamiliar subject will be unlikely to remember very much. All stoma care nurses will know of patients who do not remember being told that they would wake up after their operation with a stoma, despite the fact that they received the most careful pre-operative counselling. People being given information about polyposis are no different and they will not remember everything they have been told. It is because of this that nurses and other health care workers can play a very important role.

A nurse who is looking after a patient with FAP and who has an understanding of the inheritance pattern of the disease will be able to offer, or reinforce, advice about which relatives need to be screened. The majority of patients grow to trust the nurse who is looking after them and will respect the advice that is given. Nurses often come into contact with other members of the patient's family and an understanding of the premalignant nature of polyposis will enable the nurse to encourage a reluctant relative to make, and keep, an appointment with the clinician.

Dr Dukes's statement that a polyposis family is an ideal field in which to exercise cancer control was very prescient. Cancer can be controlled only if a person knows that he or she is at risk of inheriting a premalignant condition and is then offered and encouraged to undergo screening. Those who inherit FAP need surgical treatment and lifelong surveillance. They will in turn endure the emotional stress of knowing that their own children are at risk. These patients and their unaffected relatives need constant understanding and support from all health care workers.

REFERENCES

Berk, T., Cohen, Z., Mcleod, R.S. and Stern, H.S. (1992) Management of mesenteric desmoid tumours in familial adenomatous polyposis. *Canadian Journal of Surgery*, **35** (4): 393.

Bodmer, W.F., Bailey, C.J., Bodmer, J., et al. (1987) Localization of the gene for familial adenomatous polyposis on chromosome 5. *Nature,* **328**: 614–16.

Bulow S. (1987) Familial polyposis coli. A clinical and epidemiological study. *Danish Medical Bulletin*, **34**: 1–15.

Bulow, S., Holm, N.W. and Mellemgaard, A. (1988) Papillary thyroid carcinoma in Danish patients with familial adenomatous polyposis. *International Journal of Colorectal Disease*, **3**: 29.

Bussey, H.J.R. (1975) *Familial Polyposis Coli.* Johns Hopkins University Press: Baltimore & London.

Chapman, P.D., Church, W., Burn, J. and Gunn, A. (1989) Congenital hypertrophy of retinal pigment epithelium: a sign of familial adenomatous polyposis. *British Medical Journal*, **298**: 353–4.

Domizio, P., Talbot, I.C., Spigelman, A.D., Williams, C.B. and Phillips, R.K.S. (1990) Upper gastrointestinal pathology in familial adenomatous polyposis: results from a prospective study of 102 patients. *Journal of Clinical Pathology,* **43**: 738–43.

Dukes, C.E. (1958) Cancer control in familial polyposis of the colon. *Diseases of the Colon and Rectum*, **1**: 413–23.

Gardner, E.J. and Richards, R.C. (1953) Multiple cutaneous and subcutaneous lesions occurring simultaneously with hereditary polyposis and osteomatosis. *American Journal of Human Genetics*, **5**: 139–48.

Jagelman, D.G., DeCosse, J.J. and Bussey, H.J.R. (1988) Upper gastrointestinal cancer in familial adenomatous polyposis. *Lancet*, **2**: 1149–51.

Jarvinen, H.J. (1992) Epidemiology of familial adenomatous polyposis in Finland. *Gut*, **33**: 357–60.

Jones, I.T., Fazio, V.W., Weakley, F.L., Jagelman, D.G., Lavery, I.C. and McGannon, E. (1986) Desmoid tumours in familial polyposis coli. *Annals of Surgery*, **204**: 94–7.

Lockhart-Mummery, J.P. and Dukes, C.E. (1939) Familial adenomatosis of the colon and rectum: its relationship to cancer. *Lancet*, **2**: 586–9.

Madden, M.V., Neale, K.F., Nicholls, R.J., et al. (1991) Comparison of morbidity and function after colectomy with ileorectal anastomosis or restorative proctocolectomy for familial adenomatous polyposis. *British Journal of Surgery*, **78**: 789–92.

Miyoshi, Y., Ando, H., Nagase, H., et al. (1992) Germ-line mutations of the APC gene in 53 familial adenomatous polyposis patients. *Proceedings of the National Academy of Sciences, USA*, **89**: 4452–6.

Nugent, K.P. and Phillips, R.K.S. (1992) Rectal cancer risk in older patients with familial adenomatous polyposis and an ileorectal anastomosis: a cause for concern. *British Journal of Surgery*, **79**: 1204–6.

Phillips, R.K.S., Spigelman, A.D. and Thomson, J.P.S. (1987) *Familial Adenomatous Polyposis and Other Polyposis Syndromes*. Edward Arnold: London.

Plail, R.O., Bussey, H.J.R., Glazer, F. and Thomson, J.P.S. (1994) Adenomatous polyposis: an association with carcinoma of the thyroid. *British Journal of Surgery*, **74**: 372–80.

Spigelman, A.D., Farmer, K.C.R., James, M., Richman, P.I. and Phillips, R.K.S. (1991) Tumours of the liver, bile ducts, pancreas and duodenum in a single patient with familial adenomatous polyposis. *British Journal of Surgery*, **78**: 979–80.

Patient information booklets

These are available from The Polyposis Registry, St Mark's Hospital, Northwick Park, Watford Road, Harrow, Middx HA1 3UJ.

2 Physiology

Peter B. Loder

INTRODUCTION

Assessment of patients in the physiology laboratory has become an important part of modern coloproctology. Appropriate treatment depends on a proper understanding of pathology and insight into the physiological effects of the different treatment options. Physiological measurements of anorectal function may give significant information about the disease process that is causing symptoms and about the likely outcome of treatment. Furthermore, research based on anorectal physiological studies has given us an understanding of both normal and abnormal function of the anus and rectum. It is upon these principles that the foundations of current management rest.

PATIENTS REFERRED FOR ANORECTAL PHYSIOLOGICAL INVESTIGATION

For most patients, the reason for referral to the anorectal physiology laboratory falls into one of several major categories: as an aid to diagnosis, to provide an objective record of function, to assist in the assessment of prognosis, to assess the effect of treatment, for research or for biofeedback retraining.

Aid to diagnosis

Usually, a careful clinical history and physical examination will be paramount in making a diagnosis. In cases of clinical doubt, especially when the different potential diagnoses could lead to major differences in treatment, anorectal physiology may be indispensable. Rarely, unexpected findings during physiological testing may suggest a diagnosis that was not considered despite careful clinical assessment.

An objective record

All clinical assessment is to some extent subjective. An accurate objective recording will allow comparisons to be made, and will help to assess progress at some future time if necessary. Unfortunately, even laboratory assessment is not without some subjective variability. Therefore, its use in such cases must be with some caution, especially if any future comparison is made employing different techniques or within the same unit.

Many clinicians would consider an objective record to be mandatory in cases where there has been previous surgical treatment or injury to the rectum or anal canal and where planned treatment carries a risk of impaired function. Physiological data may be indispensable in medico-legal cases.

Assessment of prognosis

There are some conditions in which the outcome of treatment may vary considerably. Physiological measurements may have some value in predicting how likely it is that treatment will be successful. With the benefit of this information, the clinician and the patient may choose not to proceed with a course of treatment that is unlikely to result in improvement.

Effect of treatment

Clinical outcome is the ultimate arbiter of success of any treatment. With complex problems, however, it may be useful to assess the effect that a treatment has had on physiological aspects, independent of any change in symptomatology. In cases of unsuccessful treatment, this may help to detect the causes of failure.

Research

Studies of both normal subjects and patients have been essential to our understanding of the mechanisms of normal continence and defaecation and in defining the causes of dysfunction. The late Sir Alan Parks, who was a consultant surgeon at St Mark's Hospital, realized the potential importance of such research and established the unit that is now named in his memory.

Biofeedback training

In some patients, the anus and rectum are anatomically normal but function is disordered. This may be the result of neurological input from higher centres. Such patients may be assisted to regain normal function by using physiological measurement apparatus to allow the patient to distinguish normal from abnormal muscle activity.

NORMAL PHYSIOLOGICAL FUNCTION OF THE RECTUM AND ANUS

This section gives a brief outline of the important features of physiological function and is intended only as an introduction to facilitate understanding of physiological investigations. Considerable uncertainty remains concerning many detailed aspects of anorectal function and the interested reader should refer to the literature on this subject for more information.

The anus, rectum and pelvic floor function together as a unit and their separation for the purpose of description is somewhat artificial if unavoidable. Together, theirs is among the most complex tasks undertaken by any organ system. Normal social and physical functioning require that they complete their tasks with a high degree of success.

The colon may present the rectum with various quantities of gas, liquid or solid material in circumstances that may range from a crowded train to a strenuous tennis match. The nature of the contents must be discerned and the appropriateness of allowing their egress assessed. When release of contents is inappropriate, complete continence should be preserved for as long as is necessary. Evacuation, when appropriate, should be rapid, complete and with minimal straining.

The rectum

The rectum is the terminal portion of the large bowel. It is approximately 15 cm long and lies within the pelvis. At its lower end, it is angulated posteriorly to become the anal canal at the level of the muscular pelvic floor. This angulation may be important in preserving continence. The junction with the sigmoid colon at its upper end is usually marked by a forward angulation but this may be indistinct.

Functionally, the rectum acts as a reservoir. It is compliant, meaning that it can distend easily. The three rectal folds that are visible on sigmoidoscopy may slow the passage of faecal matter as it enters the rectum. In normal circumstances, the increase in pressure within the rectum as it fills will be limited and will not overcome the sphincter mechanism.

The rectum also has an important sensory function, both to allow for appropriate behavioural responses to rectal filling and to enable normal reflexes to function, preventing spontaneous evacuation. Receptors in the rectal wall and in the fat that surrounds the lower rectum may be important in this regard.

During evacuation, the pressure within the rectum increases because of contraction of the abdominal wall and pelvic floor muscles. There may be some additional contribution from the involuntary muscle in the rectal wall.

Muscles of the pelvic floor

Examination of the bony pelvis from below reveals a large opening. In life, the abdominal contents are prevented from falling through this hole by a series of muscles which together are known as the levator anti, pelvic diaphragm or pelvic floor. Of these muscles, it is the puborectalis that has the most important role in normal continence and defaecation. This muscle attaches to the pubic bones anteriorly and passes behind the anorectal junction posteriorly as a sling. As a consequence, the anorectal angle is held forward, maintaining the angle between the rectum and the anal canal. This angulation was believed to be important in normal continence; however, recent evidence does not support this concept. The contribution of puborectalis to pressure in the upper anal canal and, in particular, reflex contraction during increases in intra-abdominal pressure is, without doubt, extremely important.

During defaecation, the puborectalis normally relaxes, reducing pressure in the upper anal canal and straightening the angle between the rectum and the anus. In some patients, the puborectalis may fail to relax or may even contract during attempts to evacuate. The terms 'anismus' and 'puborectalis paradox' have been used to describe this abnormality.

Although the other muscles of the pelvic floor may not make such a prominent individual contribution to anorectal function, they remain important for normal rectal, urinary and sexual function. During normal evacuation, co-ordinated contraction of the posterior elements of the pelvic floor may make an important contribution to the increase in pressure in the rectum.

The anus

The anus is the most distal part of the gastrointestinal tract where the rectum forms a narrow canal which leaves the body. In its upper part, the anal canal is lined by epithelium, which is similar to that of the rectum. This is relatively insensitive to touch and pain sensation. More distally, the anal canal is lined by modified, hairless skin which is highly sensitive. Its upper boundary is marked by a crenated line known as the dentate line. Immediately above the dentate line the anal transitional zone extends for approximately 1–1.5 cm. This appears to have a highly specialized sensation, which has the role of distinguishing gaseous rectal contents from liquid and solid matter.

Deep to the lining of the anal canal is a specialized plexus of veins with a supporting network of fibrous connective tissue and smooth muscle. The plexus is usually concentrated in three regions around the circumference of the anal canal to form the anal cushions. This arrangement is important in providing a seal to the anus, yet allowing a large degree of dilatation during defaecation. The role of these cushions in continence may be likened to the function of a washer in a tap; failure is more likely to result in minor leakage than major incontinence. Haemorrhoids (piles) are the result of distal displacement of these cushions.

The anal sphincter mechanism comprises two types of muscle.

Innermost is the internal anal sphincter, formed by a thickening of the lowermost portion of the circularly orientated (smooth) muscle of the rectum. This layer is responsible for maintaining the anus in its normally closed state, and generates most of the pressure measured in the anal canal at rest. When the rectum is distended, the internal sphincter relaxes. This is mediated by nerves within the rectal wall and is known as the rectosphincteric reflex. It has been postulated that this allows rectal contents to come into contact with the specialized receptors in the anal transitional zone, thus allowing their nature to be discerned. As a result, this phenomenon is sometimes called sampling. However, there is considerable disagreement among researchers and this term is best avoided. Patients with the congenital condition of Hirschsprung's disease lack the nerves responsible for mediating this reflex.

Surrounding the internal sphincter there is a ring of voluntary (striated) muscle, the external anal sphincter. It is continuous above with the puborectalis muscle, which was described with the muscles of the pelvic floor. These muscles function together as a unit. They contribute part of the resting tone of the anus but have a more important role in generating increased pressure for short periods as required. They are activated either by voluntary 'squeezing' of the anus or by reflex contraction. Voluntary contraction may occur when contents have entered the rectum, causing reflex relaxation of the internal sphincter and generating a sensation of an urge to evacuate. If evacuation is inappropriate, voluntary contraction will normally prevent passage of rectal contents until internal sphincter tone is restored (as the rectum adapts to its new degree of distension) or until it is appropriate to allow egress of the rectal contents.

Reflex contraction of the external anal sphincter most commonly occurs in response to increases in intra-abdominal pressure during such events as coughing or lifting a heavy object. Were this mechanism not present, such activities would result in elevation of the pressure in the rectum to levels above the resting pressure in the anus and allow rectal contents to escape.

The external anal sphincter receives its nerve supply from the pudendal nerve. This nerve passes along the side wall of the pelvis within a fibrous canal. It is liable to injury at the point where it leaves this canal either because of stretching during straining at stool or during childbirth. This is known as pudendal neuropathy.

INVESTIGATIONS PERFORMED IN THE PHYSIOLOGY LABORATORY

Clinical history

Time and patient discomfort do not permit every available test to be performed in every case. The choice of investigations must be tailored to the clinical situation. Also, for tests performed in the physiology laboratory, even normal individuals may vary greatly. As a result, appropriate interpretation of findings can be made only in the context of the clinical setting.

For these reasons, physiological tests should always be preceded by a thorough clinical history. Besides a thorough description of the presenting problem, precise details of the patient's bowel habit and continence to flatus, liquid and solids are sought. Previous medical and surgical history and obstetric history are thoroughly explored and the patient is questioned about medications that may affect colonic or anorectal function. It is also helpful to know the findings of a thorough clinical examination, but this should not be done immediately before performing manometry because the findings may be affected.

Manometry

Anorectal manometry is the measurement of pressure within the rectum and anal canal. Several different types of manometry equipment may be used, each having some advantages and some disadvantages. Table 2.1 summarizes the advantages and disadvantages of the most commonly used manometry devices. In addition to different types of manometry apparatus, different laboratories may diverge in the technique of measurement (Table 2.2) and in the interpretation of pressure tracings. As a result, findings in one laboratory cannot be compared directly with those of another. It follows that repeated measurements in one patient to assess progress or the effect of an intervention (such as an operation) will be valuable only if performed in the same laboratory.

The technique that will be described is that used in the Sir Alan Parks Physiology Unit at St Mark's Hospital. The method uses a water-filled microballoon, employing a 'station pull-through' technique. This method is simple, rapid and reproducible, yielding clinically useful results. Other techniques may have particular advantages in some research applications.

Equipment

The probe is a 4-mm diameter latex microballoon fastened to the end of a ureteric catheter. A three-way tap connects this to a pressure transducer. The semi-disposable type used for monitoring blood pressure during anaesthesia and in intensive care is ideal. Air is excluded by filling the system with water. Output from the transducer is amplified and displayed on a chart recorder. Figure 2.1 diagrammatically displays the important components.

Technique

After checking that all air has been excluded, the system is calibrated by adjusting the pen deflection as the balloon is raised through a set height (e.g. 20 cm). Elevation of the balloon through 1 centimetre creates a pressure of 1 cmH$_2$O. After placing the patient in the left lateral position, the system is zeroed with the balloon at the level of the anal canal. Lubricating jelly is applied to the balloon which is then inserted into the rectum and the pressure noted.

Slowly, the probe is withdrawn until the first significant upward

Table 2.1 Apparatus used for anorectal manometry

Apparatus	Advantages	Disadvantages
Water-filled microballoon	Simple Inexpensive Easily calibrated Good overall assessment	Measures at one level only Affected by balloon size No directional information
Larger diameter balloons (historical interest only)	Simple Inexpensive Allow use of simple transducers	Balloon size influences pressures
Air-filled microballoon	Simple Inexpensive Portable Zero to atmosphere	Inaccurate at high pressures Averages pressure over longer distance Less rapid response to pressure changes May be influenced by warming of air
Open-ended tube	Minimal stimulation	Frequent tube blockage
Perfused tubes	Allow assessment at multiple levels Directional information	Water may cause stimulation Expensive Technical difficulties Difficulty in interpretation of multiple level, directional information
Catheter-mounted solid state microtransducers	Zero to atmosphere Directional information Suitable for ambulatory measurement	Expensive Fragile Bulky if multiple transducers

Table 2.2 Techniques of anorectal manometry

Technique	Description	Assessment
Laboratory – station pull-through	Patient studied in the left lateral position over a period of some minutes. The probe is inserted into the rectum and then withdrawn at intervals of 0.5–1 cm. The pressure is recorded at each level after sufficient time to allow stabilization. After measuring resting pressure, the procedure is repeated for voluntary contraction	Limited to laboratory, but provides accurate, reproducible information, including fluctuations in pressure
Laboratory – continuous pull-through	After stabilization, the probe is withdrawn in a continuous manner at a fixed rate by a motorized device. The position within the anal canal is indicated by the time after commencement of withdrawal	Sensation of the movement in the anal canal may cause reflex contraction of the external sphincter. Unable to assess pressure fluctuations
Laboratory – stationary, simultaneous multi-level	The probe is placed with the sensors at known positions in the anal canal and rectum. Recordings are made over several minutes	Limited to laboratory and may not record events associated with symptoms. Can record pressure fluctuations at several levels simultaneously
Ambulatory – stationary, simultaneous multi-level	The probe is placed in a known position in the anal canal, within the laboratory. Continuous recording occurs over several hours (usually 24) while the patient engages in normal activities, or those which normally precipitate symptoms	

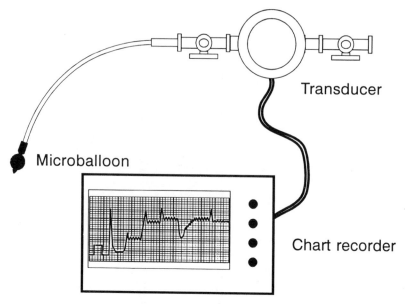

Fig. 2.1 The basic apparatus for anorectal manometry using the water-filled microballoon. The latex microballoon has a diameter of 4 mm. It is secured to a ureteric catheter. Air is excluded from the balloon and catheter during the preparation; the three-way taps allow flushing of the transducer chamber. For optimum responsiveness, the volume of water within the tubing should be minimized.

deflection of pressure is noted. At this point, the balloon is at the upper limit of the functional anal canal. The physiologist marks the position of the anal verge on the catheter. Upon withdrawal of the balloon, the distance between this point and the centre of the balloon is measured to give the manometric anal canal length.

From the upper limit of the anal canal, the balloon is withdrawn in steps of 0.5–1.0 cm. A tracing is recorded at each of these 'stations', allowing sufficient time for the pressure to stabilize. The maximum resting pressure is the largest of the pressures so recorded (Fig. 2.2).

In most resting pressure traces, regular pressure fluctuations may be observed. The most rapid of these is a vascular pulsation in time with the heart beat. Slow waves are pressure fluctuations of variable height occurring with a frequency of 15–20 per minute. They may be observed in most patients and are caused by rhythmic contractions of the internal anal sphincter. Abnormal patterns of pressure fluctuation may be observed. In patients with coloanal or ileoanal anastomoses, slow waves may be large and irregular. Particularly in subjects with increased resting pressure such as those with anal fissure or haemorrhoids, a large, very slow rhythmical contraction may be observed. These ultraslow waves occur with a frequency of less than three per minute. Sometimes, they may disappear after a few cycles, when they are known as fading ultraslow waves. Another abnormality which may be observed is that of waxing and waning slow

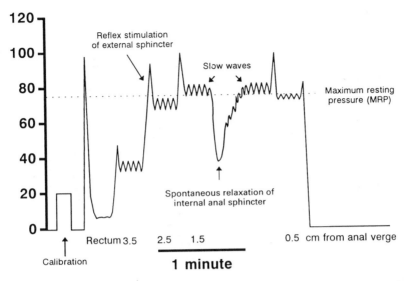

Fig. 2.2 A diagrammatic illustration of a typical resting pressure tracing showing recordings at 1 cm stations. The spontaneous internal anal sphincter relaxation would not be seen during the time period of most laboratory studies. At this time, the patient may report the desire to pass flatus. Stimulation caused by movement of the balloon between stations results in a reflex contraction of the external sphincter, causing a temporary increase in pressure.

waves. Figure 2.3 illustrates these phenomena diagrammatically. Their origin is unknown.

After recording the resting pressure trace, the balloon is reinserted into the rectum and again withdrawn in steps. After the pressure trace has stabilized at each station, the patient is asked to 'squeeze' the balloon as firmly as possible, holding the contraction for 10–15 seconds. The patient is asked to give a solid cough or alternatively to blow against a set pressure. These manoeuvres, which cause reflex contraction of the puborectalis and external anal sphincter, can enable poor effort to be distinguished from genuine muscle dysfunction.

There is considerable variability in the way in which this test may be reported, and caution must be exercised in comparing results from different laboratories. In the Sir Alan Parks Physiology Unit, the maximum increment above resting pressure is reported as the voluntary contraction pressure. Other units use the same term to describe the maximum total pressure generated during voluntary contraction. 'Maximum anal pressure' may be a better term, which avoids confusion. It should be noted that the maximum anal pressure may not be the same as the sum of the voluntary contraction pressure and the maximum resting pressure because the maximum resting pressure and the maximum voluntary contraction pressure are often recorded at different levels of the anal canal. We prefer to report the increment, however, because it gives the best guide to the function of the external anal sphincter and the puborectalis. The total

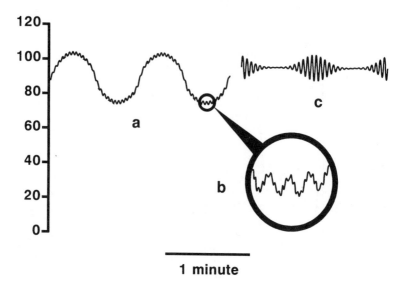

Fig. 2.3 Variations in pressure during resting manometry. (a) Ultraslow waves. These are large pressure variations superimposed on the slow wave variation occurring with a frequency of less than 1.5 per minute. (b) Vascular pressure waves. Magnification of a portion of the trace reveals these, usually small fluctuations in time with the heart beat. (c) Waxing and waning slow waves. Like ultraslow waves, these occur more frequently in patients with increased resting pressure.

pressure generated, however, may be a better reflection of the likelihood of an incontinence episode during a rise in rectal pressure. A typical tracing is illustrated in Fig. 2.4.

Perineometry

The St Mark's perineometer (Fig. 2.5) is a device for measuring the position of the pelvic floor. With the patient lying in the left lateral position, the 'feet' of the perineometer are placed on the ischial tuberosities (the bones on which we sit). By adjusting the position of the glass slide so that it is touching the anal verge, the position of the perineum above (positive) or below (negative) the level of the ischial tuberosities is measured. Resting and straining measurements are taken. Abnormal perineal descent is noted when the position of the perineum is below the ischial tuberosities either at rest or with straining.

Sensation

Normal sensation is vital for proper function of the anus and rectum. There are no tests available specifically to examine specialized anal

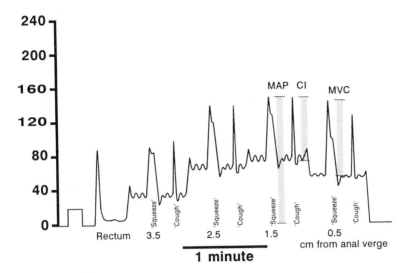

Fig. 2.4 A typical tracing to show voluntary contraction and cough increment. MAP = maximum anal pressure, the total pressure generated during a voluntary 'squeeze'; CI = cough increment, the increased pressure generated during a cough; MVC = maximum voluntary contraction, the highest increase in pressure during a voluntary contraction. Note that, in this case, maximum anal pressure ≠ maximum resting pressure + maximum voluntary contraction.

sensation. The three commonly used techniques will detect markedly impaired sensory function.

Electrosensitivity

This technique measures the amount of current required to produce a sensation and is used to assess sensation in both the anus and the rectum. Current is produced by an electrical pulse generator with an adjustable current output. The contact with the mucosal surface is through a ring electrode attached to a small Foley catheter. A built-in mechanism ensures that contact between the electrode and the mucosal surface is satisfactory and that the set current is delivered accurately. The sensation that the patient is expected to feel is demonstrated ('tapping' in the anal canal or 'vague discomfort' in the rectum), following which threshold current (current at which the patient is first aware of the sensation) is recorded.

Increased mucosal electrosensitivity threshold indicates impaired sensation, which may occur with neurological disease. In our laboratory, anal electrosensitivity is measured in the mid-anal canal only. In contrast to some others, it is our experience that the 1 cm separation between the components of the ring electrode renders separate assessment in the distal, middle and proximal anal canals meaningless because of the large amount of overlap in most patients.

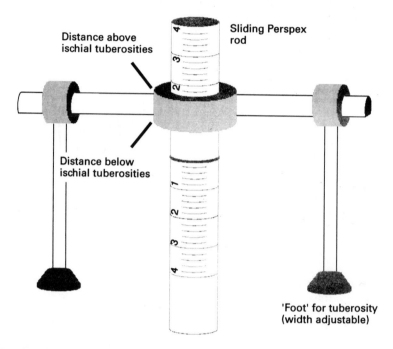

Fig. 2.5 The St Mark's perineometer used for measuring perineal position at rest and during straining.

Balloon distension

Using nothing more sophisticated than a party balloon secured to some plastic tubing and a three-way tap, the smallest volume that can be sensed in the rectum (sensory threshold volume), the volume required to produce an urge to defaecate (urge volume) and the largest volume that may be tolerated (maximum tolerated volume) are measured. To perform the test, the balloon is placed within the rectum 6 cm above the sphincters. Correct placement is ensured by inflating the balloon with 60 ml air and deflating before commencing measurement. Using a syringe, air is injected slowly and the volumes at which each of the above sensations is reported are recorded.

Increased volumes may indicate sensory impairment or an unusually large rectum (megarectum). Reduced volumes may occur with disuse after diverting colostomy, as a result of inflammatory bowel disease or after radiation therapy. Accuracy may be improved to a small extent by using a standard balloon (e.g. a 10 cm condom) or by distending with water.

Temperature sensation

It has been proposed that part of the special sensation of the anal canal is mediated through changes in temperature. This has prompted some investigators to examine the sensory threshold to change in temperature using a heater probe. There is scant evidence to support the role of temperature in anal special sensation and the test is not widely available. Nevertheless, it remains a useful technique for assessing general sensation.

Rectoanal inhibition

Distension of the rectum normally causes a reflex relaxation of the internal anal sphincter. This phenomenon is known as the rectoanal inhibitory reflex or rectosphincteric reflex. To display the reflex, anal pressure is recorded while a balloon in the rectum is rapidly inflated with 50 ml air and then deflated. A normal result is that the anal pressure will fall and then return to its previous level within one minute (Fig. 2.6). If the pressure fails to return to the preinflation level, the probe may have moved and the result is not valid. When the reflex cannot be shown with 50 ml air, it should be repeated with successively larger volumes until the sensory threshold volume is exceeded. Failure to do so may lead to a false

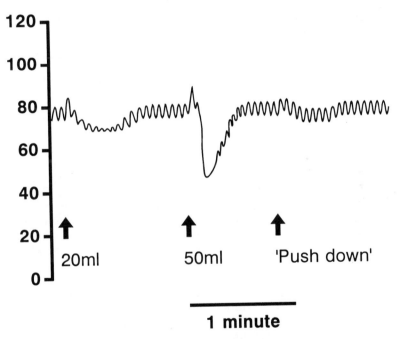

Fig. 2.6 A manometry tracing demonstrating the rectoanal inhibitory reflex and normal inhibition of the external anal sphincter with straining. At first the rectal balloon has been inflated with 20 ml air and immediately deflated. Partial inhibition is demonstrated. In the middle part of the tracing, 50 ml air has been used with much greater inhibition. Note that in both cases there is a small initial increase in pressure because of reflex contraction of the external anal sphincter. The right-hand part of the tracing demonstrates the normal fall in pressure when a subject is asked to push down. Note that there is minimal change in the amplitude of the slow waves.

diagnosis of Hirschsprung's disease in cases of idiopathic megarectum. In cases of difficulty, inhibition may be produced by stimulating the rectum with an electrical current.

Clinically, all that is important is whether or not the reflex can be demonstrated. Characteristics such as the lowest volume at which inhibition can be shown, the volume at which inhibition is maximal and the residual pressure with maximal inhibition are mainly of interest in the research setting. For such measurements to be valid, a rigidly standard technique must be used.

Neural latencies

These techniques assess the velocity of transmission of nerve impulses. Most nerves are formed from a collection of several different types of nerve fibre. These differ in their function (sensory or motor), their size and their velocity of transmission. The larger, myelinated fibres generally have faster conduction velocities and are most susceptible to damage from injury or disease. As a result, slowing of nerve conduction is a common finding in nerve injury.

Pudendal nerve terminal motor latency (PNTML) is the most commonly performed test of this type. It assesses conduction along the pudendal nerve to the external anal sphincter by measuring the time taken for a contraction of the muscle to begin after the nerve is stimulated adjacent to the ischial spine (the point where the nerve leaves its fibrous canal). The St Mark' s Pudendal Electrode (Dantec Electronics Limited, Bristol, UK) allows simultaneous stimulation of the pudendal nerve and recording of the electrical activity of the external anal sphincter. It is affixed to the index finger of a gloved hand. The ischial spine is palpated through the rectum so that the stimulating electrodes at the tip of the finger are overlying the pudendal nerve. At the base of the finger, lying within the anal canal, the recording electrodes allow detection of the motor response. An appropriate neurophysiological apparatus provides the stimulating current and displays the output from the recording electrode (Figs. 2.7 and 2.8).

Other latencies may be relevant to anorectal dysfunction. Spinal latencies record the time taken for a stimulus applied over the spine to initiate a contraction of the external anal sphincter. Because this test is difficult to perform and very uncomfortable for the patient, it is appropriate only when the clinical findings suggest a spinal neurological lesion. Perineal nerve latencies assess conduction along the perineal branch of the pudendal nerve, which supplies the striated muscle of the urethral sphincter. In this test, the pudendal nerve is stimulated in the same manner as for pudendal latencies, while the response is recorded from an electrode in the urethra.

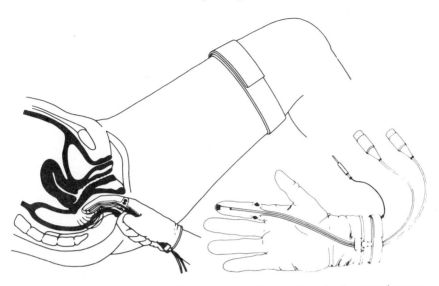

Fig. 2.7 Technique of determining pudendal nerve terminal motor latency. Using the St Mark's Pudendal Electrode® (Dantec Electronics Limited, Bristol), the pudendal nerve is stimulated at the level of the ischial spine, which is palpated from within the rectum. (From Fowler, C.J. (1991) Pelvic floor neurophysiology. *Methods in Clinical Neurophysiology*, **2**: 1–24, with permission from the publisher, Dantec Electronics Limited, Bristol.)

Electromyography (EMG)

Several investigations that examine the electrical activity of muscles are included within this section. They may provide information ranging from a simple measure of muscle activity to a complex analysis of muscle and nerve function. Operator experience may affect the reliability of results, as accurate placement of the recording electrode is essential.

Surface EMG

This, the simplest of EMG techniques, uses either a plug electrode or adhesive tabs to detect muscle electrical activity. The signal obtained is amplified electronically and the output is by means of either a loud-speaker or an oscilloscope screen. Most cases of paradoxical contraction of the external sphincter during straining may be demonstrated by this method. As a result, it is useful for biofeedback training and, because it creates little patient discomfort, it is the preferred method for this application.

Bipolar EMG

Two fine wires placed within the muscle to be examined act as the record-ing electrode. These are usually positioned in the muscle with the aid of a small hypodermic needle. The output may be through a loudspeaker or a chart recorder. The loudness of the sound or the amplitude of the pen

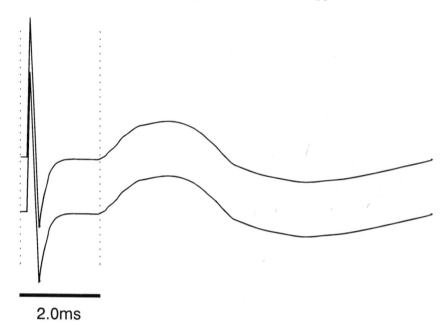

2.0ms

Fig. 2.8 A typical tracing from stimulation of the right pudendal nerve. In this case, the pudendal nerve terminal motor latency (PNTML) was 2.0 ms. Stimulation of the left pudendal nerve results in a downward deflection.

deflection correlates with the strength of the contraction but no truly quantitative data are obtained. It is particularly useful for simultaneous recording of electrical activity during manometry, for which it may be applied in the laboratory or during ambulatory recording.

Although primarily used for recording the activity of skeletal (striated) muscle of the external anal sphincter and the puborectalis, the technique may also be used to examine the electrical activity of the smooth (involuntary) muscle of the internal anal sphincter.

Concentric needle EMG

This is a valuable technique using a needle electrode that samples a relatively discrete region of muscle. Detailed analysis of the output may be useful in the diagnosis of denervation. However, as other techniques may more readily give this information, such analyses are rarely performed.

The concentric needle is most reliable for its precise anatomical localization. Consequently, this electrode is useful for mapping defects in the external anal sphincter. In this technique, the operator sequentially places the needle in multiple positions in the anatomical region of the external anal sphincter to detect the presence of electrical activity. An electrically quiet sector indicates the position of a defect in the external anal sphincter, such as that which may occur as a result of an obstetric injury. The technique may also be useful in locating the external anal sphincter muscle when planning surgical correction of such developmental abnormalities as ectopic anus. Because the anal sphincters may now be imaged accurately by anal endosonography, the need for thorough mapping has diminished.

Single-fibre EMG

The single-fibre EMG electrode records from a very small region – the territory of merely a few muscle fibres – and gives details of the electrical activity of single muscle fibres. Fibre density is the most frequently reported parameter. This is an index of the number of muscle fibres, within the sampling region of the electrode, which are supplied by a single motor neurone. Nerve damage, followed by reinnervation of the muscle, causes an increase in the fibre density. At least 20 samples must be taken – the fibre density is the average number of phases recorded (Fig. 2.9). This method is the most sensitive test for pudendal nerve damage,

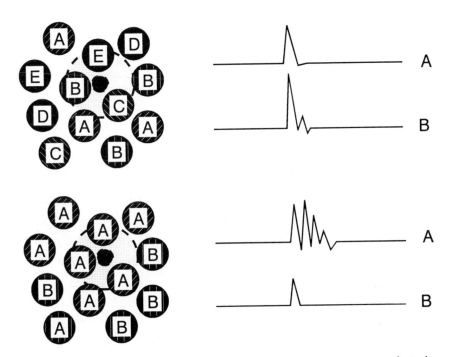

Fig. 2.9 Single fibre EMG. The upper diagram illustrates a normal study. On the left-hand side of the diagram, multiple muscle fibres are shown, each labelled to indicate the nerve fibre supplying it. The shaded area within the broken circle is the region of recording for the single fibre electrode. An impulse along nerve fibre A will result in the upper recording (one phase), fibre B the lower recording (two phases). The average number of phases over 20 recordings (= fibre density) is less than 1.5. The lower diagram illustrates the result of denervation and subsequent reinnervation. Unlike the normal situation, adjacent nerves are supplied by the same neurone. Many recordings will show polyphasic potentials like the upper trace (four phases). The fibre density is greater than 1.5.

but requires some experience to perform and is dependent on there being a significant amount of reinnervation after nerve injury.

Balloon expulsion

Assessment of defaecation in the laboratory remains an extraordinarily difficult problem. In our laboratory, a simple balloon expulsion test is favoured. The same balloon used for testing sensation to rectal distension is inflated with 50 ml water and gentle traction applied to the tubing. Most normal subjects can expel the balloon upon request. Patients with obstructed defaecation are rarely successful unless a large amount of traction is applied to the tubing. Electromyography may be used during this examination to establish whether the external anal sphincter and puborectalis are relaxing normally.

Of course, lying in the left lateral position attempting to expel a water-filled balloon under the watchful gaze of an anorectal physiologist is quite unlike normal defaecation. To minimize this problem, some investigators use a gel-filled artificial stool and allow the subject to sit on a commode in privacy.

Rectal or pouch compliance

The importance of a compliant reservoir for normal continence has already been outlined. Compliance may be measured in the laboratory by recording pressure within the rectum (or ileoanal pouch) during distension of a water-filled rectal balloon. The precise details of the technique may differ. At St Mark's, a 10-cm long condom is tied to a double-lumen catheter of the type used for central venous access. The distal port is connected to a peristaltic pump which is set to infuse water at 50 ml per minute. Pressure within the balloon is recorded through a pressure transducer attached to the more proximally opening lumen. If the paper speed of the chart recorder is adjusted to 5 cm per minute, the amount of water infused may be read as 10 ml per centimetre (10 ml/cm). Before placing the balloon in the rectum, a tracing is made of the compliance of the balloon alone. Rectal pressure is calculated as the difference between the pressure obtained in the rectum and the pressure in the balloon at the same volume of distension.

Compliance is calculated by taking the inverse slope of the line (volume change divided by pressure change). Thus a steeply sloping tracing represents a low compliance, and a flat tracing a high compliance. This investigation has a limited role in the assessment of patients with anorectal dysfunction because there is a very large range of normal values. Only patients with very extreme values may be said to be abnormal. However, after restorative proctocolectomy with ileoanal pouch, compliance has been found to be a useful predictor of function. Generally, those patients with higher compliance values have better function with fewer pouch evacuations per day and less leakage. Figure 2.10 illustrates typical com-

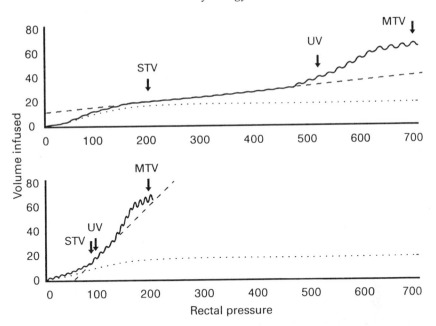

Fig. 2.10 Ileoanal pouch compliance. The upper tracing illustrates a high-compliance pouch, the lower tracing a low-compliance pouch. Balloon pressure is shown by the dotted line. This is subtracted from the total pressure to obtain the pouch pressure. The slope of the line is illustrated by the broken line; a high compliance is demonstrated by a lower slope. MTV = maximum tolerated volume; STV = sensory threshold volume; UV = urge volume.

pliance curves from a high-compliance, well-functioning pouch and from a low-compliance pouch.

Saline continence test

This test was developed to distinguish finer disorders of continence and to assess rectal motility. It is performed by placing a catheter into the rectum and infusing saline at a constant rate. Rectal and anal pressures are recorded during the infusion; the volume and rectal pressure at which leakage occurs are noted. Most normal subjects can retain 1500 ml before leakage occurs.

Despite initial enthusiasm for this test, its results have not been as reliable as expected. The amount of patient discomfort and the embarrassment caused by the test have meant that it has been largely abandoned.

Other techniques

Ambulatory studies

Advances in electronics have enabled the collection and storage of large amounts of information using portable equipment. Solid state pressure transducers may record pressures continuously in the anal canal, the rectum and at other levels while the subject undertakes normal activities. Simultaneous electromyography may be recorded using implanted bipolar wire electrodes or surface patches. All the information obtained is stored in a small box, not much larger than a 'Walkman' music cassette player. Event buttons on the recording box enable the subject to record such activities as eating, passing flatus, pain or incontinence episodes. After the completion of the recording time (usually 6 or 24 hours), the data are downloaded onto a computer for analysis.

These studies are useful for several reasons. First the physiology laboratory is far from a normal environment. In some situations, it is possible that these abnormal surroundings may influence the findings. Secondly, as many complaints are intermittent, the abnormality being sought may not be apparent during the limited duration of the investigation. Thirdly, many 'abnormal' findings may be present in asymptomatic subjects and thus their occurrence in symptomatic patients need not be related to the symptoms. To be certain that such findings are related to the complaint being investigated, it may be necessary to demonstrate that the abnormality occurs at the time of the symptoms.

With all these advantages, why do we still perform 'static' manometry in the laboratory? There are several reasons but most important are the expense and the time-consuming nature of ambulatory studies. A single unit can perform eight to ten physiological investigations in one working day using standard laboratory-based techniques. With two ambulatory systems, it would be impossible to complete this number of investigations in one week. In addition, the solid state transducers are expensive and may be easily damaged.

Despite its limitations, the physiology laboratory provides a controlled environment in which many factors, including patient movement and probe position, may be regulated precisely. It remains the mainstay of investigation into anorectal function.

Radiology and nuclear medicine

Many radiological investigations are employed in the diagnosis of gastrointestinal disease. These will not be discussed in detail except where they specifically complement physiological investigation.

Anal endosonography is indispensable in the diagnosis of sphincteric injury, which may result from childbirth, impalement injuries, sexual penetration, fistula surgery or other anal operations. The technique may also image other abnormalities such as myopathy of the internal anal sphincter, abscesses and fistulae.

Colonic transit studies assess the time taken for faecal matter to pass through the colon. They enable constipated patients to be divided into those with 'slow transit' and those with 'outlet obstruction'. Many patients have some features of both these types and thus a colonic transit study forms part of the normal investigation of severely constipated patients. Different protocols are used by different units. The St Mark's method employs three different shaped radio-opaque markers (rings, rods and cubes). Gelatin capsules each containing twenty markers of one known type are taken on three consecutive days followed by a single abdominal X-ray on the sixth day. The radiologist counts the number and distribution of each shaped marker to establish whether transit is normal or delayed.

Evacuation proctography has a limited place in the assessment of defaecatory disorders. Seated on a special commode, the patient is asked to evacuate a specially prepared radio-opaque paste that has been instilled into the rectum. Radiographic screening is recorded on videotape to allow for later interpretation in slow motion and in freeze frame. Simultaneous manometry and electromyography during evacuation proctography are techniques that may aid interpretation of the significance of radiographic findings.

Radioisotope transit studies are being used increasingly to study the passage of contents through the gastrointestinal (GI) tract under circumstances which as near as possible resemble normal physiological conditions. Accurate quantification of transit throughout the entire gut is possible with this technique. Because many patients with abnormal gut function have abnormalities in more than one region of the gastrointestinal tract, this ability to examine the passage of material from mouth to anus is important. Furthermore, by using different radioactive isotopes, it is possible to examine the individual passage of solids and liquids simultaneously.

Investigation of other parts of the GI tract

The realization that abnormalities of colonic function may be accompanied by abnormalities of other regions of the gastrointestinal tract has prompted anorectal physiologists to broaden their interest in gastrointestinal motility. All regions of the gastrointestinal tract are amenable to study either using tubes inserted through the nose or the anus, or, rarely, using radiotelemetry capsules. By recording pressure simultaneously at several points along the gastrointestinal tract, the progression of gut contractions can be assessed.

The oesophagus may be examined by passing a tube via the nasogastric route. In the laboratory, a tube with perfused side holes at multiple levels is used in most cases. Ambulatory oesophageal manometry employs a tube with several solid state transducers. These tubes may also incorporate a sensor to detect the reflux of acid from the stomach into the oesophagus.

A long intestinal tube may be positioned in the small intestine with the aid of X-rays to confirm its position. Such studies are usually performed using ambulatory equipment because it is necessary to study motility during both fed and fasting states. Smooth muscle electromyography may be recorded in addition to pressure. Normally there are specific patterns of activity recognisable after meals (postprandial period) and between meals (interdigestive period). The interdigestive period is characterized by four distinct phases of activity, which may be distorted in certain conditions. Patients with types of chronic intestinal pseudo-obstruction and other motility disorders may have an abnormality predominantly of the smooth muscle (myopathy) or of the nervous control (neuropathy). Myopathy is characterized by impaired muscle contraction giving low pressures on manometry. Patients with neuropathy, on the other hand, display normal increases in pressure with gut contraction but poor propagation of these contractions to more distal sites.

Colonic motility may be assessed by a tube placed in the colon at colonoscopy. Patients with slow transit constipation have a decreased frequency of contractions and poor propagation of contractions along the colon. It can be shown that administration of a stimulant laxative increases the frequency and the distance of propagation of contractions.

These studies will almost certainly have an increasing role in diagnosis in the future. They are invaluable in assessing the effect of medications on gastrointestinal motility and may eventually enable effective drugs to be developed for the treatment of major motility disorders. Demonstration of a generalized motility disorder may help to warn of the futility of operations directed at improving symptoms attributable to one region of the gut only.

Biofeedback training

This technique has proved successful in the treatment of many patients with obstructed defaecation and paradoxical contraction of the external anal sphincter and puborectalis. It has also been used for the treatment of certain types of incontinence and anal pain, with limited success. The principle behind the technique is that the patient, given appropriate information about the activity of his or her anal musculature, can modify inappropriate actions. Electromyography or manometry with oscilloscope, auditory or digital output is used to display activity in the external anal sphincter during squeezing and straining exercises.

The details of the treatment protocol may vary. Either a portable system which the patient may use at home or a series of laboratory sessions may be used. Success depends on proper selection of patients and a rapport between the well-motivated patient and an enthusiastic therapist.

THE CLINICAL ROLE OF THE PHYSIOLOGY LABORATORY

Having given a general overview of the principles of normal physiology and the investigative techniques available, the clinical conditions most frequently referred to the physiology laboratory are now discussed briefly.

Incontinence

The many factors that contribute to normal continence have been outlined above. Anorectal physiological investigations may yield information about diagnosis, prognosis and the effect of treatment. Such information may be invaluable in deciding between alternative management strategies.

Manometry provides the most useful diagnostic information. Most incontinent patients have decreased anal pressures. Diminished resting pressure usually implies dysfunction of the internal anal sphincter and is often associated with passive leakage and flatus incontinence. This may occur as a result of injury, neurological disease or primary disease of the smooth muscle.

External anal sphincter dysfunction is usually reflected in decreased voluntary contraction pressure and cough increment. Injury (mostly obstetric or surgical), neurological disease and, rarely, muscle disease are the possible causes. Diagnosis of sphincter injury is important because such patients may benefit from surgical repair. Anal endosonography and EMG mapping are able to locate such injuries. Some investigators have found that, when a sphincter injury is present in patients with pudendal neuropathy (diagnosed by prolonged pudendal nerve latencies or by increased fibre density) the results of sphincter repair are frequently poor. A defunctioning colostomy may be performed at the time of sphincter repair, especially if the sphincteric injury is associated with infection, inflammatory bowel disease or a rectovaginal fistula. Manometry is usually performed before closure of the colostomy to assess the effectiveness of repair and to predict potential function after restoration of bowel continuity.

Neuropathy without sphincter injury has been treated by several different operations which aim to 'tighten up' the anal sphincters, lengthen the anal canal and restore the anorectal angle. One such operation is the postanal repair described by Sir Alan Parks. Although providing relief for many patients, in the long term many patients deteriorate. Abnormal descent of the perineum is a frequent finding, and this may contribute to progressive pudendal nerve injury with deteriorating function.

Abnormal sensation by balloon distension and electrosensitivity testing may suggest a neurological abnormality such as a spinal tumour or multiple sclerosis. Spinal latencies may confirm the site of such lesions but generally imaging tests such as magnetic resonance imaging of the spine will be required.

Sometimes standard investigations are normal in patients presenting with incontinence. Ambulatory studies may be useful to distinguish those patients who have intermittent abnormalities such as episodic elevation of rectal pressure or prolonged spontaneous relaxations of the internal anal sphincter. If such relaxations have a mechanical cause such as rectal intussusception, surgical treatment may be successful. High rectal pressures may occur during hypertonic contractions of the colon in patients with the irritable bowel syndrome. New medications are being developed which may be able to reduce such contraction. Ambulatory manometry may be vital in assessing their efficacy.

A group of patients will remain, however, in whom all investigations are normal. Some of these patients have a psychological cause for their symptoms and it is vital that clinicians be aware of this possibility. The clinical features of psychological disturbance should be sought in all patients with bowel dysfunction so as to avoid overinvestigation and to allow appropriate early intervention.

Constipation

Constipation is a common complaint with many different causes. It is appropriate to investigate those cases that are long-standing, severe and resistant to standard dietary advice and simple laxatives. When the onset has been recent, it is important to exclude colorectal cancer, serious metabolic illnesses and medications as causes. Physiological investigations are aimed at distinguishing slow transit constipation, obstructed defaecation and Hirschsprung's disease.

Manometry is usually normal in constipated patients. A normal rectoanal inhibitory reflex excludes the diagnosis of Hirschsprung's disease. Large balloon distension volumes may suggest a diagnosis of idiopathic megarectum (or megacolon), which should be confirmed by a barium enema. Patients with this condition often have a good result from surgery.

Some patients with obstructed defaecation have abnormal contraction of the puborectalis muscle during defaecation. This is best shown by increased EMG activity in the external anal sphincter and puborectalis during straining while attempting to expel a balloon, or by an increase in anal pressure during straining or increased angulation at the anorectal junction during evacuation proctography. Biofeedback retraining may reverse this abnormality and allow normal defaecation.

Slow transit constipation is usually diagnosed by a radio-opaque marker transit study. Evacuation proctography is useful when the clinical features suggest a specific anatomical abnormality as a cause of obstructed defaecation. Rectocele and rectal intussusception, when causing symptoms, may be surgically corrected with good results.

Solitary rectal ulcer syndrome

This is a distressing condition usually characterized by excessive straining at stool. Patients with this affliction often experience an almost constant desire to defaecate, causing them to spend many unsuccessful hours at the lavatory. Blood and mucus are frequently passed and there may be an area of inflammation or ulceration in the lower rectum. Physiological studies will often show paradoxical contraction of the external anal sphincter and the puborectalis. In long-standing cases, abnormal perineal descent and pudendal neuropathy may be present. A partial or complete prolapse of the rectum is often demonstrated using evacuation proctography. Biofeedback therapy may reduce the risk of recurrence after surgery.

Rectal prolapse

In this condition, the rectum periodically invaginates and protrudes through the anus. Many patients are incontinent, adding to the distress of the complaint. Anorectal physiology studies before surgical correction allow assessment of sphincteric function and may help to predict whether incontinence will improve postoperatively.

Preoperative assessment

An objective assessment of sphincter function may be valuable in the planning of operative management. Manometry before closure of an intestinal stoma may help predict whether a reasonable degree of continence can be expected, especially in cases where the stoma has been formed to protect an anal operation. When an operation carries a risk of incontinence, it may be useful to assess this risk by preoperative manometry. This is particularly important if there has been previous surgery, injury or disease, or if there is a potential for future litigation.

Low rectal carcinoma may present the surgeon with a choice between a very low anterior resection with a coloanal anastomosis or an abdominoperineal excision of the rectum with a permanent end colostomy. A high degree of sphincteric function is necessary for acceptable continence after coloanal anastomosis.

Ileoanal pouch operations

A successful restorative proctocolectomy with an ileoanal pouch anastomosis may give a very good functional result in patients who would otherwise require a permanent ileostomy. Unfortunately, not all patients have a good functional result from this operation. Several factors are important for a good result. These include good sphincteric function, a large volume, high compliance and an absence of outlet obstruction. Anorectal physiology testing may help in the selection of suitable patients for this operation and to help find the cause of unsatisfactory pouch function. Where a cause can be found, revisional surgery may enable a good function to be achieved.

Anal pain

Most patients with anal pain, for which no cause is apparent on physical examination, have normal anorectal physiology studies. Rarely, causes such as spinal cord pathology or overactivity of the internal anal sphincter may be diagnosed by anorectal physiology studies. One cause of internal sphincter overactivity is a hereditary myopathy. This is characterized by a high resting pressure with bizarre fluctuation and an abnormally thickened internal sphincter on anal endosonography.

Anal fissure is a common cause of anal pain. It is usually associated with an increase in the maximum resting pressure, often with ultraslow waves. The diagnosis is usually made on the clinical features. Treatment, by dividing part of the internal anal sphincter (lateral anal sphincterotomy), is usually successful. However, in unsuccessful cases, anorectal physiology should be examined before repeated attempts to reduce anal pressure.

Haemorrhoids

Patients with symptomatic haemorrhoids frequently display increased resting pressure, ultraslow waves and decreased anal sensation. It is not known whether these abnormalities have a role in the causation of haemorrhoids or are secondary phenomena. Clinically, investigations rarely assist with diagnosis or selection of treatment. An exception is the patient with an unusual combination of symptoms, especially if elderly. Haemorrhoidectomy in such patients may lead to incontinence if there is inadequate sphincter function.

CONCLUSION

An understanding of the normal physiology and of the altered physiology in disease states of the entire gastrointestinal tract is vital to modern colorectal surgical practice. Anorectal physiology testing and investigation of other regions of the gut have been essential in the development of our current understanding of normal and abnormal functioning of the gut. These investigations now have an important place in the management of gastrointestinal disease.

This overview has outlined the basic physiology of continence and defaecation, and briefly described most of the investigations that are available to examine the function of the anus, rectum and other regions of the gastrointestinal tract. The study of gastrointestinal motility is a complex and expanding field. Gradually, the puzzle of how the gut works is being pieced together. Undoubtedly, as the picture nears completion, new investigations and novel treatments will become available for the relief of some of these most distressing complaints.

FURTHER READING

Henry, M.M. and Swash, M. (Eds) (1992) *Coloproctology and the Pelvic Floor*, 2nd edn. Oxford: Butterworth-Heinemann.

Kumar, D. and Gustavsson, S. (Eds) (1988) *An Illustrated Guide to Gastrointestinal Motility*. John Wiley: Chichester.

Miller, R. and Mortensen, N.J. (1989) Anorectal physiology. *Surgery Annual*, **21**: 303–26.

3 Medical management of Crohn's disease and ulcerative colitis

Michael J.G. Farthing

INTRODUCTION

Inflammatory bowel disease (IBD) is an 'umbrella' term that encompasses *specific* inflammatory disorders of the gastrointestinal tract in which the aetiology is known and the *non-specific* disorders such as Crohn's disease (CD), ulcerative colitis (UC) and the rarer forms of inflammatory bowel disease such as collagenous colitis and microscopic colitis. Intestinal infections are common in both the industrialized and the developing world and can mimic non-specific inflammatory bowel disease, particularly when they present as bloody diarrhoea (Table 3.1). In some parts of the UK abdominal tuberculosis is as common as CD although almost exclusively limited to immigrants from the Indian subcontinent. It is therefore essential to exclude infection in a patient presenting for the first time with symptoms suggestive of non-specific inflammatory bowel disease and also to ensure that coincident infection is not present in a patient with established inflammatory bowel disease in relapse.

CD and UC can occur at any age but most commonly present between the third and sixth decades of life (Jayanthi, Probert and Mayberry 1991). The incidence and prevalence of UC and CD vary with geographic loca-

Table 3.1 Enteropathogens causing bloody diarrhoea

Bacteria	*Shigella* spp.
	Salmonella spp.
	Enteroinvasive *Escherichia coli* (EIEC)
	Enterohaemorrhagic *E. coli* (EHEC)
	Campylobacter jejuni
	Yersinia enterocolitica
	Mycobacterium tuberculosis
	Aeromonas spp.
	Plesiomonas spp.
Protozoa	*Entamoeba histolytica*
	Balantidium coli
Viruses	Cytomegalovirus (immunocompromised)
Helminths	*Schistosoma* spp.
	Trichuris trichiura

tion (Table 3.2), but both disorders are more common in the industrial-ized world. However, UC is known to occur in many countries in the developing world, where CD is at present extremely rare. However, CD is now known to occur in Asian immigrants to the UK, suggesting that environmental factors are important in aetiopathogenesis. Both UC and CD are more common in the Jewish community compared with non-Jews, and IBD is more common in whites than non-whites. There is consider-able additional evidence to support an important genetic component in the risk of developing IBD. The familial incidence of CD and UC is 10–15%, occurring mainly in first-degree relatives. As yet there is no clear genetic marker for these diseases although HLA antigens appear to be helpful in some populations, particularly the Japanese.

Table 3.2 Incidence and prevalence (per 100 000) of ulcerative colitis and Crohn's disease

	Incidence		Prevalence	
	UC	CD	UC	CD
Denmark	9.5–20.3	117–157	3.6–4.1	–
France	3.0	4.2	–	–
Iceland	7.4	0.9	122	–
Israel	6.9	3.1	138	19.5
Italy	1.9	0.8	–	–
Norway	12.8–14.8	–	5.2	–
Sweden	4.7–13.1	234	4.2–6.1	146
UK	7.2–11.3	–	6.7–8.3	–
USA	10.9–16.0	225	4.0–7.0	90.5

– = no data

The causes of UC and CD are not known. However, a number of envi-ronmental factors have been identified which may be important in the pathogenesis and possibly the aetiology of these disorders (Table 3.3). In CD the possibility that a transmissible agent is responsible has been con-sidered for many decades (Ljungh 1992). Current interest focuses on atyp-ical mycobacteria particularly *Mycobacterium paratuberculosis*. More recently there have been suggestions that the measles virus might be responsible but, despite finding these organisms in Crohn's tissue, there is as yet no evidence to causally link the virus with the disease. Similarly, UC has long been thought to be an infectious disorder although no single enteropathogen has yet been identified. There is some evidence to associate a type of enteroadhesive *Escherichia coli* with UC, although again there is no evidence to suggest that this organism is the primary cause of the disease (Shanahan 1993).

Dietary factors – particularly exclusion of milk in UC and administra-tion of an elemental diet in CD – suggest that dietary antigens may influ-ence disease activity although it seems unlikely that they are primary factors. Non-smokers have a two- to sixfold increase in the incidence of

Table 3.3 Environmental factors that may influence the aetiopathogenesis of inflammatory bowel disease

		UC	CD
Infective agents	Adhesive *E. coli*	?	–
	Mycobacterium paratuberculosis	–	?
	Measles virus	–	?
Diet	Milk	+	?
	Liquid diet:		
	elemental	–	+
	polymeric	–	+
Smoking*		+	+

*Decreases activity in UC; increases activity in CD.
? = possible/controversial role

UC, whereas CD is two to four times more common in smokers (Shanahan 1993). There is a small increased relative risk (1.5–2) of developing UC or CD in women taking the oral contraceptive pill.

The host response to an environmental 'trigger' is also likely to be important. It has been suggested that intestinal barrier function, as demonstrated by increased intestinal permeability, may be a precursor of CD which might be under genetic control. However, this remains controversial and not all studies can confirm this observation.

Whatever the environmental trigger may be, both CD and UC are characterized by intestinal inflammation that involves both humoral and cellular immune responses. There is some evidence to suggest that UC may be an autoimmune disorder, as circulating, disease-specific autoantibodies against colonocytes have been detected (Shanahan 1993). In UC and CD there may be a subtle immunoregulatory disorder that permits chronic inflammation to persist and be amplified by a variety of other inflammatory mediators released from cells taking part in the inflammatory response, including cytokines, prostaglandins, leukotrienes, platelet-activating factor, reactive oxygen metabolites and a variety of vasoactive substances including kinins.

DEFINITIONS

UC is an inflammatory disorder of the colon which usually begins in the rectum and extends in continuity to involve the more proximal colon to variable extents. The small intestine is never affected. There is an acute inflammatory response in the more superficial layers of the bowel wall. CD can involve any part of the gastrointestinal tract, disease areas generally not being in continuity. Inflammation may involve the entire thickness of the bowel wall, resulting in deep ulceration and fistula formation. Chronic inflammatory cells are often organized as granulomas which are the pathognomonic feature of CD.

DIAGNOSIS

Before appropriate treatment can be initiated it is essential to establish a firm diagnosis of non-specific inflammatory bowel disease, to attempt to distinguish between UC and CD and to make an assessment of the extent and severity of the disease.

Clinical assessment

Common symptoms of UC and CD are summarized in Table 3.4. The first symptoms of colitis are usually bleeding and diarrhoea. In patients with proctitis, bleeding is accompanied by increased mucus production, and constipation is the rule rather than diarrhoea. The severity of the diarrhoea correlates well with the extent of colonic inflammation. Thus, with a mild proctosigmoiditis, stools are often formed or semi-formed, whereas in extensive colitis it is usual to have loose or watery stools. Bowel looseness and frequency may be associated with urgency of defaecation which sometimes may result in incontinence.

IBD is often associated with other abdominal symptoms, particularly pain. Left-sided lower abdominal pain is common and this is generally relieved by defaecation. It may also occur following a meal but again is relieved by defaecation. Abdominal pain may also be obstructive in character, again usually occurring after a meal, often located in the centre of the abdomen, cramping in character and occurring in waves. Obstructive abdominal pain is often associated with abdominal distension and loud abdominal sounds (borborygmi).

Bowel symptoms are often accompanied by symptoms of a systemic illness, which may include fever, loss of appetite and weight loss. In young children and adolescents retardation of growth and development is an extremely important complication of IBD due to a variety of factors including reduced food intake, abdominal pain on eating and possibly humoral mechanisms involving cytokines which reduce appetite. Extraintestinal manifestations of IBD are also common, involving the skin (erythema nodosum, pyoderma gangrenosum), the joints (ankylosing spondylitis, arthritis), the eyes (episcleritis, iritis) and the liver (sclerosing cholangitis, other mild inflammatory disorders).

The clinical differentiation between UC and CD can be difficult; in

Table 3.4 Symptoms of inflammatory bowel disease

	UC	CD
Diarrhoea	++	++
Rectal bleeding	+++	+
Abdominal pain	±	++
Anal lesions	–	++
Weight loss	±	+
Fever	±	+
Fistula	–	+

approximately 10–15% of cases it may be impossible clinically, endo-scopically or histologically to distinguish between the two. However, there are certain clinical features that are highly suggestive of CD, notably anal and perianal disease (ulceration, fissures, fistulae), the presence of an abdominal mass (usually in the right iliac fossa) and enterocutaneous fis-tulae. Rectal bleeding almost always accompanies UC, but may be absent in Crohn's colitis. Another typical feature of CD is the presence of inflam-matory lesions of the lips, in which there is swelling of one or both lips often accompanied by ulceration of the mouth and tongue. In children and adolescents this may be the only manifestation of CD. Internal fistu-lation in CD may be extensive, involving adjacent segments of bowel, the bladder and the internal genital organs, particularly the vagina.

Microbiology

Intestinal infections are extremely common in both the industrialized and the developing world and may masquerade as non-specific IBD, and in some instances can occur in patients with established IBD. A variety of organisms are known to cause bloody diarrhoea (see Table 3.1) but watery diarrhoea due to infection may also be confused with IBD (Table 3.5). These infections are often self-limiting although some, particularly dysen-teric shigellosis, *M. tuberculosis* and amoebiasis, require specific anti-microbial chemotherapy. It is thus essential that appropriate measures are taken to exclude infection prior to starting treatment of non-specific IBD. Three faecal specimens should be collected on separate days and exam-ined by direct light microscopy as a saline wet mount and submitted to routine culture for conventional gut pathogens, ensuring that conditions for isolation of *Campylobacter jejuni* and *Yersinia enterocolitica* are included. Microscopy of a saline wet mount may reveal the typical, highly motile *C. jejuni* on direct dark-field or phase-contrast microscopy or the erythrophagic trophozoites of *Entamoeba histolytica*. Concentration tech-niques may be required to isolate cysts of intestinal parasites. The oocysts of *Cryptosporidium parvum* can also be identified on direct microscopy using a modified Ziehl–Neelsen or other special stain. Rectal swabs taken at proctoscopy are also needed to isolate *Neisseria gonorrhoeae* by

Table 3.5 Microbial enteropathogens responsible for acute watery diarrhoea

Bacteria	Enterotoxigenic *E. coli* (ETEC)
	Salmonella enteritidis
	Shigella spp. (early phase of infection)
	Vibrio cholerae
	Vibrio parahaemolyticus
Viruses	Rotavirus
	Enteric adenovirus (types 40 and 41)
	Norwalk and related viruses
Protozoa	*Cryptosporidium parvum*

culture but chlamydia usually require the use of special tissue culture cell lines for identification.

Serological testing is also used to diagnose intestinal infection but in clinical practice is usually restricted to the diagnosis of yersiniosis and amoebiasis. It is also possible to detect toxins in the stools of patients with antibiotic-associated colitis, particularly that due to *Clostridium difficile*. New diagnostic techniques are emerging including faecal antigen detection assays in which specific antibodies are used to identify pathogen-specific antigens in stool. DNA probes have been developed that can detect the genes of specific virulence factors such as genes encoding for enterotoxins, invasion antigens or other species-specific antigens; ultimately, this approach may replace conventional culture techniques for screening for gut pathogens. Faecal culture, however, will be required for the foreseeable future to determine the antibiotic sensitivity of any organisms isolated.

Endoscopy

Examination of the rectum and anal canal should be regarded as routine in any patient suspected of having non-specific IBD. Rigid sigmoidoscopy can be performed simply and rapidly in an outpatient clinic and requires no bowel preparation. In UC the rectum is usually abnormal, with a range of abnormalities from diffuse erythema with loss of the normal vascular pattern in the rectal mucosa, progressing to bleeding on contact with the mucosa, to spontaneous bleeding and ultimately to discrete ulceration. Despite the name, ulcerative colitis, overt ulceration is uncommon except in the severe forms of the disease. In CD and a variety of other conditions the rectum may be normal, although a rectal biopsy should always be taken because histology may reveal the granulomas of CD or possibly the features of microscopic colitis or collagenous colitis (Table 3.6). The use of topical steroid preparations, however, can confuse the endoscopist by promoting healing of the rectum in patients with UC but leaving more proximal inflammation not accessible to the enema or the sigmoidoscope.

Table 3.6 Infections and inflammatory conditions of the colon in which the rectum may be spared

Infections	Amoebiasis
	Pseudo-membranous colitis
	Yersiniosis
	Campylobacter jejuni
	Tuberculosis
	Cryptosporidiosis
	Salmonellosis
	Shigellosis
Inflammatory conditions	Crohn's disease
	Ulcerative colitis
	Microscopic colitis
	Collagenous colitis
	Behçet's disease

In CD the earliest lesion is diffuse patchy erythema between areas of normal vascular pattern. Multiple aphthoid ulceration strongly suggests but is not pathognomonic of CD. Ulceration in the rectum can become progressively more severe from superficial ulcers through to deep serpiginous ulcers, ultimately resulting in the cobblestone appearance typical of CD. Fibrotic strictures in the rectum occur more commonly in CD but can be found in patients with UC. Rectal ulceration is not limited to UC and CD but may be a feature of a variety of other disorders, particularly specific IBD due to infection (Tables 3.7 and 3.8).

After rigid sigmoidoscopy, the anal canal should be examined with a proctoscope. The narrow 'medical' sigmoidoscope does not provide an adequate view of the anal canal, when fissures and fistulae can easily be missed.

When the rectum is normal or when the upper limit of disease cannot be defined, examination of the entire colon and distal ileum is indicated. For total colonoscopy the bowel should be prepared ideally with a hypertonic balanced electrolyte solution containing polyethylene glycol or mannitol, or a non-absorbed osmotically active salt such as sodium picosulphate. These solutions can be drunk slowly or administered rapidly via nasogastric tubes. In UC the endoscopic abnormalities in the colon usually diminish in severity as the disease proceeds proximally and the pathological changes are always in continuity. In contrast, in CD discontinuity is the rule with erythema, aphthoid ulcers or deep ulcers being immediately adjacent to normal-looking mucosa. Disease activity may be most apparent in the right colon. It is often possible to enter the terminal ileum and confirm whether the disease involves the small intestine, which is highly suggestive of CD. Biopsies should be taken from ileum and throughout the colon to confirm the endoscopic diagnosis. If there is

Table 3.7 Diseases producing 'specific' abnormalities in the rectum

Deep ulcers	Crohn's disease
	Amoebiasis
	Tuberculosis
	Syphilis
Pseudo-membrane	*Clostridium difficile*
Vesicles	Herpes simplex virus
Beads of pus	Gonorrhoea

Table 3.8 Microbial agents causing proctitis

Neisseria gonorrhoeae
Chlamydia trachomatis:
   LGV
   non-LGV
Treponema pallidum
Herpes simplex virus

LGV, lymphogranuloma venereum

any concern that the appearances might have an infective aetiology (see Tables 3.1, 3.5 and 3.7), tissue should be sent for microbiological culture including *Mycobacterium tuberculosis*, Ziehl–Neelsen stain and possibly for DNA analysis by polymerase chain reaction.

Radiology and cross-sectional imaging

For decades, barium radiology has been the cornerstone of the radiological diagnosis of IBD. Double-contrast barium enema, in which the barium–air interface is used to examine the bowel mucosa and the overall configuration of the colon, has been partially replaced by colonoscopy. In experienced hands the two techniques have similar accuracy but colonoscopy has the advantage in that it can provide mucosal biopsies for histological examination and has a valuable therapeutic component such as polypectomy and balloon dilatation of strictures. The choice between barium enema and colonoscopy may also depend on local expertise and available resources. In UC an unprepared ('instant') barium enema can be used in patients with colitis to obtain a rapid estimate of the extent and severity of the disease. The plain abdominal radiograph is also invaluable in assessing patients with acute severe colitis. The presence of air in the colon usually allows an assessment of colonic calibre, haustral pattern and the extent of disease. Inflamed colon is usually devoid of faeces and contains only air, whereas non-involved colon usually contains faecal residue. Thus, the point where faecal residue can be identified on the plain abdominal radiograph corresponds reasonably closely to the proximal limit of disease. In very severe acute colitis the abdominal radiograph will indicate whether colonic dilatation has occurred, and a chest radiograph should be obtained to ensure that there is no air under the diaphragm, indicating intestinal perforation.

Examination of the small intestine is dependent almost entirely on the barium follow-through examination – the only exception being the duodenum, proximal jejunum and distal ileum, which can often be visualized during endoscopy. The barium follow-through examination should be normal in UC but in CD may reveal a variety of abnormalities, including aphthoid ulcers, discrete ulceration, diffuse inflammatory changes with typical fold pattern abnormalities, strictures and fistulae communicating with an adjacent part of intestine or with the skin.

Barium contrast examination of the small intestine can also be achieved by performing a small bowel enema (enteroclysis) in which barium is introduced into the proximal small intestine through a tube placed in the duodenum. This can provide more detailed information on small intestinal strictures and internal fistulae, particularly when overlapping loops of bowel cannot be separated by compression. Most radiologists would not feel that this is the first-line approach for examining the small bowel.

Cross-sectional imaging with ultrasound, computed tomography (CT) and magnetic resonance (MR) can provide useful additional information because of their ability to image the bowel wall, serosa, mesentery and lymph nodes. Ultrasound examination is the first approach when intra-abdominal abscess is being considered although a negative examination does not exclude the diagnosis, in which case it may be necessary to proceed to CT. The use of cross-sectional imaging techniques has assisted the development of interventional radiological procedures such as abscess aspiration for diagnosis and microbiological culture and also placement of catheters for more prolonged drainage procedures, including irrigation. MR imaging has found a useful application in the assessment of rectal and perianal CD, particularly the mapping of fistulae and the planning of their surgical treatment.

Radionuclide scanning can be used to assess the severity and extent of IBD. White blood cells can be labelled with a variety of radionuclides and their localization in inflamed intestine can be detected by gamma-camera imaging. White cell scans correlate well with barium follow-through examinations and colonoscopy, and in some instances seem to be more sensitive. The severity of disease may also be assessed by measuring excretion of labelled white blood cells in the stool, although this test has not found wide application in clinical practice.

Histopathology

Histological confirmation of a diagnosis of IBD should be obtained whenever possible. As stated previously it is important to distinguish specific infective colitis from UC or CD because of the treatment implications and long-term prognosis. Infective colitis is characterized by large numbers of neutrophil polymorphs within the epithelium, sometimes referred to as 'cryptitis', which is more typical than the crypt abscesses of UC. Some infections have typical features such as the pseudo-membrane of antibiotic-associated colitis due to *Clostridium difficile*, and the caseating granulomata of tuberculosis. More often, however, the histological features of infective colitis merge with those of non-specific IBD and a clear distinction between the two is often impossible.

Similarly, in approximately 15% of patients with colitis the cause cannot be clearly attributed to either CD or UC. It is helpful to distinguish between these two conditions because the prognosis may be different and because certain forms of surgery (e.g. ileoanal pouch anastomosis) is not an option for patients with CD. As stated previously, the rectum may appear endoscopically normal in IBD but have microscopic changes consistent with one of the rarer forms of colitis such as collagenous colitis, microscopic colitis or lymphocytic colitis.

Histological examination of the colon is an important part of assessing cancer risk in colitis. Epithelial cell atypia or dysplasia is thought to be a precursor of cancer and, when severe, is now considered to be an indication for colectomy. Milder forms of dysplasia can occur as a result of acute inflammation, and it is suggested that repeat biopsies should be taken from these patients when the disease has entered remission. Some 25% of patients who develop cancer in colitis do not have dysplasia; thus the relationship between dysplasia and cancer is neither constant nor precise.

TREATMENT

There is a wide range of options available for the treatment of non-specific IBD. This is the usual situation when the aetiology of a disease is unknown and thus reliance is placed entirely on controlling the underlying pathological process rather than eradicating the cause of the disease. Tabe 3.9 summarizes the main therapeutic agents available for the treatment of IBD.

Table 3.9 Treatment of inflammatory bowel disease

Drugs	Corticosteroids	Hydrocortisone
		Prednisolone
		ACTH
	New steroids	Tixocortol pivalate
		Budesonide
		Fluticasone propionate
	Aminosalicylates	5-ASA (see Table 3.10)
		4-ASA
	Immunosuppressives	Azathioprine
		6-MP
		Cyclosporin
		Methotrexate
	Antimicrobial agents	Broad spectrum
		Metronidazole
		? Anti-mycobacterial
Nutrition	Oral supplements	
	Enteral nutrition	Elemental diet
		Polymeric diet
	Intravenous nutrition	

Drugs

Corticosteroids

Since the first description of ACTH therapy for IBD in 1951, a variety of corticosteroid preparations have been developed that are effective in controlling the disease. Corticosteroids are useful for treating acute relapses of UC and CD, and are active systemically and topically (Shanahan 1993; Crotty and Jewell 1992), but have no value in maintenance therapy. They do not have a single mechanism of action in IBD but have effects at many points on the immunoinflammatory cascade. Corticosteroids inhibit the function of T and B lymphocytes, which partly relates to their inhibitory effects on cytokine release. In addition, macrophage and monocyte function is impaired, reducing the ability of these cells to act as antigen-presenting cells. Corticosteroids also affect the production of prostaglandins and leukotrienes in the intestinal mucosa, compounds that are important for amplifying the immune/inflammatory response. Corticosteroids have a number of unwanted effects, including cushingoid appearance, skin changes, osteoporosis, exacerbation of diabetes mellitus and osteonecrosis; in children and adolescents, they can inhibit growth and promote epiphyseal closure.

Aminosalicylates

The prototype in this class of drug is sulphasalazine, originally developed for the treatment of rheumatoid arthritis (Baron et al. 1962; Crotty and Jewell 1992; Carpani de Kaski and Hodgson 1993). The drug has two components, a salicylate moiety linked by an azo bond to a sulphonamide, sulphapyridine. Colonic bacteria contain an azo reductase which liberates the salicylate moiety into the colonic lumen, where it acts as an anti-inflammatory agent. More recently it has become apparent that 4-ASA (para-aminosalicylic acid) also has anti-inflammatory properties and is as effective as 5-ASA in the treatment of IBD (O'Donnell et al. 1992). The presence of the sulphonamide moiety in sulphasalazine has limited its use (see below) and a series of other 5-ASA preparations have therefore been developed (Table 3.10). When 5-ASA is given orally it is rapidly absorbed by the small intestine and is therefore not available to treat colonic inflammation. To prevent absorption in the small intestine, 5-ASA has been formulated as a variety of resin-coated preparations to provide slow or delayed release of the 5-ASA. It has also been produced as a dimer (olsalazine) or linked by an azo bond to an innocuous carrier molecule (balsalazide). The mechanism of action of the aminosalicylates is not fully understood although these drugs are known to act at several key points in the arachidonic acid pathway, thereby inhibiting production of prostaglandins and leukotrienes. They are also scavengers of free oxygen radicals. There is evidence that ASA drugs can modulate the effect of cytokines in the intestinal mucosa. Many of the adverse effects of sulphasalazine such as headache, nausea, skin rashes, haemolytic anaemia and male infertility have been overcome with the new 5-ASA drugs. However, other problems have emerged with these drugs including diarrhoea (most commonly reported with olsalazine) and occasional impairment of renal function.

Table 3.10 5-ASA preparations for treatment of inflammatory bowel disease

Delivery mode	Drug	Formulation
Azo-linked	Sulphasalazine	Sulphapyridine
	Olsalazine	5-ASA dimer
	Balsalazide	Alanine-linked
	Ipsalazaide	Glycine-linked
	Polyasa	Sulphanilamide
Coated preparations of mesalazine		
Delayed release	Asacol	Eudragit S (pH 7.0)
	Rowasa	5-ASA/resin
Slow release	Pentasa	Ethylcellulose microgranules
	Claversal	Eudragit L (pH 6.0)
	Salofalk	Eudragit L (pH 6.0)

Immunosuppressives

Several immunosuppressive drugs have been shown to play an important part in the management of IBD, particularly in maintenance therapy (Table 3.10). The first drugs to find a place in the management of IBD were azathioprine and its metabolite, 6-mercaptopurine (6-MP) (Crotty and Jewell 1992; Carpani de Kaski and Hodgson 1993). Both drugs are effective in maintaining remission in UC and CD, thereby acting as steroid-sparing agents (Willoughby et al. 1971; O'Donoghue et al. 1978). The effects of these drugs in IBD are thought to be predominantly due to their inhibitory effects on T lymphocytes but they have also been shown to affect B lymphocyte function and natural killer cell activity. Azathioprine (and 6-MP) has a number of important and potentially serious adverse effects, including bone marrow suppression, pancreatitis and polyneuritis. These adverse effects are almost always an indication for immediate withdrawal of the drug. Occasionally, after 10–14 days of taking azathioprine, patients may experience an influenza-like illness with fever and myalgia. This is usually a self-limiting illness and patients are generally advised to continue taking the medication, as the symptoms will usually resolve in a few days. There are long-term concerns about neoplasia but these seem to be largely restricted to transplant recipients taking the drug. A limited study suggests that azathioprine is safe in pregnancy.

Cyclosporin was introduced to prevent rejection of renal transplants. Because of its potent immunosuppressive properties it has been used in a variety of immune-mediated disorders, including IBD. Although initial studies in CD were encouraging, a recent multi-centre placebo controlled trial has indicated that it is not of value in CD, either for inducing or maintaining remission. However, there is increasing evidence to suggest that cyclosporin can induce remission in patients with severe acute UC and that it will maintain remission in some of these individuals (Crotty and Jewell 1992; Carpani de Kaski and Hodgson 1993). Further work is required to confirm these encouraging observations. Cyclosporin has also been shown to be active in distal UC when administered as an enema. Cyclosporin is a potent inhibitor of CD4 T lymphocyte activation and reduces the responsiveness of these lymphocytes to the cytokine interleukin 2 (IL-2). Cyclosporin also reduces the production of cytokines, interferon-gamma and IL-2 by helper CD8 T lymphocytes. Finally, cyclosporin has an inhibitory effect on antigen-presenting cells such as macrophages. Cyclosporin has a number of unwanted side effects of which nephrotoxicity is a major concern. Others include paraesthesiae, hypertrichosis, gingival hyperplasia and hypertension. Monitoring of drug concentrations in plasma is essential to prevent toxic effects.

Another immunosuppressive drug, methotrexate, has been used in the treatment of refractory CD and UC; preliminary reports suggest that it may find a place in the management of IBD. Further controlled studies are required before this drug can be incorporated into routine clinical practice.

Antimicrobial agents

There is little evidence to suggest that antimicrobial chemotherapy has a major part to play in either the treatment of acute attacks or the maintenance of remission in IBD. One study has suggested that the antibiotic tobramycin, when given with conventional steroid medication, induced remission more rapidly than steroids alone. Further studies are required to establish the role of antibiotics in UC. There is, however, evidence to suggest that metronidazole, which is effective against anaerobic bacteria, is also useful in the management of colonic and perianal CD. This drug has immunosuppressive as well as antibacterial properties and thus its precise mode of action is unclear. Long-term use is limited because of peripheral neuropathy. There has been considerable interest in the possibility that CD may be caused by one of the atypical mycobacteria such as *Mycobacterium paratuberculosis*. Although initial uncontrolled studies of antimycobacterial chemotherapy in CD were encouraging, controlled studies even with quadruple chemotherapy have failed to prove conclusively that these drugs are of value in CD. For the present, the use of these drugs should be restricted to evaluation in controlled clinical trials.

Nutritional therapy

Reversal of undernutrition is an important part of the overall management of patients with IBD. However, there is evidence that enteral nutrition with elemental or polymeric liquid diets can induce remission in CD as effectively as corticosteroids. Interestingly, 'bowel rest' using solely intravenous nutrition is not an effective primary therapy for CD. Nutritional therapy in UC administered either enterally or parenterally does not appear to influence disease activity but, as in CD, may be of value in replacing nutritional deficits.

TREATMENT OF ULCERATIVE COLITIS – PRACTICAL GUIDELINES

The principles of the treatment of UC are threefold: the prompt and appropriate treatment of acute attacks of colitis, the introduction of appropriate maintenance therapy to reduce the risk of further attacks and the timely selection of patients requiring colectomy.

Acute attack

The two major considerations when treating an acute attack of UC are the severity and the extent of the disease. The severity of an attack can be defined on the basis of symptoms, clinical features and laboratory investigations (Table 3.11). Particularly sinister signs in a severe attack include fever, tachycardia and anaemia. A severe attack should be treated

Table 3.11 Defining the severity of an attack of ulcerative colitis

	Mild	Moderate	Severe
Bowel frequency (no. per day)	<4	4–6	>6
Blood in stool	±	+	++
Temperature	Normal	Intermediate	>37.8°C on 2 of 4 days
Pulse rate (beats/min)	Normal	Intermediate	>90
Haemoglobin	Normal	Intermediate	<75%
ESR (mm in 1st hour)	<30	Intermediate	>30

in hospital by an intravenous regimen of fluids and corticosteroids (hydrocortisone or prednisolone). Anti-diarrhoeal drugs such as codeine phosphate and loperamide are best avoided during a severe acute attack. Other supportive measures such as blood transfusion may be required. Patients must be carefully monitored during a severe attack because of the risk of toxic megacolon and perforation. A daily plain abdominal radiograph is the only safe way to exclude this complication. Failure to respond to this intensive regimen after 5–7 days is usually taken as an indication for colectomy. If there are no absolute indications for colectomy and the patient particularly wishes to pursue medical therapy, it may be reasonable to offer a trial of intravenous cyclosporin (4 mg/kg), as this drug can induce remission in some apparently steroid-resistant cases.

Mild or moderate attacks of UC can usually be managed on an outpatient basis with prednisolone (20–40 mg daily) in combination with an oral 5-ASA drug designed to treat colonic disease (mesalazine, olsalazine) (Hanauer 1993). Depending on the extent of colitis, topical therapy as a corticosteroid or 5-ASA retention enema may also be appropriate. Mild attacks of UC may respond to a 5-ASA drug alone, but this may have to be given in high dosage to achieve a good therapeutic response. The extent of the disease often has a major impact on the choice of therapeutic regimen in acute UC.

Proctitis

Disease that is localized to the rectum can usually be treated topically either with corticosteroid suppositories or foam or with 5-ASA suppositories. Occasionally in resistant cases it is worth trying acetarsol suppositories, although these are not widely available. Constipation is a common associated feature of proctitis and is often helped by the addition of a bulking agent to the diet.

Distal colitis

UC involving only the rectum and sigmoid colon can often be managed with topical therapy alone. Foam-based steroid enemas travel retrogradely in the colon and will often treat the entire sigmoid colon, despite their low volume. Alternatively, aqueous enemas (corticosteroid or 5-ASA) can be used. Because of their extremely low mass, foam enemas are often better tolerated than aqueous enemas. For acute severe distal UC, systemic corticosteroid therapy may be necessary.

Extensive colitis

UC involving the hepatic flexure and beyond almost invariably requires systemic therapy. Topical therapy to the rectum may be added if there is marked frequency and urgency, indicating severe distal disease. Thus, oral corticosteroid with a 5-ASA drug, combined with topical therapy in the form of a foam or aqueous enema, often proves to be the most efficacious approach.

Maintenance treatment

There are no special dietary considerations in the maintenance therapy of UC although a few patients have benefited from a milk-free diet. Despite the clear efficacy of corticosteroid medication in the treatment of acute attacks, it has no part to play in maintenance therapy of UC. Long-term use of corticosteroids puts patients at increased risk of developing complications without any proven beneficial effects. 5-ASA drugs and immunosuppressives, however, have been shown to offer long-term benefit in maintaining remission in UC.

5-ASA

Early controlled clinical trials of sulphasalazine showed unequivocally that this drug was able to reduce substantially the risk of relapse in UC. Up to 15% of patients, however, are unable to tolerate this drug because of the dose-related side effects such as headache, nausea and malaise. The newer 5-ASA preparations have proved to be highly acceptable and all have been shown to be as effective in maintaining remission as sulphasalazine (see Table 3.10). The efficacy of maintenance therapy is dose-related although the higher doses often required to induce remission during an acute attack are generally not required for maintenance therapy. Once the diagnosis of UC has been firmly established (i.e. episodic, recurrent attacks of colitis), it is reasonable to consider maintenance therapy with a 5-ASA drug for life. However, in practice, many patients who have been well for a number of years often gradually withdraw maintenance medication. There are no clear guidelines as to how one might predict whether relapse is likely to occur after many years in remission.

Immunosuppressives

There is now convincing evidence that azathioprine (2 mg/kg) is effective in maintaining remission in UC. This drug is used as a second-line maintenance agent and is generally introduced only after relapse while taking a maintenance 5-ASA drug at an appropriate dose. Patients need to be carefully monitored to minimize the risks of developing bone marrow suppression.

TREATMENT OF CROHN'S DISEASE – PRACTICAL GUIDELINES

The goals for the management of a patient with CD are principally to control symptoms such that the patient may maintain as normal a lifestyle as possible. In children and adolescents achievement of full growth potential continues to be a major therapeutic objective (Farmer and Michener 1979; Farthing 1991). Symptom patterns are more diverse in CD than in UC and, unlike UC, the disease is not cured by surgery. Thus a patient with CD has to face, at least for the time being, a lifetime with the disease – which inevitably has a major influence on that individual's approach to life. Many patients do not always express their long-term fears about the disease, the majority being extremely stoical, often minimizing symptoms when consulting their general practitioner or hospital specialist. Nutritional support is a vital component of the management of many patients with CD but this usually needs to be combined with drug therapy in both the acute and the maintenance phases of the illness.

Nutritional therapy

Although many patients would like to find a dietary solution to CD, no specific diet has yet been identified that has a long-term effect on the natural history of the disease (Greenberg et al. 1988). However, nutritional therapy does play an important part in replacing nutritional deficits, promoting growth and development in children and adolescents, treating acute relapses of CD and, in some cases, providing symptomatic relief.

Replacement of nutritional deficits

Many patients with CD lose weight during the acute phase of the disease, mainly because of anorexia and reduced food intake. Malabsorption is an uncommon cause of weight loss in CD and is probably physiologically relevant only in the patients with diffuse jejunoileitis or after extensive small intestinal resection. Nutritional support may be provided by supplementing oral intake, by nasogastric tube feeding or, when indicated, by intravenous nutrition. Overnight tube feeding controlled by means of a simple rotary pump can supplement normal food taken during the day. Specific nutritional deficits may need to be corrected. For example, vitamin B_{12} deficiency can occur following resection of more than 100 cm of distal ileum; magnesium deficiency commonly occurs in patients with a short small intestine.

Promotion of growth and development

About 30% of children and adolescents with CD experience some degree of growth retardation. Maintenance of adequate nutritional intake is an important factor in the management of growth retardation combined with measures directed towards controlling inflammatory activity (Belli et al. 1988). One approach that tackles these objectives simultaneously uses an elemental diet as the sole source of nutrition. These diets generally require administration by a nasogastric tube and are usually given for at least 4–6 weeks. In certain cases it may be worth considering more prolonged therapy, particularly in diffuse small intestinal disease that is responding poorly to anti-inflammatory drugs.

Control of inflammation

Elemental diet (and possibly polymeric diet) can reduce inflammatory markers in CD and induce remission with efficacy similar to corticosteroids (O'Morain, Segal and Levi 1984; Gorard et al. 1993). However, up to 30–40% of patients find this therapeutic approach unacceptable and are unable to tolerate the diet. Some patients are able to drink elemental diets when served chilled or flavoured; this is probably most valuable in children and adolescents with growth retardation. Withdrawal of elemental diet is associated with relapse of CD, and long-term follow-up at one year suggests that the relapse rate is in fact higher in patients treated with elemental diet than in those receiving conventional therapy with corticosteroids (Gorard et al. 1993).

Symptom control

Withdrawal of certain foods in individual patients may improve symptoms although there are no specific general recommendations that one can make in CD. Diarrhoea may be exacerbated by spicy and high-fibre foods; many patients have a preference for a bland diet consisting of fish, chicken, rice and potatoes, etc. Patients with obstructive symptoms due to small intestinal strictures are generally advised to avoid particularly indigestible foods such as fibrous vegetables, nuts, etc., as these may exacerbate obstructive pain. A liquid diet can often completely relieve symptoms of intestinal obstruction.

Drug therapy

Active disease

Severe acute CD is treated in a similar way to severe UC, with an intravenous regimen of corticosteroids sometimes combined with broad-spectrum antibiotics including metronidazole. Intravenous nutritional support may be required, although if tolerated this is probably better provided by an elemental diet administered by nasogastric tube. For moderate acute disease, oral prednisolone 40 mg daily should be given for at least 1–2 weeks and not be reduced until symptomatic improvement has been observed. It is a mistake to withdraw corticosteroid therapy too rapidly before a remission has really become established. Mild attacks may respond to a 5-ASA drug alone although in CD this class of drug is considerably less potent than corticosteroids. Asacol (mesalazine) and olsalazine are recommended for colonic disease, and Pentasa for small intestinal disease because of its slow release profile. Metronidazole is as effective as sulphasalazine in controlling colonic disease.

Maintenance therapy

There is no evidence that corticosteroid medication has any role in the maintenance treatment of CD, so ideally these drugs should be withdrawn completely following treatment of an acute relapse. However, there seems to be a group of patients who note a deterioration in their symptoms even following withdrawal of relatively small doses of corticosteroid, and clinical impression continues to support the view that such patients may have a steroid-dependent remission. It should be stressed, however, that there is no controlled clinical trial evidence to support this observation.

There is increasing evidence that 5-ASA drugs have a role in maintenance therapy in CD and results of further clinical trials will become available in the near future (International Mesalazine Study Group 1990). Even though we do not have the final answer on the role of these drugs in CD, it seems reasonable to offer patients therapy with a 5-ASA drug while the results of these trials are awaited.

Azathioprine or 6-MP has an important part to play in the maintenance therapy of some patients with CD who repeatedly relapse following the withdrawal of corticosteroid or other treatment following an acute attack (Willoughby et al. 1971; O'Donoghue et al. 1978). However, these drugs are not without side effects and the patient needs to be counselled carefully about the risks and benefits of taking such medication. Monitoring of the blood count at regular intervals is recommended during azathioprine therapy although bone marrow suppression can still occur within the monitoring interval and thus not be detected by such a surveillance programme.

Cyclosporin does not seem to have a role in the maintenance therapy of CD although other immunosuppressive drugs as such methotrexate may prove to be of value in the future.

Drug therapy after intestinal resection

It is now well established that within a year of an intestinal resection endoscopic surveillance confirms that more than 90% of patients have evidence of recurrent CD, often without symptoms. In view of the evidence that 5-ASA drugs have a modest but nevertheless significant effect in maintaining CD in remission, these drugs might be considered following ileal resection.

Symptom control

Diarrhoea in CD is not always related to active disease but may relate to previous surgery, such as right hemicolectomy. This may be treated more appropriately with an anti-diarrhoeal drug such as loperamide or codeine phosphate, or the bile salt-binding resin, cholestyramine, which binds bile salts that would otherwise enter the colon following ileal resection and exacerbate diarrhoea.

Special problems in Crohn's disease

As CD can affect any part of the alimentary tract, its clinical manifestations are diverse and often pose challenging management problems. The following summarizes some of the author's personal views on the management of special problems of CD in different regions of the gastrointestinal tract.

Orolabial

The so-called thick lip syndrome is an uncommon manifestation of CD, but particularly troublesome in adolescents and young adults. It may be the only evidence of the disease initially, and can be associated with a fissure in the lip and more extensive aphthous ulceration in the mouth. Treatment centres around the use of anti-inflammatory drugs, but the response is often disappointing and the disease seems to wax and wane in a relatively independent manner. Steroid tablets may be dissolved slowly in the mouth or given as a mouthwash using prednisolone-21-phosphate. Alternatively, steroid cream may be applied locally. The response to systemic steroids is similarly disappointing. Orolabial CD in adolescents often improves as the individual enters adulthood.

Gastroduodenal

Symptoms may be similar to those of a peptic ulcer but response to acid inhibitory drugs is usually less dramatic. Treatment is similar to that of CD elsewhere in the gastrointestinal tract but additional symptomatic relief can often be provided by an H_2-receptor antagonist or a proton pump inhibitor. In duodenal CD, vomiting commonly accompanies acute exacerbations of the disease, but once the inflammatory process is under control this usually subsides. Stricturing disease does occur, in which case a gastrojejunostomy may be required to bypass the obstruction.

Diffuse jejunoileitis

This is a particularly sinister form of CD which commonly affects the young. The entire small intestine may be involved initially with a diffuse inflammatory process followed later by multiple strictures. Surgery should be restricted to the management of obstructing strictures and should always be conservative. The disease may respond poorly to anti-inflammatory drugs. High-dose corticosteroids combined with an immunosuppressive drug such as azathioprine may be required for long periods of time. In adolescents with growth potential it may be worth considering long-term nasogastric feeding with elemental diet for periods of many months. Maintenance therapy may be enhanced by addition of the 5-ASA drug, Pentasa, which is released in the small intestine.

Ileocaecal

This is the classic site for CD and accounts for more than 60% of cases.

Medical treatment of CD in this region follows the usual guidelines; when this disease is localized, early surgery should be considered – particularly if there are other complications such as stricture or internal fistulation. Psoas abscess may complicate CD in this region of the intestinal tract.

Colitis

In approximately 15% of patients with colitis it may be impossible to distinguish between CD and UC. CD colitis is sometimes slower to go into remission than UC. The complications requiring urgent surgery are less common in CD. In CD the colitis may remain persistently active, resulting in chronic diarrhoea and chronic ill health. Medical treatment with corticosteroids, 5-ASA drugs and metronidazole can often control the disease for many years. If difficulties are encountered in withdrawing prednisolone, a trial of azathioprine or 6-MP is warranted.

Anorectal

The anal lesions of CD may be critical in distinguishing CD from UC. Chronic fistulation, discharging sinuses, fissures and active rectal ulceration with strictures are the typical features. Although a variety of treatments such as topical steroids or 5-ASA drugs can relieve symptoms in the short term, there is no treatment that will reliably alter the natural history of destructive anorectal CD. Intermittent courses of antibiotics including metronidazole, however, can control symptoms but surgery may be required to drain abscesses that are not discharging spontaneously. Involvement and ultimately destruction of the sphincters compounds the problem and leads to incontinence. Patients will often continue with severe symptoms because of their fears of rectal excision and a stoma. Once the decision is taken to proceed with surgery, patients often feel a sense of liberation from the morbidity of this aspect of their disease.

Anorectal disease may be complicated by a low rectal stricture (which may require regular dilatation) or fistulation into the genital tract (vagina or prostate). These complications may hasten the need for rectal excision.

REFERENCES

Baron, J.H., Connell, A.M., Lennard-Jones, J.E. and Avery Jones, F. (1962) Sulphasalazine and salicylazo-sulphadimidine in ulcerative colitis. *Lancet*, **1**: 1094–9.

Belli, D.C., Seidman, E., Bouthilier, L., et al. (1988) Chronic intermittent elemental diet improves growth failure in children with Crohn's disease. *Gastroenterology*, **94**: 603–10.

Carpani de Kaski, M. and Hodgson, H.J.F. (1993) Inflammatory bowel disease. *Alimentary Pharmacology andTherapeutics,* **7**: 567–79.

Crotty, B. and Jewell, D.P. (1992) Drug therapy of ulcerative colitis. *British Journal of Clinical Pharmacology*, **34**: 189–98.

Farmer, R.G. and Michener, W.M. (1979) Prognosis of Crohn's disease with onset in childhood or adolescence. *Digestive Diseases and Sciences*, **24**: 752–7.

Farthing, M.J.G. (1991) Crohn's disease in childhood and adolescence. In: Anagnostides, A.A., Hodgson, H.J.F. and Kirsner, J.B. (Eds) *Inflammatory Bowel Disease*. Chapman & Hall: London, pp. 12–25.

Gorard, D.A., Hunt, J.B., Payne-James, J.J., et al. (1993) Initial response and subsequent course of Crohn's disease treated with elemental diet or prednisolone. *Gut*, **47**: 155–9.

Greenberg, G.R., Fleming, C.R., Jeejeebhoy, K.N., Rosenberg, I.H., Sales, D. and Tremaine, W.J. (1988) Controlled trial of bowel rest and nutritional support in the management of Crohn's disease. *Gut*, **29**: 1309–15.

Hanauer, S. (1993) Medical therapy of ulcerative colitis. *Lancet*, **342**: 412–17.

International Mesalazine Study Group. (1990) Coated oral 5-aminosalicylic acid versus placebo in maintaining remission of inactive Crohn's disease. *Alimentary Pharmacology and Therapeutics*, **4**: 55–64.

Jayanthi, V., Probert, C.S.J. and Mayberry, J.F. (1991) Epidemiology of inflammatory bowel disease. *Quarterly Journal of Medicine*, **78**: 5–12.

Ljungh, A. (1992) Microbiological aspects of inflammatory bowel disease. In: Jarnerot, G., Lennard-Jones, J., Truelove, S. (Eds) *Inflammatory Bowel Disease*. Corona AB: Malmo, pp. 73–89.

O'Donnell, L.J.D., Arvind, A.S., Hoang, P., et al. (1992) Double-bind controlled trial of 4-aminosalicylic acid and prednisolone enemas in distal ulcerative colitis. *Gut*, **33**: 947–9.

O'Donoghue, D.P., Dawson, A.M., Powell-Tuck, J., Bown, R.L. and Lennard-Jones, J.E. (1978) Double-blind withdrawal trial of azathioprine as maintenance treatment for Crohn's disease. *Lancet*, **2**: 955–7.

O'Morain, C., Segal, A.M. and Levi, A.J. (1984) Elemental diet as primary treatment of acute Crohn's disease: a controlled trial. *British Medical Journal*, **288**: 1859–62.

Shanahan, F. (1993) Pathogenesis of ulcerative colitis. *Lancet*, **342**: 407–11.

Willoughby, J.M.T., Kumar, P.J., Beckett, J. and Dawson, A.M. (1971) Controlled trial of azathioprine in Crohn's disease. *Lancet*, **2**: 944–7.

4 Enterocutaneous fistulae and their management

Alastair Forbes and Celia Myers

INTRODUCTION

Enterocutaneous fistulae are abnormal openings between the intestine and the skin (usually that of the anterior abdominal wall). They occur most often following abdominal surgery in which the bowel has been opened. They are particularly associated with surgery for Crohn's disease, but also occur as a complication of diverticular disease and in combination with a range of rarer diagnoses. Gunshot wounds to the abdomen are, fortunately, an unusual cause in the UK. The enterocutaneous fistula represents the breakdown of a penetrating bowel disorder with an adherent abscess, and as such is almost always associated with local sepsis at least initially.

CLASSIFICATION

The management of enterocutaneous fistulae is markedly influenced by the anatomical classification of the fistula, as to a large extent this determines the likelihood of spontaneous resolution. Fistulae may be simple, multiple or complicated, and any of these may be obstructed (Fig. 4.1). It will be appreciated that the simple single fistula with no obstruction (Fig. 4.1a) stands a greater chance of closing, with good supportive care, than multiple complex fistulae (Fig. 4.1b); where the two ends of bowel have become separated or communicate only via an abscess cavity, (Fig. 4.1c) resolution without further surgery is most unlikely, and if there is distal obstruction (Fig. 4.1d) conservative therapy is bound to fail.

POSTOPERATIVE FISTULAE

Postoperative fistulae are considered by most surgeons to be a surgical failing. Whilst this is not usually the case, it may be, and has perpetuated a critical attitude that has had the unfortunate effect that very few surgeons are prepared to share their experience in public. In consequence, we lack good data as to the true incidence. In a large study of postoper-

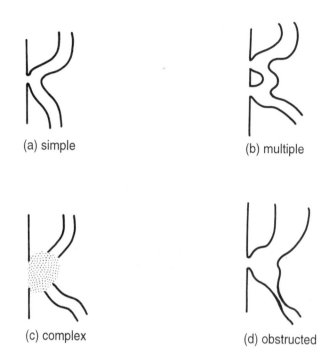

(a) simple

(b) multiple

(c) complex

(d) obstructed

Fig. 4.1 Classification of fistulae.

ative fistulae referred for specialist help, Lévy et al. (1989) considered 335 consecutive cases. Crohn's disease was present in 6.3% of the patients, compared to a frequency in ulcerative colitis (a condition not normally linked with fistula formation) of 4.2%. This was obviously not a controlled study and the incidence and attributable risk from surgery of different types in different conditions remain unclear. For postoperative fistulae over all, a spontaneous closure rate of around 50% can be anticipated if the Paris data (Lévy et al. 1989) are representative. Fistulae are not themselves often responsible for fatality but affect sick patients, and Lévy found a 4% in-hospital mortality rate.

FISTULAE IN CROHN'S DISEASE

Enterocutaneous fistulae affect around 15% of patients with Crohn's disease at some time in their lives (Rinsema et al. 1990), although nearer one-third of those with perianal manifestations of the disease are likely to be affected. Some 85% of the fistulae occur in the postoperative period, and extrapolation from published series suggests that about 25% of laparotomies have in the past been complicated by fistula formation. Such fistulae are nearly always through or close to the line of incision. Simple drainage is effective in some patients, but in about a third there will be an associated abscess which necessitates a more definitive surgical approach if medical management fails. The mortality of enterocutaneous fistulae complicating surgery for Crohn's is nearly double that of non-Crohn's cases, emphasizing the poor condition of many of these patients rather than a direct effect of the fistulous process.

When considering fistulae in Crohn's disease, it is helpful to distinguish anastomotic-type fistulae from fistulae of diseased bowel. The former may conveniently be thought of as those that might follow any intestinal surgery whereas the latter are dependent on the coexistence of Crohn's disease. This has clinical relevance as the former will often heal spontaneously while the latter rarely will, which largely explains the apparently contradictory reports in the literature of spontaneous healing in anything from 0 to 60% – like has not been compared with like.

The Calgary group (Kelly and Preshaw 1989) have provided a useful account of their experience with fistulae in Crohn's disease. Because it considers all patients having surgery for the disease at a single centre, it is probably the nearest we have to true incidence data. Inevitably, however, with the long period of data collection, some of the interventions and results may not now be considered optimal. They reported a total of 236 resections for Crohn's disease, of which almost half (109) were re-operations in patients with prior surgery for the disease. Sixty patients had a fistula (or fistulae), of which only 15 were enterocutaneous. The sites are summarized in Table 4.1. The 11 patients with previous surgery fell into one of two groups according to the timing of the previous surgery. One group presented early (2–6 months after surgery), and all had a fistula originating at a dehiscence of the anastomosis; six (75%) had no active Crohn's disease. These patients can reasonably be considered to belong to the perioperative/anastomotic group similar to patients with other surgical conditions suggested above. The second group presented late (3–5 years after surgery): all had recurrent, and usually stenotic, Crohn's disease at the intestinal end of the fistula. Whatever the relation to the timing of previous surgery, the fistula opened via the old scar in every case.

The patient with previously undiagnosed Crohn's disease who presents

Table 4.1 Enterocutaneous fistulae in Crohn's patients

	Spontaneous*	Operated*
Ileocutaneous	1	2
Ileoileal + ileocutaneous	1	1
Ileocolic + ileocutaneous	1	0
Colocutaneous	1	0
Anastomosis–skin	0	7
Anastomosis–ileum–skin	0	1
Total	4	11 (all via scar)

*The spontaneous column refers to patients who had had no previous abdominal surgery; all those in the operated group had had previous surgery for Crohn's disease.
Data from Kelly and Preshaw (1989).

with apparent acute appendicitis raises an interesting question in respect of fistula risk. A gridiron incision in the right iliac fossa has been made, but the appendix is normal and the ileocaecal area is involved by Crohn's disease. With this scar it will always be believed that the appendix has been removed, which is potentially dangerous if appendicitis subsequently develops. However, if the appendix is removed, will there not be a very high risk of fistula formation? The answer lies in the nature of the fistulous process which appears never to transfer disease to a new structure. Although appendicectomy may well be complicated by enterocutaneous fistula, if a fistula occurs it is ileal and not from the operated area on the caecum. In other words the fistula is provoked by the laparotomy and not by the appendicectomy. In our view, surgeons unexpectedly finding Crohn's disease at gridiron incision should remove the appendix. Hopefully, this problem will soon disappear with the increasing use of diagnostic laparoscopy in patients with abdominal pain.

IMAGING OF ENTEROCUTANEOUS FISTULAE

The imaging of enterocutaneous fistulae is far from ideal. Abdominal ultrasound scanning may reveal areas of abnormal intestine and associated abscesses but is not likely to show the fistulous track itself. Plain abdominal radiographs similarly (though even less often) may demonstrate a fluid level within an abscess cavity but contribute little. Imaging of the gastrointestinal tract from within, using barium (and a number of alternative contrast agents), is the mainstay of investigation of fistulae in most hospitals. Careful screening of the contrast agent as it traverses the intestine is essential, as the sequence of the appearance of contrast at different levels will often be crucial to correct interpretation. The fistulous track(s) will often but not always be shown. Complementary to the intestinal contrast study is the 'fistulogram' in which a contrast agent is injected (often requiring considerable pressure) through a small catheter previously inserted into the fistulous opening. Use of an occlusion balloon inflated just below the skin allows the necessary pressure with less tendency for the contrast to spill ineffectually.

Endoscopic examination is rarely directly helpful in fistula assessment, as fistulous openings (even those that can be reached) are often invisible endoscopically. Endoscopy may, however, help to establish whether there is underlying Crohn's disease or diverticulosis and to document the sites of these. Contrast-enhanced computed tomography (CT) scan is increasingly helpful in the assessment of fistulae, but again frequently fails to show the fistulous openings and is best at demonstrating associated abscesses; retroperitoneal disease is less likely to be missed than with ultrasound scanning. The most promising modality for imaging of abdominal fistulae is magnetic resonance imaging (MRI), which has great potential to discriminate normal and diseased tissues. Few scanners are available in the UK as yet, but early data indicate that, in addition to virtually all the information provided by ultrasound and CT, in 75% of cases MRI also demonstrates all fistulous orifices.

FACTORS IMPEDING CLOSURE

It will already have been inferred that a number of factors impede spontaneous closure of enterocutaneous fistulae. These are conveniently grouped in Table 4.2, but this should not be considered to be a comprehensive list. Clearly these factors are relative rather than absolute, but a patient with several of them is most unlikely to respond completely to medical therapy.

Table 4.2 Factors impeding closure of fistulae

General factors	Sepsis
	Malnutrition
Gastrointestinal pathology	Crohn's disease
	Focal malignancy
	Radiation enteritis
Anatomical factors	Distal obstruction
	Bowel discontinuity
	Abscess
	Mucocutaneous continuity

IMMEDIATE MANAGEMENT OF THE ENTEROCUTANEOUS FISTULA

The immediate management of the enterocutaneous fistula follows standard practice with initial assessment and resuscitation of the patient. This is likely to require fluid replacement, the drainage of abscesses, and transfusion when appropriate. It is never too soon to begin taking very great care of the skin around the fistulous opening, especially when the fistula is from high in the bowel and the effluent rich in enzymes (and probably acidic also). This is probably one of the greatest challenges for the stoma care therapist. Important, though less immediate, is the need for nutritional support of the patient. Total parenteral nutrition (TPN) will often be required with the patient kept 'nil-by-mouth', but surprisingly often (and usually if the highest fistula is in the lower ileum) enteral feeding will allow sufficient bowel rest without either the hazards of TPN or the loss of the important health-preserving (trophic) effects of luminal nutrients on the small bowel mucosa.

The patient with a high enterocutaneous fistula (or stoma) presents particular problems. First, it may be very difficult to assess fluid balance. The unstable patient may well need a central venous line to monitor venous filling pressures and a urinary catheter to permit accurate measurement of urine volume. All such patients must be weighed daily if at all possible. It is to be expected that the fluid requirement will be in excess of 5 litres per day and this should be anticipated. If the patient is drinking, it will probably be necessary to curtail oral fluid intake. This apparently paradoxical advice stems from the absence of sodium in all commonly consumed drinks. The intestinal response to receipt of sodium-free liquids is to secrete sodium into the bowel; water follows the salt, thus leading to potentially huge extra volumes of fluid finding their way into the intestinal lumen. In a normal person this extra fluid is readily reabsorbed in the lower ileum and the colon. The patient with a high fistula does not have this opportunity, and the losses of fluid and electrolytes readily become life-threatening. Fortunately, knowledge about the coupling of sodium, glucose and water transport in the intestine helps us to overcome this problem by the use of balanced electrolyte solutions – exactly as promoted for acute diarrhoeal illnesses in small children. If a solution containing at least 60 mmol sodium per litre is used liberally for thirst, and free (sodium-lacking) fluids limited to no more than 500 ml a day, most patients with more than 1 metre of reasonably normal intestine above the fistula will retain rather than lose body water. Sodium status can, and should, be monitored by regular measurement of the urinary sodium. These need not be timed samples – all that is required is knowledge that the concentration is no less than 30 mmol/l. Daily weights provide useful general data on nutrition but more particularly reflect the patient's fluid balance.

Tetany in intestinal disease is more often the result of magnesium deficiency than calcium deficiency, and when both coexist it will usually require correction of the magnesium level before hypocalcaemia can be overcome. As magnesium deficiency is common in the patient with a short bowel or high fistula, it should be actively sought with preventative intent.

SPECIFIC MANAGEMENT OF ENTEROCUTANEOUS FISTULAE IN CROHN'S DISEASE

The specific management of enterocutaneous fistulae in Crohn's disease may sensibly be divided between that of patients presenting in the early postoperative period and those with spontaneous fistulae or fistulae presenting many months or years after surgery.

In the postoperative group, general medical and nursing care will continue, with particular attention to skin care (see below). Nutritional support will be required and this will often need to comprise a period nil-by-mouth on parenteral nutrition. If the fistula is low in the bowel, however, enteral feeding may be feasible, and is always desirable if possible. Spontaneous closure of a single fistula may be expected in about 50% of patients over 4–6 weeks. If any of the adverse factors alluded to elsewhere obtain, this figure will be substantially reduced. It should be noted, however, that the apparent closure rate is very much greater, as it is common for the skin opening to close over, but without resolution of, the underlying fistula between the bowel and the (internal) abdominal wall. Perhaps one-third of all 'closures' with medical therapy reopen within 3 months (Driscoll and Rosenberg 1978). Debate continues over the value or otherwise of immunosuppressive agents such as azathioprine and cyclosporin. Steroids are not absolutely contraindicated in the management of patients with Crohn's-related fistulae, as they can be helpful if there is continuing active Crohn's disease, but they will tend to impair healing and cannot be considered at all satisfactory in the management of the fistula itself.

True spontaneous fistulae are very rare in Crohn's disease; indeed, Crohn himself never saw one! They usually arise from an embryological remnant of the urachus running to the umbilicus, and account for about 4% of all umbilical fistulae (Greenstein et al. 1984). For all practical purposes these never close without surgery. We believe that late postoperative fistulae in Crohn's share most of their behaviour with those characteristic of the spontaneous fistula, and anticipate a need for surgery.

Surgery for enterocutaneous fistula is likely to be successful if there is localized disease and if it is possible to excise both the involved bowel and the fistulous track in their entirety. Naturally, any surgery should be preceded by full resuscitation if it is to have the best chance of success. Surgery can be considered strongly indicated if the fistula is spontaneous, if a jejunal site is involved or if the fistula includes a communication with the bladder. Surgery gives poorer results if the colon is involved or, unsurprisingly, when there is extensive disease and/or complex multiple fistulae. Closure of interrupted bowel should probably not be attempted without a proximal defunctioning stoma; in general, surgery is best avoided if there is extensive disease, already a functionally short bowel or risk of this, and when the fistula is well tolerated.

NON-SURGICAL INTERVENTION IN FISTULA MANAGEMENT

In addition to the general supportive measures already outlined, and full nutritional provision – intravenously or enterally as appropriate – an 'antisecretory' regimen will usually be indicated. Typically this will comprise oral loperamide, and an H_2 blocker (such as cimetidine or ranitidine) or omeprazole. The loperamide acts mainly by slowing intestinal transit and (to a lesser extent) by reducing intestinal secretion, and is preferred to codeine phosphate or diphenoxylate as it avoids sedation and anticholinergic side effects such as blurred vision and dry mouth (although some authors believe that an anticholinergic is helpful in this context). The omeprazole or H_2 blocker is used not to reduce gastric acid secretion but to benefit from the reduction (by about 500 ml per day) of the volume of gastric secretion which goes along with the suppression of acid.

There are anecdotal reports, but no controlled data, that azathioprine (or its metabolite 6-mercaptopurine) is helpful in fistula management. As it acts on developing cells, no response would be expected for 4–6 weeks, so this will often be irrelevant anyway. Impaired healing as a result of its use does not, however, appear to be a problem. Steroids are relatively contraindicated because of their effects on wound healing and infection risk, and are inappropriate if an abscess is associated with the fistula. They may be of value if there is active Crohn's disease and surgery is inappropriate at the time. Again, there are no controlled data on which to base firm advice.

Cyclosporin, a relatively new immunosuppressant with a major role in the prevention of rejection of transplanted organs, has been assessed provisionally in fistula therapy. At a standard dose of 4 mg/kg per day it was given intravenously to four patients with a total of eight fistulae, all of whom were unresponsive to prednisolone, azathioprine and experimental therapy with antibodies (Hanauer and Stathopoulos 1991). All the fistulae improved and six of the eight closed. Although one enterocutaneous fistula recurred later, this was above a new distal stricture. These promising data await confirmation by other groups.

Somatostatin and its analogue octreotide are also showing considerable promise. Somatostatin is an intestinal hormone that has inhibitory effects on a whole range of functions, including the reduction of secretion from the stomach, intestine and pancreas, and slowing the speed of intestinal transit. As it also increases water and electrolyte absorption, it is understandable that it has been thought potentially valuable in patients with fistulae and short gut syndrome. There are, however, two important effects that may not be so advantageous in this context: absorption of nutrients is diminished, and intestinal/splanchnic blood flow is reduced with potential impairment of healing as a result. Somatostatin itself is very unstable and needs to be given by a continuous infusion (with no gap even when the infusion set needs changing) if the effect is to be maintained. Octreotide is an eight amino acid peptide that retains the activity of the larger somatostatin molecule, but is also much more stable and can be given as intermittent subcutaneous injections (usually three times daily). Either will reduce fistula output reliably and reproducibly by about 500 ml per day (Nubiola et al. 1987). Unfortunately, this effect lasts only for as long as the patient is on the drug. There are anecdotal but quite convincing data from several units (including our own) that octreotide will also speed the closure of fistulae. However, to date it has not appeared that it will increase the percentage of fistulae that close, merely the speed at which they do so. Octreotide is quite a painful injection for many patients; if this is a problem, the drug may be given by continuous subcutaneous infusion or intravenously.

The use of octreotide specifically in Crohn's disease-related fistulae has not been adequately assessed. Our impression is that it helps in preoperative management but does not itself increase the frequency of spontaneous closure; this accords with provisional data from other units (Scott, Finnegan and Irving 1990).

ENTEROCUTANEOUS FISTULA – SUMMARY

The first step in the management of enterocutaneous fistulae (Table 4.3) must always be to resuscitate the patient. This is followed by classification of the nature and aetiology of the fistula(e), as these have bearing on the likely outcome with or without surgery. If fistulae are spontaneous, high jejunal, involving the bladder or Crohn's related, surgery should be considered and probably planned for. If fistulae are postoperative without complicating factors, a successful non-surgical result may be anticipated in about 50%. While awaiting surgery, or if the patient is not

Table 4.3 Enterocutaneous fistula: summary

Resuscitate and classify

If spontaneous, high jejunal, involving bladder, or Crohn's related:
  consider/plan surgery

If post-operative without complicating factor:
  anticipate successful non-surgical result in 50%

While awaiting or if not for surgery:
  Bowel rest + careful fluid and sodium balance
  Anti-secretory regimen
  Consider drug therapy of Crohn's as relevant
  Consider octreotide

thought an appropriate candidate for surgery, the bowel should be rested (parenteral or defined enteral feeding, depending on fistula site) with careful attention paid to fluid and sodium balance. An anti-secretory regimen (e.g. loperamide and omeprazole) should be started, and specific drug therapy considered if there is active Crohn's disease. In the difficult case there may be a place for administration of octreotide.

NURSING MANAGEMENT

Many factors are responsible for the morbidity suffered by patients with enterocutaneous fistulae. The physical discomfort caused by corrosive small bowel fluid and the appliances needed to cope with this are coupled with the mental trauma of a postoperative complication and the sight of small bowel fluid leaking uncontrollably from the abdomen. The need for frequent changing of the patient's night clothes and bed linen removes any sense of independence and morale deteriorates rapidly. When oral fluids are withheld, further psychological problems may develop. Some patients experience cravings for food and may have visual and olfactory hallucinations, which abate after the reintroduction of a normal diet. To obtain optimum results, great care must be taken to ensure effective management of fistulae, including meticulous skin care and collection of the drainage to assess loss so that correct fluid and electrolyte replacements can be given.

Every effort must be made to ensure the well-being of patients at all times. They may suffer the unfortunate consequences of malnutrition and, apart from the obvious weight loss and unhealthy looking appearance, may have to contend with dry skin and hair loss. If patients have been moved to a specialist centre for management, there may be feelings of isolation and loneliness to cope with. Some of these patients may, as a result, become demanding and dependent on the nursing staff, and a great deal of patient and family support and encouragement can be necessary (McIntyre et al. 1984).

Aim of care

The aim of care is to restore the physical comfort and well-being of the patient. A feeling of trust and security and improved morale will develop from the ultimate control of leakage and odour. Guidelines for care are outlined below.

Assessment

Assessment is the key to a well-applied adhesive appliance.

Total area involved and the site of the fistula

Care must be taken to choose an appliance that is large enough and appropriate for extensive wound areas; for example, a large clear wound drainage appliance (e.g CliniMed) or a large wound manager (Convatec). If other small areas are leaking (such as old drain sites) and it is not possible to include them in the whole procedure, a small paediatric appliance (Wetland, Convatec or Hollister) should be tried. It is important that any drainage from these areas is collected because the exudate can rapidly soak the main appliance, causing soreness, eventual leakage and certain odour breakthrough. This type of leakage is avoidable, and its control and collection will prevent unnecessary stress and anxiety to the patient.

Assessment of the drainage is important and will influence the type of appliance selected. If drainage is of large volume from the small bowel content of a thin consistency, an appliance with secondary drainage is most appropriate. With even body contours, a 57 mm, 70 mm or 100 mm Stomahesive flange with a urostomy pouch is an ideal choice (Fig. 4.2).

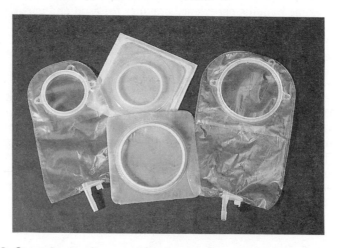

Fig. 4.2 Stomahesive flange with urostomy pouch suitable for secondary drainage with even body contours.

The thin drainage easily passes into an attached catheter drainage bag. This method prevents the appliance from overflowing or bursting, so the patient feels reassured and secure. Stomahesive flanges are very durable in the presence of corrosive small bowel effluent.

With a thicker output such as that from the large bowel or with infected material, the appliance should have a wider outlet or an access window. This type can be flushed through two or three times a day with warm saline and (optional) added deodorant drops, eliminating the tenacious material and keeping the appliance clean and fresh. This is a task with which relatives or the patient may wish to be involved. The appliance ultimately stays in place for longer as there will be no unpleasant odour to require its removal.

Assessment of the skin and equipment required

Intact and healthy skin is a bonus: keeping the skin in good condition is one of the biggest challenges to be faced by the nurse caring for a patient with an enterocutaneous fistula. Once the appropriate appliance has been chosen, on the basis of the type of drainage and the size of the fistula, consideration should be given to its suitability for the patient's skin, whether there is a need for extra skin protection and whether body contours could be a potential source of leakage.

Intact skin can tolerate Stomahesive paste which can be 'piped' into skin creases and crevices with a syringe. It is then gently warmed with a hairdryer to harden off, when it can be moulded and patted into skin crevices to give a sound, hard surface on which more paste can be applied if necessary. In this way good appliance adhesion can be obtained. If multiple small openings need an appliance and the choice is restricted to only one type, applying Orobase paste with a spatula to the skin between the fistula openings will keep it healthy between appliance changes.

If a low area of granulating skin is near a large crater, the crater should be filled with Granuflex paste to skin level and then piped over with Stomahesive paste which is allowed to harden. This will provide a good surface area for appliance adhesion and a better opportunity for granulation.

Edges of craters and large fistulae can benefit from a thin flattened-out application of Orobase paste. This cures soreness and, if an appliance has access points, can be reapplied without disrupting the appliance. When creases, crevices and contours arising from old drain sites and scars have been built to skin level, it may be appropriate to apply a sheet of Comfeel (Fig. 4.3), which will give an even and flat surface. A small quantity of Stomahesive paste piped on top of the Comfeel around the fistula will prevent seepage between the two surfaces. If there is leakage from groin and loin areas because of excessive weight loss, it may be necessary to fill in craters with Cohesive washers, moulded and rolled to skin level. The appliances needed in these areas are usually small and it is important to select one with an appropriate outlet. Some patients with terminal disease may be allowed a normal diet, which may produce a thicker than normal output from a fistulous small bowel with an opening in the loin area. Selecting an appliance may be difficult because the output needs to be

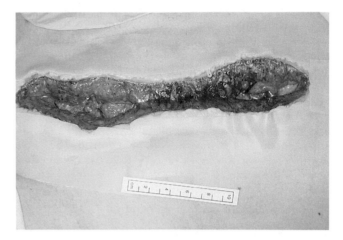

Fig. 4.3 The use of Comfeel to produce an even surface for application of the appliance.

channelled so that it is not obstructed by the patient in the resting position. Convatec (developed by Craig Medical) has a wide-bore outlet and comes with secondary drainage facilities. This appliance will fit onto System 2 flanges and can be unhinged so that changes of patient position can be accommodated (Fig. 4.4).

Bile drainage coming into contact with the skin quickly causes inflammation and excoriation. This is exacerbated by the frequent dressing changes required if leakage is constant. An effective procedure to manage this situation requires two people, one of whom should use suction to collect the leakage. This permits the partner to wash the skin with warm water and then dry it with a hairdryer on a low setting. A good sticking surface can be achieved by using a larger than required Stomahesive flange to which a urostomy bag is attached. (This can be connected to sec-

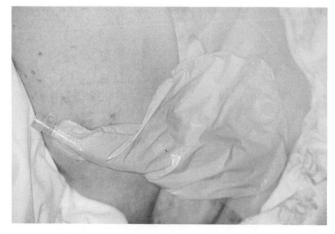

Fig. 4.4 High output system suitable for wide-bore drainage.

ondary drainage if the loss is copious.) Directional emptying is advantageous with thin consistency output; this prevents bile staining of clothes, which is extremely difficult to remove.

Further preparation can be carried out if the skin is intact. Patients who are very sick, unable to bath or shower, or who have been pyrexial develop greasy/oily skin which causes loss of adhesion of the appliance – the edges curl and leakage occurs. To resolve this problem, the skin should be clean, warm and dry. A light layer of tincture of benzoin will facilitate adhesion. If the skin is pruritic, causing the patient to scratch, a simple remedy that will enhance adhesion and improve quality of life is a thin layer of Caladryl lotion. If the skin is very painful and inflamed, gentle irrigation with water followed by meticulous atraumatic drying with a hairdryer is necessary. Applying Comfeel or extra-thin Granuflex sheets to the warm dry skin will provide an excellent surface from which to proceed.

Suction equipment should be used appropriately as an integral part of the process of skin care and appliance application, so that the fistula output does not come into contact with the skin and care can be carried out without risk of leakage or contamination. It is not usually possible for one person to use suction and carry out additional care effectively, so another member of staff or, if appropriate, the patient or a relative should assist in the procedure.

Any urine-producing fistula can be well controlled by using warm water and a hairdryer to warm and dry the skin and to promote appliance adhesion. The fistula site should be kept free of hair to optimize adhesion, reduce discomfort and prevent infection of hair follicles. On unbroken skin, tincture of benzoin can be applied to dry the surface and help the appliance remain in place. Stomahesive paste and Cohesive washers can be used, but the most valuable product in the presence of urine is Relia Seal – a large, double-sided, thin and malleable adhesive washer. The most awkward leaks can be controlled using this with a Coloplast one-piece urostomy appliance and secondary drainage.

Perhaps most difficult to manage is a jejunostomy below the skin surface in a large open wound. If the patient can tolerate a light general anaesthetic, Coloshield (Fig. 4.5) (used for anastomotic protection) can be sutured to the jejunostomy, and seepage prevented by applying Stomahesive paste to the suture line. Comfeel applied to the skin edges with a light dressing permits the Coloshield to be placed in a 24-hour specimen container which facilitates accurate assessment of output and healing. The Coloshield will stay in place for 7–10 days before it is shed. To ensure continued healing, it may be necessary to use it for 4–6 weeks.

Principles of effective practice

1. Allow sufficient time to carry out the procedure.
2. Prepare the patient in advance with careful explanation of the procedure, using a professional and caring attitude.
3. Ensure that everything necessary is available.

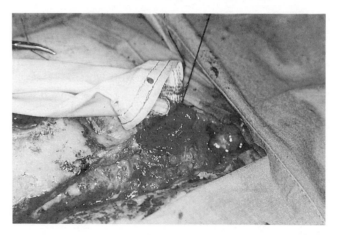

Fig. 4.5 Coloshield being applied to a jejunostomy in the middle of a deep wound crater.

4. Enlist the assistance of an appropriate helper, who may be a member of the care team or the patient or a relative if appropriate.
5. Ensure that all documentation is completed meticulously so that other members of the ward team can follow procedures with the same degree of success.

The well-applied adhesive appliance

The advantages of a well-applied adhesive appliance are many:

1. The patient can rest.
2. The skin is protected.
3. Risk of cross-infection is minimized.
4. Unpleasant odours are removed.
5. Patient mobility is assured.
6. Accurate assessment of losses and correct replacement is simplified.
7. Nursing time is saved.
8. Waste of bed linen, pads, padding and dressings is minimized.
9. For the majority of patients, dignity is preserved.
10. In terminal cases, the patient achieves peace and rest.

Once an appliance is successfully applied, the patient should be encouraged to rest in bed for at least an hour to promote adhesion. The patient is also advised that certain movements such as bending need a hand placed across the appliance for support, and that overfilling and swinging of the appliance about the abdomen should be avoided at all times because this inevitably leads to leakage.

Regular inspection of the appliance is vital – it should never be assumed that the appliance will 'look after itself'. Painstaking, meticulous care and a team approach are major factors in successful management, and even in extreme cases a regular pattern of appliance changes is advantageous.

Appliances and adhesives wear out quickly in the presence of alkaline proteolytic secretions which cause erosion, skin ulceration, bacterial colonization, pain and discomfort. It is essential that patching of a leaking appliance is discouraged. If the appliance is looking 'tired' with obvious seepage, it must be changed at once.

Fistula management, when taught correctly, can be rewarding because it undoubtedly improves the care and well-being of patients, offering comfort, eliminating the sense of 'odour always being around' and restoring dignity throughout a difficult time.

REFERENCES

Driscoll, R.H. Jr and Rosenberg, I.H. (1978) Total parenteral nutrition in inflammatory bowel disease. *Medical Clinics of North America,* **62**: 185–201.

Greenstein, A.J., Sachar, D., Tzakis, A., et al. (1984) Course of enterovesical fistulae in Crohn's disease. *American Journal of Surgery,* **147**: 788–92.

Hanauer, S.B. and Stathopoulos, G. (1991) Risk benefit assessment of drugs used in the treatment of inflammatory bowel disease. *Drug Safety,* **6**: 192–219.

Kelly, J.K. and Preshaw, R.M. (1989) Origin of fistulae in Crohn's disease. *Journal of Clinical Gastroenterology,* **11**: 193–6.

Lévy, E., Frileux, P., Cugnenc, P.H., Honiger, J., Ollivier, J.M. and Parc, R. (1989) High output external fistulae of the small bowel: management with continuous enteral nutrition. *British Journal of Surgery,* **76**: 676–9.

McIntyre, D., Richie, J., Hawley, P., Bartram, C. and Lennard-Jones, J. (1984) Management of enterocutaneous fistulas: a review of 132 cases. *British Journal of Surgery,* **71**: 293–6.

Nubiola, P., Sancho, J., Seguira, M. et al. (1987) Blind evaluation of the effect of octreotide (SMS 201-995), a somatostatin analogue, on small bowel fistula output. *Lancet,* **2**: 672–4.

Rinsema, W., Gouma, D.J., von Meyenfeldt, M.F., van der Linden, C.J. and Soeters, P.B. (1990) Primary conservative management of external small-bowel fistulas. *Acta Chirurgica Scandinavica,* **156**: 457–62.

Scott, N.A., Finnegan, S. and Irving, M.H. (1990) Octreotide and gastrointestinal fistulae. *Digestion,* **45**, suppl 1: 66–71.

5 Nutrition and the short bowel syndrome

Susanne Wood

INTRODUCTION

Of all the disorders arising from gastrointestinal disease, the short bowel syndrome is one of the most difficult to manage. Patients are faced with a daily life circumscribed by the constraints of their illness and its treatment. There is a need to be always close to a lavatory, either to empty the large volumes of fluid from the stoma appliance or, if the bowel is in continuity with the rectum, in case of an urgent call to stool. Fluid and electrolyte losses pose a constant risk of life-threatening metabolic disturbance and, together with the malabsorption of nutrients, can lead to a physical weakness that makes even the most basic of activities a major undertaking. Depression arising from the physical changes is often compounded by the frustration of having to comply with a rigorous dietary and medication regimen and by the inability of relatives and friends to understand this rather uncommon condition.

Many patients feel a sense of physical, emotional and social isolation and, on turning to health care professionals, often receive conflicting advice. The complexity of the short bowel syndrome requires a cohesive programme of care with doctors, nurses, including stoma care specialists, dietitians and pharmacists working with the patient towards the common goal of devising a treatment programme acceptable to the patient in its application and outcome. Although the possibility of enhancing intestinal adaptation by drugs and safer small bowel transplantation lie in the future, for most patients this will be a life-long condition with all the associated problems of chronic disability.

DEFINITION AND CAUSES

The short bowel syndrome is caused by a reduction in the capacity of the small intestine to digest and absorb adequate amounts of nutrients. In addition to the malabsorption of food and drink, excessive quantities of water and electrolytes may be lost due to impaired reabsorption of gastrointestinal secretions. The term 'short bowel syndrome' is misleading, as the symptoms can occur not only following massive small bowel resection but also in the presence of extensive inflammation or disorders of motility in an intestine of otherwise satisfactory length. 'Intestinal failure' is therefore a more accurate description.

Common underlying diseases are outlined in Table 5.1. Some of these may lead to both massive resection and continuing disease within the remaining bowel. Assessment of current intestinal anatomy and the presence of residual disease (either during surgery or by radiological examination) and understanding how normal physiological processes have been altered by any changes comprise an essential first step towards developing a logical plan of care.

Early identification of inflammation, obstruction or intra-abdominal sepsis allows timely treatment and reduces the influence on intestinal function.

Table 5.1 Common causes of the short bowel syndrome

Massive intestinal resection	Crohn's disease
	Small bowel infarction
	Radiation enteritis
Extensive intestinal disease	Crohn's disease
	Radiation enteritis
Disordered motility	Pseudo-obstruction
	Scleroderma

PHYSIOLOGICAL CHANGES

Motility

The transit of nutrients and upper gastrointestinal secretions is most rapid through the jejunum, slower in the ileum and slowest in the colon. The ileum, ileocaecal valve and colon play important roles in controlling transit time (Ricotta et al. 1981). The length of time nutrients are in contact with a healthy intestinal absorptive surface has a major impact on outcome. Resection of the ileum and colon with the formation of an end-jejunostomy results in very rapid transit owing to the loss of controlling mechanisms. The presence of any colon in continuity with remaining small bowel slows transit, an effect enhanced by retention of the ileocaecal valve.

Water and sodium absorption

Every day, in addition to food and drink, approximately 3.5–5 litres of fluid enters the jejunum. This fluid is composed of saliva, gastric and pancreatic secretions and bile. There are important differences in the physiology of fluid and sodium absorption between the jejunum, ileum and colon. Within the jejunum the sodium concentration of the intraluminal contents is maintained at approximately 90 mmol/l by the ready absorption and secretion of sodium through the loose intercellular junctions of the jejunal mucosa. The absorption of sodium is dependent not only on its intraluminal concentration but also on the presence of glucose (Fortran 1975). Water absorption is controlled by the osmolality of intraluminal fluid.

Within the ileum, sodium absorption is able to take place against a concentration gradient and the absorption of water results in only about 1 litre of effluent passing through the ileocaecal valve every day. The colon readily absorbs both sodium and water.

Understanding the physiology of sodium and water absorption is critical in the management of patients with short bowel syndrome. The entry into the jejunum of hypotonic drinks, such as water or tea, stimulates the secretion of sodium and fluid which, in the presence of an end-jejunostomy, is washed straight out of the body (Newton et al. 1985). In clinical practice it is convenient to estimate the sodium concentration of jejunal effluent as 100 mmol/l. As sodium is lost, the patient experiences thirst and may drink increasing amounts of water and other hypotonic fluids, causing further sodium depletion. The physical effects are usually apparent before major changes occur in blood chemistry. Lethargy, cramps, sunken dark-ringed eyes, reduced skin turgor, rapid low volume pulse, dizziness on standing due to postural hypotension and rapidly decreasing body weight are all important warning signs. Because of the influence of the renin angiotensin mechanism, the sodium concentration of plasma often remains within the normal range of values until body stores are severely reduced (Ladefoged and Olgaard 1979). The conservation of sodium in the kidney reduces urinary losses, and a concentration of less than 20 mmol of sodium per litre of urine measured in a random specimen is indicative of sodium depletion. The concomitant increase in urinary potassium losses results in declining plasma values. Without attention to the physical signs and a knowledge of the urine chemistry, plasma electrolyte measurements that reveal normal concentrations of sodium but reduced levels of potassium may result in inadequate treatment with potassium replacement alone.

Owing to the capacity of the colon to readily absorb water and sodium, the presence of even a short length of colon in continuity with the bowel can greatly enhance water and sodium balance.

The third element that causes particular concern in patients with short bowel syndrome is magnesium. Impaired mental concentration, paraesthesia, tetany (unresponsive to calcium injection), cardiac arrythmia and convulsions all occur as plasma levels decline.

Nutrient absorption

Most nutrients are absorbed within the first 150–200 cm of jejunum, the exception being fats which continue to be absorbed throughout the small intestine. Bile salts are reabsorbed in the terminal ileum, which is also the site of receptor cells for vitamin B_{12}. Massive ileal resections may result in fat malabsorption due to a reduction in both the absorptive surface and the bile acid pool. The presence in the colon of undigested fats promotes the absorption of oxylate. As the urine volume of patients with short bowel syndrome is often very low, this leads to a high concentration of urinary oxylate and the risk of renal oxylate calculi (Dowling, Rose and Sutor 1971).

HOW MUCH BOWEL IS NEEDED?

In order to absorb sufficient amounts of water, electrolytes and nutrients to survive without the need for parenteral support, about 50 cm of jejunum is required, provided it is in continuity with the colon. The colon slows transit through the remaining jejunum, thus promoting nutrient absorption, and is responsible for absorbing water and sodium. Loss of the colon and formation of an end-jejunostomy removes these advantages and such patients require approximately 1 metre of jejunum in order to achieve satisfactory absorption (Nightingale et al. 1992). Adaptation of the remaining small bowel can occur over several years following massive resection. This process is stimulated by the passage of food through the gut.

AIMS OF CARE

Maintenance of fluid and electrolyte balance

Excessive daily intestinal losses pose a constant threat of dangerous metabolic disturbance and vascular collapse. Monitoring and management of fluid and electrolyte status therefore take priority over all other aspects of care. The often rapid development of complications requires vigilance and a constant awareness of the risk.

Maintenance of adequate nutritional status

The effects of nutrient malabsorption take longer to become apparent than those of excessive fluid losses. For many patients it is difficult to achieve an ideal body weight and aiming to do so adds to their anxiety. Acceptable functional parameters such as stamina and mental concentration are more realistic goals.

Social rehabilitation

The complex treatment necessary to maintain the life of a patient with short bowel syndrome can add to the social isolation. To provide effective help, professionals need skills in advocacy, counselling, patient education and practical organization.

DEVELOPING THE TREATMENT PLAN

Assessment

In order to obtain a clear understanding of the wide range of problems arising from the short bowel syndrome, detailed physical and laboratory investigations must be performed. This may seem a daunting task but when organized in a logical fashion provides invaluable information on which to base the treatment plan. Details of clinical and laboratory investigations are given in Table 5.2.

Table 5.2 Assessment of patients with the short bowel syndrome

Intestinal length	At surgery – the length and anatomy of gut remaining, rather than that removed, should be recorded By radiology – if surgical details are unavailable, a contrast follow-through examination is helpful
Intestinal transit	The time taken for food to appear in the effluent after being eaten: an important guide to the effectiveness of therapy

Fluid and sodium balance	Fluid balance records
	Daily body weight
	Blood pressure when lying and when standing
	Blood urea, serum electrolytes
	Random urine sodium concentration
	Clinical signs of sodium depletion:
	    Thirst
	    Lethargy
	    Cramps
	    Sunken, dark-ringed eyes
	    Rapid low-volume pulse rate
	    Dizziness on standing – due to postural hypotension

Magnesium status	Serum levels
	Clinical signs of depletion:
	    Poor mental concentration
	    Tetany
	    Cardiac arrhythmia
	    Convulsions

Nutritional status	Body weight – noting presence of oedema or dehydration Presence of fat stores/muscle mass Stamina Mood Signs of specific nutrient deficiencies Serum albumin and total protein Calcium, phosphate, alkaline phosphate Haemoglobin, mean corpuscular volume Vitamin B_{12} and folate Serum ferritin

The importance of the role played by the nurse in this assessment process cannot be overemphasized. Without accurate records of body weight – measured at the same time and on the same weighing scales every day – and fluid intake and output, inappropriate treatment may be prescribed by the doctor. For the patient with a high-output stoma, an accurate measurement of daily effluent losses is critical in order to calculate the amount of sodium that needs to be replaced. Frequent leakage due to poorly fitting bags or a poorly constructed stoma can lead to inaccurate information and inadequate treatment.

Intervention

A successful therapeutic regimen can be achieved only by careful evaluation of the effects of each intervention. Patients should be warned at the outset that frequent alterations to drug and dietary therapy may be required in order to establish the best course of action for each individual. This prevents patients losing confidence in their medical attendants if frequent adjustments to therapy are required.

The treatment plan for the patient with short bowel syndrome can be divided into four progressive stages, which are outlined in Table 5.3.

Establishing stability

The type of treatment at this stage will depend on the extent of any existing deficiencies and the volume of intestinal losses. The first consideration for a patient with high losses, particularly from a jejunostomy, will be to reduce jejunal secretions by restricting oral intake to 500 ml of fluid daily. This may be any type of fluid. Reliable venous access is particularly important: if peripheral veins are inaccessible, this should be through a central venous catheter. To replete a patient already deficient in sodium and fluid, sodium chloride 0.9% should be infused intravenously until the concentration of sodium in the urine is greater than 20 mmol/l. This should be measured in a random specimen of urine on every alternate day during repletion and twice weekly thereafter while the patient is in hospital. The severe thirst, due to sodium depletion, will resolve as intravenous replacement restores equilibrium. Careful explanation of the rationale for fluid restriction and close supervision are essential in order to prevent covert drinking. Frequent mouthwashes must be provided.

When fluid and sodium balance have been restored, a maintenance regimen should be established before transition to the intake of fluids and nutrients by mouth. Daily intravenous fluid requirements may be calculated from fluid intake and output and body weight records. Rapid changes in body weight are a reflection of alterations in fluid balance (1 kg = 1 litre). Similarly intravenous sodium requirements can be calculated by allowing 100 mmol for every litre of the previous day's stomal effluent to which is added 80 mmol for insensible losses. These requirements may be increased if the patient is pyrexial. Therefore a patient with daily stoma losses of 3 litres will require approximately 400 mmol of sodium in the following 24-hour period. Provided that sodium replacement is adequate,

Table 5.3 A treatment plan for a patient with short bowel syndrome and high intestinal losses

---

Stage I   *Establish stability*
Restrict oral fluids to 500 ml daily
Achieve reliable venous access
Administer sodium chloride 0.9% intravenously until the concentration of sodium in the urine is greater than 20 mmol/litre
Maintain equilibrium by infusing:

fluid	calculated from previous day's losses and daily body weight records (1 kg = 1 litre)
sodium	100 mmol for every litre of previous day's intestinal losses plus 80 mmol (increased if there are excessive insensible losses)
potassium	60–80 mmol daily
magnesium	8–14 mmol daily

calories, protein, vitamins, trace elements – if enteral absorption is inadequate

Stage II *Transfer to oral intake*
Continue intravenous maintenance therapy
Start low-fibre meals
Start anti-diarrhoeal drugs – 30–60 minutes before meals, and gastric anti-secretory drugs
Commence oral rehydration solution. Discourage fluids around meal times (sauces, gravy, custard and small amounts of fluid may be taken with the meal)
Restrict the intake of non-electrolyte drinks to 1 litre daily
Encourage snacks and supplementary nourishing drinks (within the oral fluid restriction). Consider the need for enteral tube feeding
Commence oral magnesium oxide capsules 12–16 mmol daily (3–4 capsules)
If intestinal losses remain high, commence octreotide (a somatostatin analogue)
Gradually withdraw intravenous therapy

Stage III *Rehabilitation*
The patient and family should understand the physiological changes that have occurred and the rationale for treatment
Detailed stoma care for patients with high-output stomas
Referral to community continence service for patients with intestinal continuity and incontinence due to liquid stools
Referral to medical social worker for assistance with social security benefits
If intravenous therapy cannot be withdrawn owing to continuing high intestinal losses (persistently greater than 2 litres daily), teach the patient to perform intravenous therapy at home

Stage IV *Long-term care*
Regular monitoring and review of therapy
Vitamin B_{12} replacement if more than 1 metre of terminal ileum resected
Other nutrients that require particular attention – zinc, iron, folic acid, fat-soluble vitamins

---

there are no excessive requirements for intravenous potassium. Magnesium should be included in the intravenous regimen to maintain normal plasma levels (0.7–1.0 mmol/l) and 8–14 mmol daily is usually adequate. If the patient is malnourished and/or it is known that a slow transition to adequate enteral absorption will be likely, calories, protein, vitamins and trace elements should also be included in the intravenous regimen.

Transfer to oral intake of food and drink

Intravenous maintenance therapy should be continued throughout this stage until adequate enteral absorption has been established. While continuing to restrict oral fluid intake to 500 ml daily, the patient may be allowed low-fibre meals. Controversy exists concerning the type of food such patients should eat. Clearly any food that encourages rapid transit through the intestine is best avoided. Patients who have a colon should be advised to limit the intake of oxylate in the diet (chocolate, rhubarb, tomatoes, spinach, tea). Unless there are distressing symptoms from steatorrhoea, fat intake need not be restricted as it provides an excellent form of calories and helps to make the diet more palatable. Cholestyramine may help to relieve some of the bloating, wind and watery diarrhoea caused by fat malabsorption in such patients. Patients unable to digest lactose may be helped by restricting milk-based products.

Anti-diarrhoeal drugs should be started gradually and administered in increasing doses. It is usual to give codeine phosphate up to 60 mg four times daily and loperamide up to 4 mg 30–60 minutes before meals. A gastric antisecretory drug such as omeprazole 40 mg daily may also be helpful. To promote absorption of once-only daily drugs, they should be administered at the time of day when intestinal transit is slowest – i.e. at bed time.

All enteral sodium should be provided with a carbohydrate source in order to promote absorption. Salt may be sprinkled liberally on to meals; for patients with jejunal or ileal losses of greater than 1 litre per day an oral rehydration solution should be sipped throughout the day. Although patients with colon are normally able to absorb sufficient amounts of sodium from food, urine sodium concentrations should still be monitored and electrolyte solution prescribed as necessary. In order to promote absorption and limit secretion of sodium and fluid in the jejunum, oral sodium replacement is best taken as an iso-osmolar glucose electrolyte solution containing between 60 and 120 mmol of sodium per litre. A modification of the World Health Organization oral rehydration solution (glucose 20 g, sodium chloride 3.5 g, sodium bicarbonate or citrate 2.5 g added to 1 litre of tap water) is suitable. Palatability may be increased by flavouring with small amounts of fruit juice. Most patients are able to tolerate between 1 and 1.5 litres of this solution, which provides 90 mmol of sodium per litre daily. Non-electrolyte oral fluids should remain restricted to less than 1 litre daily. Avoiding fluids at meal times slows the transit of food, promotes nutrient absorption and reduces intestinal losses.

In order to increase nutrient intake, liquid supplements may be taken within the oral fluid restriction. Elemental diets are best avoided as their high osmolarity increases fluid and sodium losses from the gut. In addition, no advantage has been demonstrated in the short bowel syndrome by the administration of an elemental diet when compared with a more acceptable whole protein, polymeric diet. In some instances, it is helpful to raise nutritional intake by giving an overnight enteral feed by nasogastric or gastrostomy tube, in addition to food by day. In this manner the small intestine is used day and night. Salt can be added to such a feed, reducing the need for oral rehydration solution.

Magnesium may be replaced orally in the form of magnesium oxide capsules (1 capsule = 4 mmol of magnesium). Two to four capsules are taken as a single dose at bed time.

If, despite the dietary and drug regimen described above, intestinal losses remain greater than about 3 litres daily, octreotide (a somatostatin analogue) 50 µg by subcutaneous injection twice or three times daily may be of some help.

Rehabilitation

For successful long-term rehabilitation it is vital that the patient and family understand the physiological changes that have occurred and the rationale for the treatment prescribed. Changes in metabolic status can occur so rapidly due to sudden increase in intestinal losses that the patient must be able to recognize the clinical signs and know how to adjust therapy or whom to contact for advice. Good stoma care is essential for the patient with a high-output stoma whereas those patients whose intestine is in continuity and have large volumes of liquid stool should be referred to a community continence adviser for the supply of suitable incontinence pads. Many patients find it hard to explain the nature of their condition to friends, neighbours and employers. In particular, others find it very difficult to understand how the patient can be eating large amounts of food and yet often remain very thin. Supplying simple written information can help the patient communicate more effectively with other people.

Many patients with short bowel syndrome find it very difficult to achieve an ideal body weight and often it is necessary to accept a compromise where stamina and mental functions are adequate even though body weight may be very low. Patients are often very distressed by their body image. Lack of body fat leads to increased awareness of low temperatures with the need for increased heating within the home. Patients should be referred to a medical social worker to ensure that all the social security benefits to which they are entitled are obtained.

If it has been impossible to achieve the therapeutic goals detailed in Table 5.4 and withdraw intravenous therapy completely, long-term intravenous support at home will be required. If so, the patient should undertake a formal training programme and explicit arrangements should be made for the supply and funding of feed and equipment in the community.

Table 5.4 Desired therapeutic outcomes

Daily intestinal losses less than 2 litres
Daily urine output greater than 1 litre
Urine sodium concentration greater than 20 mmol/litre
Serum magnesium concentration within normal limits (0.7–1.0 mmol/litre)
Body weight and stamina acceptable to patient

Long-term care

All patients with short bowel syndrome, whether receiving community intravenous therapy or not, require frequent and regular formal monitoring and review of their condition. There should be a key health worker at the hospital – doctor, dietitian, nurse, stoma care specialist or nutrition nurse specialist – who knows the patient and will be the main contact person if urgent problems arise.

CONCLUSION

Short bowel syndrome is a condition that can lead to severe disability and isolation for the patient. It is a complex disorder, the successful management of which requires a thorough understanding of normal physiology, how that has been altered in the individual patient, careful assessment and a well structured treatment programme with attention to monitoring and regular evaluation. It is a serious condition which can be life-threatening, and health professionals caring for such people need to be constantly aware of their responsibilities not only in protecting patients from complications but also in helping them achieve some acceptable quality of life.

REFERENCES

Dowling, R.H., Rose, G.A. and Sutor, D.J. (1971) Hyperoxaluria and renal calculi in ileal disease. *Lancet* **1**: 1103–6.

Fortran, J.S. (1975) Stimulation of active and passive sodium transport by sugars in the human jejunum. *Journal of Clinical Investigation* **55**: 728–37.

Ladefoged, K. and Olgaard, K. (1979) Fluid and electrolyte absorption and renin–angiotensin–aldosterone axis in patients with severe short bowel syndrome. *Scandinavian Journal of Gastroenterology*, **14**: 729–35.

Newton, C.R., McIntyre, P.B., Lennard-Jones, J.E., Gonvers, J.J. and Preston, D.M. (1985) Effect of different drinks on fluid and electrolyte losses from a jejunostomy. *Journal of the Royal Society of Medicine*, **78**: 27–34.

Nightingale, J.M.D., Lennard-Jones, J.E., Gertner, D.J., Wood, S.R. and Bartram, C.I. (1992) Colonic preservation reduces need for parenteral therapy, increases incidence of renal stones, but does not change the high prevalence of gall stones in patients with short bowel. *Gut*, **33**: 1493–7.

Ricotta, J., Zuidema, G.D., Gadacz, T.R. and Sadri, D. (1981) Construction of an ileocaecal valve and its role in massive resection of the small intestine. *Surgery, Gynecology and Obstetrics*, **152**: 310–14.

6 Surgical procedures

R. John Nicholls

INTRODUCTION

The construction of a stoma is an important part of the intestinal surgeon's work. It should always be done with the awareness that the
patient's quality of life can be profoundly affected by an unsatisfactory
stoma. Surgical developments in large bowel cancer and inflammatory
bowel disease over the last 30 years have tended to reduce the number
of stomas constructed. There is therefore the initial question of the necessity of a stoma. This is a strategic decision which should be governed by
the pathology of the disease. For example, the choice between anterior
resection and total rectal excision for rectal cancer should be determined
by an assessment of the tumour itself and not influenced by the simple
desire to avoid a stoma. If adequate surgical clearance cannot be achieved,
an attempt at anterior resection can lead to local recurrence which might
have been avoided by a total rectal excision. Local recurrence is rarely
treatable to give long-term survival.

At a technical level a poorly sited or poorly constructed stoma can make
the patient's life miserable. The surgeon must therefore achieve two
things: first, the correct indication in the light of the pathology; and secondly, a good technical result. Throughout this process, the patient must
be brought into the discussion through explanation facilitated by the team
approach in which the stoma therapist, nurse, social worker and surgeon
work in concert. Under certain circumstances, the patient's own wishes
may contribute to the decision whether or not to construct a stoma.

INDICATIONS

There are two general indications for an intestinal stoma: (1) when surgical ablation of the disease requires removal of the anal sphincter mechanism; and (2) when the surgeon wishes to defunction the bowel owing to
the presence of distal pathology.

Removal of the anal sphincter will be required under the following circumstances:

1. Low rectal cancer
2. Certain cases of anal cancer
3. Inflammatory bowel disease:
   (a) Crohn's disease affecting the anus and rectum
   (b) Ulcerative colitis not suitable for a restorative procedure
4. Trauma with severe destruction of the pelvic floor such that reconstruction is impossible
5. Functional bowel disease

The resulting stoma will be permanent and constructed from the terminal portion of the intestine. It will therefore be an 'end' stoma.

Defunctioning of the bowel owing to distal pathology may be required for the following:

1. Intestinal obstruction
2. Perforation
3. Fistulation
4. Trauma
5. Incontinence
6. Functional bowel disease
7. Protection of an anastomosis

In these circumstances the stoma (it is hoped) will be temporary. It can either be constructed as a 'loop' stoma or as an 'end' stoma with closure of the distal segment.

RECTAL CANCER

Over the last 30 years there has been a trend away from total rectal excision to sphincter-preserving procedures (Fig. 6.1). This has mainly been due to the greater use of anterior resection made possible by developments in anastomotic technique. Such technical advances include low

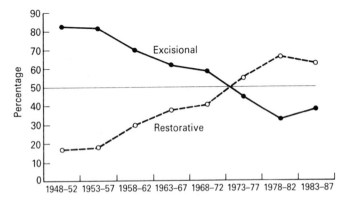

Fig. 6.1 The changing trend of restorative and excisional procedures for rectal cancer at St Mark's Hospital, from 1948 to 1987.

hand-sutured colorectal anastomosis, coloanal anastomosis and stapled anastomosis using either a purse-string to close the distal rectum (single-stapled anastomosis) or a double-stapled technique (Knight and Griffin 1980) in which the distal rectum is closed by a transverse stapler. It is now technically possible to carry out an anastomosis as distal as is anatomically possible; the important question, however, is whether this is justified on pathological grounds. A wrong decision to perform an anterior resection resulting in inadequate local clearance of the tumour is likely to lead to local recurrence, which is a disaster for the patient.

Total rectal excision versus anterior resection

Certain guidelines have evolved with time which enable the surgeon to decide between these two procedures. They are based on various pathological attributes of the tumour, which can be related to the subsequent risk of local recurrence developing.

Level of the tumour

This is the most important factor. There is a relationship between the level of survival and local recurrence. The rectum in adults becomes the sigmoid colon at about 15 cm from the anal verge. It is conventionally divided into thirds: lower 4–7 cm, middle 8–11 cm and upper 12–15 cm from the anal verge. This allows for the average length of the anal canal of about 3 cm. Survival is lower with local recurrence higher after surgical treatment of lower third tumours compared with those of the middle and upper third (Morson, Vaughan and Bussey 1963). Whilst this may not necessarily be the ultimate determining factor, it is a consideration when deciding on the type of operation.

The level of the tumour will determine the so-called margin of distal clearance. This is the length of normal rectum below the most distal point of the carcinoma as measured by the pathologist when the anterior resection specimen is examined in the laboratory. In the 1950s it was felt that a margin of 5 cm was necessary to achieve adequate clearance of the tumour. This meant that no tumour with its lower border lying below 8 cm (i.e. 3 cm for anal canal plus 5 cm for distal clearance) could be treated by anterior resection. Earlier it had been shown that the microscopic spread of cancer cells within the wall of the rectum was limited in most cases to no more than 2 cm, and further pathological studies in the 1950s confirmed this (Quer, Dahlin and Mayo 1953). The technical development of low colorectal and coloanal anastomosis then had the pathological reassurance that the margin of clearance could be less. There are now many studies which strongly suggest that a margin of 2–3 cm is acceptable (Pollett and Nicholls 1983) in that local recurrence and long-term survival rates do not appear to be compromised. The result has been that carcinomas down to 7 cm from the anal verge, and sometimes less, are now routinely treated by anterior resection (Fig. 6.2). Caution must still be exercised, however. Margins of 1 cm or less are probably associated with increased local recurrence (Phillips et al. 1984). Furthermore, it has been

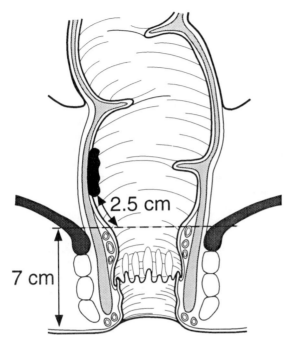

Fig. 6.2 Safe margin of distal clearance.

suggested that failure to remove all the mesorectum may also lead to increased local recurrence (Heald and Ryall 1986).

Direct local spread

It is generally accepted that carcinoma of the rectum begins from a focus of dysplasia in the mucosa which invades across the muscularis mucosae into the submucosa. The lesion grows outwards to invade the muscle wall of the rectum and then to penetrate it. When it does so, it gains access to the extrarectal tissues, including the surrounding fat and other organs (e.g. genital organs in females, urological apparatus in males and the lateral pelvic wall and sacrum in both sexes). As can be imagined, the prognosis is related to the degree of local spread. The greater the spread, the more likely that blood vessels and lymphatics are invaded, leading to metastases. The degree of local spread is also related to the subsequent development of local recurrence following surgical treatment (Dukes and Bussey 1958). For this reason it may be inappropriate to carry out an anterior resection in cases with extensive extrarectal spread. Local extent can be assessed with reasonable accuracy by digital examination and by imaging, including ultrasonography, computed tomography (CT) and magnetic resonance imaging. Where spread is extensive there may be an indication for preoperative radiotherapy (Cummings 1986) which appears to be effective in reducing the incidence of subsequent local recurrence (Gerard et al. 1988).

It would be unwise to carry out an anterior resection for a growth in the lower third of the rectum and some in the middle third where local spread is extensive.

Histological grade

The diagnosis of rectal cancer should be confirmed histologically by examination of a preoperative biopsy. This also allows the pathologist to assess the aggressiveness of the tumour, expressed on the histological grade. There is a relationship between grade and local recurrence and survival. A poorly differentiated or anaplastic growth carries a poor prognosis. When such a tumour is located in the lower third of the rectum, total rectal excision is indicated.

Local lymph node involvement

Survival and local treatment failure are influenced by the presence of regional lymph node metastases. It can be difficult to identify these preoperatively. Both digital examination and imaging by ultrasonography or CT are inaccurate. However, if identified before treatment, anterior resection is again unwise if the tumour is placed low in the rectum.

Patient's wishes

No one would want a permanent stoma. Most patients, however, appreciate the advice that one is necessary when the concept of complete and radical clearance of the tumour is explained. Because local recurrence almost always leads to death, the surgeon has a responsibility to maintain objectivity. The consequences can be disastrous when the patient insists on a sphincter-preserving operation when the pathology of the tumour is against it. It is the surgeon's first duty to offer the patient the highest chance of cure.

The criteria for total rectal excision may be less strictly applied in patients who would find a permanent stoma particularly difficult to manage. For example, old age and infirmity, poor eyesight or upper limb arthritis might influence the decision towards a restorative procedure. The surgeon still has to be realistic about the risk of local recurrence. In addition it should be remembered that bowel function after low anterior resection may be poor with the possibility of frequency and urgency and incontinence occurring for weeks to months postoperatively (Bennett 1976).

Anal sphincter

Anterior resection is contraindicated in patients with an anal sphincter considered to be too weak to maintain continence. The sphincter can be assessed clinically in the majority of cases. Anorectal physiological tests, particularly manometry, will give an objective figure of anal resting and voluntary contraction pressures.

Summary

Based on these considerations, the indications for total rectal excision with permanent colostomy in adenocarcinoma of the rectum are as follows.

1. Growth in lower rectum
2. Unless locally not extensive
3. Unless well differentiated histologically
4. Some growths in the middle rectum if:
   (a) Locally extensive
   (b) Poorly differentiated histologically

Disseminated disease

Patients with disseminated disease having a growth in the upper rectum should be treated by anterior resection. The morbidity of a high colorectal anastomosis is low and function is usually good. No defunctioning stoma is necessary in most cases. In those with a more distal tumour there is a higher chance of anastomotic breakdown with a low anastomosis (about 10–20%) which will lead to significant morbidity. The chance of breakdown is increased threefold in the palliative case. Furthermore, a temporary stoma may be thought desirable, requiring its subsequent closure a few weeks later. With or without defunctioning, acceptable bowel function may take months to be established. All these factors can mean that a low anterior resection is poor palliation in a patient whose life expectancy, owing to the dissemination, is likely to be measured in months rather than years.

A Hartmann's operation in this circumstance is a reasonable procedure to choose. It clears the tumour while avoiding the trauma of a perineal excision. All being well, it will be the only operation necessary. While the patient has a colostomy, management is straightforward in most cases, and psychologically the knowledge that the anus is still present is a comfort.

Local treatment

Local treatment, whether by local surgical excision, radiotherapy, diathermy resection or laser destruction, has a place in management. In the case of local excision and contact radiotherapy, selected small locally confined tumours can be successfully treated for cure with 5-year survival rates ranging from 70% to over 90% (Papillon and Berard 1992). These selected cases comprise around 5% of the total number of rectal carcinomas. Local excision for cure should be confined to tumours in the lower third for which a total rectal excision would otherwise be necessary. It is not an alternative to anterior resection for most proximal growths.

Palliation in patients with disseminated disease by diathermy, radiotherapy or laser destruction may relieve local symptoms of bleeding, mucus and tenesmus for a time. The overall rate of satisfactory control of symptoms is, however, poor.

Anal carcinoma

Anal carcinoma is a tumour of squamous epithelial origin, hence the term 'anal epithelioma' used by many clinicians. It can be divided into carcinoma of the anal canal itself, or carcinoma of the skin at the anal verge (anal margin carcinoma). These tumours are rare, accounting for 1–2% of all large bowel carcinomas. Regional lymphatic spread takes place to the pararectal and also to the inguinal lymph nodes. Surgery used to be the method of treatment, small carcinomas being removed by local excision, and more extensive lesions by total rectal excision. Local excision still has its place, but chemoradiotherapy has now largely replaced major ablative surgery as the first line of treatment. The results are as good, with average 5-year survival rates of 65% (Greenall et al. 1985). Today, major surgery is reserved for patients who do not respond to chemoradiotherapy. It takes the form of total rectal excision with permanent colostomy and is often complicated by delayed perianal wound healing due to the effect of the radiotherapy.

Temporary defunctioning after anterior resection

Anterior resection can be divided into 'high' and 'low'. High anterior resection is defined by a colorectal anastomosis lying above the pelvic peritoneal reflection. In low anterior resection it is below. The anastomotic leakage rate after high anterior resection is less than 5%. A temporary defunctioning stoma is not necessary except in occasional circumstances, such as where there is significant sepsis through local perforation or other viscera (e.g. the bladder) have been resected along with the primary tumour to leave a potential route of fistulation if the bowel anastomosis breaks down (Fig. 6.3). In any case, the surgeon has to assess each case on its own merits.

With low anterior resection, the anastomotic leakage rate is much higher, ranging from 5% to 30%. This appears to be surgeon-related (McArdle and Hole 1991). With coloanal anastomosis, breakdown appears to be even more likely, so it may be prudent to cover these with a defunctioning stoma. Again, this is a matter of judgement in the individual case, but general guidelines for a temporary stoma would include:

1. Technical difficulty with anastomosis
2. Incomplete 'doughnut' with stapled anastomosis
3. Significant pelvic contamination
4. Patient with cardiovascular disease

Faecal loading of the colon was previously regarded as an indication, but on-table lavage will resolve this intraoperatively.

An alternative to a formal defunctioning stoma is an intubated caecostomy. This can be inserted as part of intraoperative on-table lavage and left in place for 10 days postoperatively. It may decompress the colon above the anastomosis, but does not prevent faeces passing into the segment.

A defunctioning stoma can be constructed from the proximal transverse colon or terminal ileum. It should never be placed to the left side of the

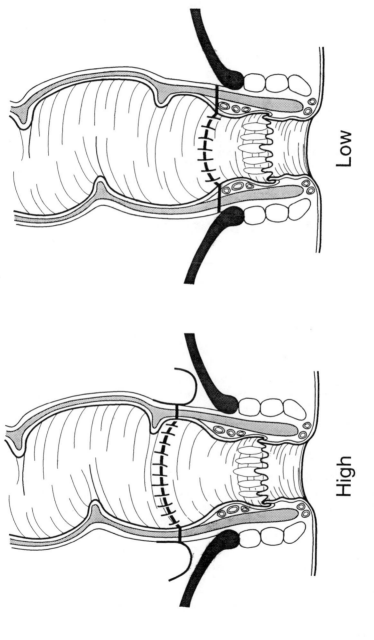

Fig. 6.3 Anterior resection related to peritoneal reflection.

middle colic vessels. In anterior resection, the left colon to the anastomosis is usually perfused only by the marginal artery. A stoma in this part of the colon can result in damage to the marginal vessels, in either its construction or its closure, leading to necrosis of the entire colon distal. Surgeons differ in the choice between a loop ileostomy or loop transverse colostomy. There may be advantages for the former, including less odour, fewer appliance changes and a lower incidence of problems (Williams et al. 1986).

Familial adenomatous polyposis

This is a special case of neoplastic disease of the intestine. The large bowel component is treated by surgery: there are three options as shown in Fig. 6.5. A conventional proctocolectomy with permanent ileostomy would be indicated only if a carcinoma in the lower rectum were present. These options are discussed below, under 'Ulcerative colitis'.

INFLAMMATORY BOWEL DISEASE

Ulcerative colitis

Surgery for ulcerative colitis can be divided into emergency and elective. Over all about 20–30% of patients with the disease come to surgery. These include chiefly those with inflammation extending beyond the splenic flexure, so-called extensive colitis. It is these patients who are more likely to suffer from acute severe colitis leading to toxic dilatation and perforation or chronic disease resulting in long-standing ill health, and for the subsequent development of carcinoma. Occasionally, a patient with left-sided colitis, and rarely with disease confined to the rectum, requires surgery. In this circumstance severe symptoms, including frequency and urgency of defaecation, are usually the indication.

Emergency surgery

The indications for emergency surgery performed at St Mark's Hospital are shown in Table 6.1. Failed medical treatment for acute severe colitis is by far the commonest and represents about 40% of patients admitted in this condition. Perforation is an absolute indication for surgery. Toxic dilatation is also regarded as such in the UK. It is noteworthy that bleed-

Table 6.1 Indications for emergency surgery in ulcerative colitis, St Mark's Hospital, 1976–1990 (106 patients)

Acute severe colitis (failed medical treatment)	71
Toxic dilatation	23
Perforation	9
Bleeding	2
Other	1

ing is a rare indication. When it occurs, the site is usually from ulceration in the rectum. In bleeding, therefore, the type of operation may need to be modified to include the rectum.

Operation It is now generally accepted that the emergency operation of choice is colectomy with terminal ileostomy and preservation of the rectal stump (Fig. 6.4). Emergency proctocolectomy in ulcerative colitis no longer has a place except in exceptional circumstances. Even when it is necessary to remove the rectum, the pelvic floor can almost always be preserved in a form of Hartmann's procedure.

Colectomy with ileostomy and preservation of the rectal stump has a mortality of less than 5%. It results in restoration of health, allowing steroid medication to be withdrawn, and leaves the therapeutic options of proctectomy, ileorectal anastomosis or ileoanal anastomosis open for the future.

It is important for technical reasons to leave a long distal stump. In practice this will include the distal sigmoid as well as the rectum. There are two reasons for this. First, it enables the distal segment to be exteriorized either as an initial manoeuvre to form a mucous fistula or for subsequent exteriorization if a closed stump leaks. Secondly, a long stump is

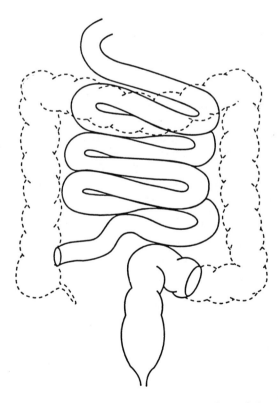

Fig. 6.4 Colectomy with ileostomy and preservation of the rectal stump.

easily found during any subsequent elective operation. This facilitates the dissection and increases safety.

The decision whether to close the distal stump or perform a mucous fistula will depend on the general condition of the patient, particularly nutritional state, and the quality of the bowel wall to hold sutures or staples. It is dangerous to close the bowel if it is friable, thickened and brittle. Although a mucous fistula can be awkward to manage, often more so than the ileostomy itself, safety should not be sacrificed by risking closure of unsuitable bowel.

Elective surgery

There are three broad indications for elective surgery in ulcerative colitis: (1) failed medical treatment, (2) retardation of growth in a child and (3) malignant or premalignant transformation.

Failed medical treatment It may be difficult for both the patient and the gastroenterologist to perceive that medical treatment is not succeeding. The chronic nature of the disease may seem so stable in itself that the difference from normality may not be obvious. Failure of medical treatment can therefore be difficult to define. General guidelines would include:

1. *Chronic ill health.* Loss of energy, anaemia, time off work, inability to lead a normal home life, low weight, poor appetite.
2. *Recurrent acute exacerbations.* Judgement is required, based on the frequency and severity, as to which surgery should be considered.
3. *Severe symptoms.* Patients may feel systemically well but be incapacitated to a degree by frequency and especially urgency of defaecation leading to incontinence. These may restrict normal living significantly.
4. *Extra-alimentary manifestations.* Inflammatory bowel disease may be associated with pathology in other organs. The commonest is the joints. There are two forms of arthropathy, including an activity-related polyarthropathy and a sacroileitis of the ankylosing spondylitis type. The former is helped by surgery, the latter is said not to be. Others include pyoderma gangrenosum (improved by proctocolectomy in about 50% of cases) and liver disease (not helped by surgery). Erythema nodosum and oral aphthous ulceration tend to be associated with Crohn's disease.

Retardation of growth in a child Chronic inflammatory bowel disease may cause retardation of growth. Paediatricians managing such cases will monitor growth according to percentile norms. Steroid medication leads to early fusion of epiphyses (occasionally it produces osteoporosis severe enough to cause pathological fractures). The clinician must therefore be aware of these facts in order to avoid this serious complication which is avoidable by timely surgery.

Malignant transformation The risk of malignant transformation is largely confined to patients with anatomically extensive disease. It is very low within the first 10 years from onset. Thereafter the cumulative incidence is about 1% per year. Thus, of 100 patients with an intact large bowel, about 10 will develop a cancer by 20 years. There is some evidence that the rate increases with the length of interval from onset.

In patients who have had an ileorectal anastomosis for ulcerative colitis, the risk of cancer developing in the rectal stump is less although significant at around 5% at 20 years.

All patients with long-standing ulcerative colitis must be monitored by endoscopy and histological examination of biopsy specimens. The histopathologist is able to identify a pre-malignant state (severe dysplasia) which, if present, constitutes an indication for surgery. A fully established malignancy is an absolute indication for surgery, the nature of which will depend on the relation of the carcinoma to the anal sphincter and the presence or absence of dissemination. The considerations are similar to those discussed for rectal cancer as to whether a restorative operation can be justified.

Choice of operation In the elective surgery of ulcerative colitis there are only three possible operations: (1) total proctocolectomy with permanent ileostomy, (2) colectomy with ileorectal anastomosis and (3) restorative proctocolectomy with ileoanal reservoir (Fig. 6.5).

In all cases a complete colectomy is carried out. Partial colectomy has no place in the surgery of ulcerative colitis owing to the high possibility of recurrent disease in the residual colon. The questions revolve around whether the rectum should be taken or not and, if so, whether the anus can be preserved.

Conventional proctocolectomy with permanent ileostomy

This was the standard operation for ulcerative colitis from the early 1950s when Brooke (1952) described the everted spout ileostomy. This transformed the surgery of ulcerative colitis by creating a stoma that could readily be managed by the patient. Up to that time, ileostomies were either flush or, if projected, covered by skin grafts to prevent contraction and stenosis. They were not satisfactory for the patient. Conventional proctocolectomy has been carried out much less frequently since the introduction of restorative proctocolectomy. It still, however, has a place in the surgery of ulcerative colitis. The present indications include:

1. *Patient preference.* After considering the advantages and disadvantages of the three options above, the patient may decide to have a single operation that will cure the disease. The morbidity and unpredictable function of a restorative proctocolectomy may be unacceptable. The decision may be influenced by the patient's age.
2. *Poor anal sphincter.* This could exclude an ileoanal procedure.
3. *Low rectal carcinoma.* The arguments for total excision or a restorative procedure are similar to those given above for rectal cancer.

When discussing the indications, the disadvantages of the operation should also be pointed out. Besides the permanent ileostomy, delayed healing of the perineal wound and complications of the ileostomy are frequent. About 25% of patients still have an unhealed perineal wound 6 months after proctocolectomy, and the cumulative surgical revision rate of the

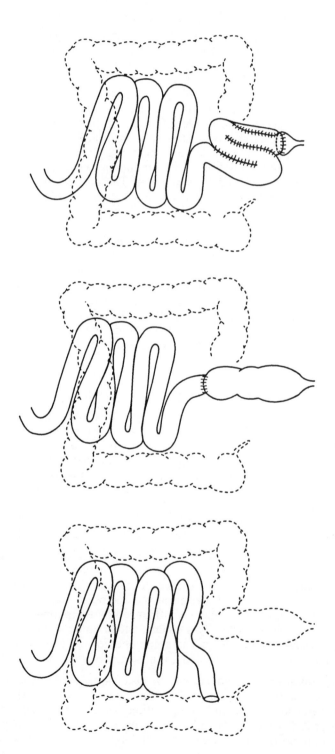

Fig. 6.5 Elective operation for ulcerative colitis or familial adenomatous polyposis.

terminal ileostomy is around 20–30% at 5 years. Intestinal obstruction due to adhesions occurs in 10–20% over the same period.

Rectal dissection can lead to pelvic nerve dysfunction. This has become a disproportionate fear in the minds of patients. In reality, using the technique of close rectal dissection combined with an intersphincteric removal of the anal canal, it can be avoided. A close rectal dissection should not be carried out in patients with dysplasia or an established cancer, but in the rest – i.e. the majority of patients – it should be the routine technique of dissection.

The Kock ileostomy

The conventional Brooke ileostomy was a major step forward in the technical development of the surgery of ulcerative colitis. It did have certain disadvantages, however. Besides the presence of an abdominal stoma, the necessity constantly to wear an appliance and to empty it at intervals during the day intruded both practically and psychologically on the quality of life of the patient. With these considerations in mind, Kock (1971) developed a terminal ileal reservoir with an artificial flutter valve system to create a continent ileostomy no longer requiring an appliance (Fig. 6.6). This procedure was applicable to patients whose anal sphincters had been removed in proctocolectomy. It consisted of an ileal reservoir into which a short length of terminal ileum had been invaginated to create a nipple valve which would retain faeces until cannulated via the abdominal stoma. The Achilles heel of the procedure was the tendency for the nipple valve to prolapse, breaking the continence mechanism. This would require

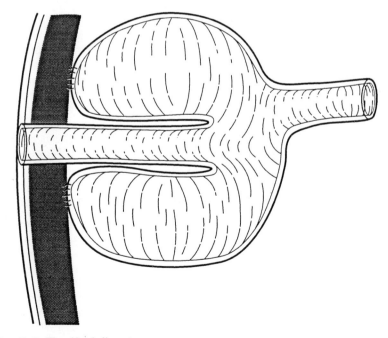

Fig. 6.6 The Kock ileostomy.

reoperation to revise the valve and was necessary in most series in 20–40% of cases, although in Kock's hands the revision rate was less than 10% (Myrvold 1987).

In patients having a proctocolectomy with anal excision who wished to avoid the constant flux of faeces and wearing of an appliance, the Kock reservoir, when successful, greatly improved the quality of life. This is especially so since the abdominal stoma is flush and placed just above the pelvic bone.

Colectomy with ileorectal anastomosis

This operation is a compromise to avoid a stoma in patients with ulcerative colitis and familial adenomatous polyposis. The diseased section is left behind but, owing to its proximity to the anal verge, is easily inspected by rigid sigmoidoscopy.

In ulcerative colitis it is indicated when the rectum is not so diseased that its reservoir function is lost, there is no dysplasia evident in the large bowel and when the anal sphincter is competent. It is also obligatory to maintain long-standing surveillance of the rectal stump and, if the patient is unlikely to comply, the operation is contraindicated.

The operation is now performed less often, following the introduction of restorative proctocolectomy which now accounts for about 10% of patients having surgery for ulcerative colitis. There is a long-term failure rate of 10–40% (Mann 1988) owing to the activity of inflammation in malignant transformation in the rectal stump. Nevertheless, in the remaining patients, function is often very acceptable and the operation itself has a low morbidity and fairly short convalescence.

In familial adenomatous polyposis, colectomy and ileorectal anastomosis remains the operation of choice in the young (<20 years) provided surveillance is assured. This will require at least twice yearly examinations of the rectum with destruction of adenomas as necessary. In older patients the cancer risk increases and those with uncontrollable or extensive adenoma formation in the rectum or with an already established carcinoma of the large bowel should have a restorative proctocolectomy. It is also apparent that, in patients having had a colectomy and ileorectal anastomosis, there is a marked increase in the occurrence of rectal cancer above the age of 50 years. More intensive surveillance of these is required and a restorative proctectomy will be necessary in some cases.

Restorative proctocolectomy (proctectomy after previous colectomy)

This operation was described by Parks to combine the aims of complete removal of disease with avoidance of a permanent ileostomy. It is suitable for selected patients with diffuse mucosal large bowel disease, including ulcerative colitis, familial adenomatous polyposis and certain cases with functional bowel disease. It is not indicated in Crohn's disease, where recurrent inflammation in the small bowel and anal fistulation are responsible for a high failure rate. Initially the operation was always covered by a temporary ileostomy (Parks, Nicholls and Belleveau 1980). More recently, some surgeons have avoided this without any apparent increase in complications (Keighley et al. 1991). However, the surgeon should select these cases carefully.

Crohn's disease

Emergency surgery

As with ulcerative colitis, Crohn's colitis may present as an emergency and the indications for urgent surgery are identical. In addition, Crohn's disease may cause local perforation with abscess formation and/or fistulation. An abscess will require drainage, and in certain circumstances defunctioning of the bowel should be considered. This may be carried out as part of a colectomy when resection is considered necessary owing to involvement of the colon. Alternatively, it may involve a simple defunctioning with drainage of the abscess. The split ileostomy technique has been advocated in the latter circumstance. The terminal ileum is divided and exteriorized proximally as an end everted ileostomy and distally as a mucous fistula. In this way, the distal bowel is completely defunctioned and is also accessible for the intraluminal administration of medication. The technique has been used for severe anorectal sepsis or rectovaginal fistula. Whilst it is hoped that such defunctioning is only temporary, in practice only about 20% of patients are subsequently able to have the stoma closed (Harper et al. 1983).

Elective surgery

The general indications for elective surgery are the same as for ulcerative colitis. The cancer risk, although present, is considerably lower in Crohn's disease. A permanent stoma will be necessary when removal of the anal sphincter mechanism is necessary. The indications for proctectomy include:

1. Severe rectal disease
2. Severe anal disease
3. Both 1 and 2.

Patients with severe rectal disease have a high incidence of simultaneous anal disease. When either is the indication for surgery, there is little chance of avoiding a permanent stoma.

The incidence of anal Crohn's disease is greater the more distal the intestinal involvement. When it is confined to the small intestine, the incidence is 10–15% compared with 50–80% with rectal involvement (Hellers et al. 1980). Anal disease on its own is the main indication for proctectomy in only 5–15% of all patients with an anal lesion. It is the combination of anal and rectal disease that raises the likelihood of surgery being necessary.

Total rectal excision with a terminal colostomy is justified when the colon above is not affected. Long-term recurrence after this operation is infrequent, with a cumulative reoperation rate for further disease of around 10–20% at 5 years (Ritchie and Lockhart-Mummery 1973).

Proctocolectomy is the operation of choice when anorectal disease is combined with colonic involvement. Again, the reoperation rate for recurrence is low, being reported as between 10% and 30% at 5 years.

In 50% of patients with large bowel Crohn's disease there is rectal sparing. For these a colectomy with ileorectal anastomosis is suitable. The recurrence rate requiring further surgery is, however, high: around 50% at 5 years (Allan et al. 1977; Flint et al. 1977). Recurrence, when it occurs, is usually in the terminal ileum up to the anastomosis. It may be possible therefore to resect and reanastomose healthy small intestine to the rectum. Thus, recurrence after ileorectal anastomosis does not necessarily involve removal of the rectum with formation of a stoma.

Patients with aggressive Crohn's disease requiring several resections of small bowel and having had a proctocolectomy may be left with a small intestinal stoma of the upper ileum or jejunum. In this circumstance, they are at risk of water and electrolyte imbalance and nutritional deficiency of protein and calories, and also vitamins (e.g. vitamin B_{12}). Management of a high output ileostomy is discussed in Chapter 4.

OTHER INDICATIONS FOR STOMA FORMATION

Obstruction

Large bowel obstruction presenting as an emergency is most commonly due to a carcinoma (Fig. 6.7). Less frequent causes include diverticular disease, volvulus, sliding inguinal hernia and adhesions (which are much more likely to cause small bowel obstruction). In infants, imperforate anus or Hirschsprung's disease may be the cause.

Patients with an obstructing carcinoma are often old and presentation may be delayed. The choice of surgery will depend on the general condition. If poor, an intubated caecostomy under local anaesthetic may relieve the obstruction and allow the general condition to improve. If the patient is fit for a laparotomy, which is usually the case after a period of preoperative water and electrolyte replacement, it is now generally agreed that resection of the primary tumour should be aimed for. The question then arises whether a primary anastomosis should be made or whether the bowel should be exteriorized as in Hartmann's procedure. If this latter course is followed, a subsequent operation to restore intestinal continuity is anticipated. Unfortunately, owing to age, frailty, postoperative complications and the patient's own wishes, this happens only in about 50% of cases. Resection with primary anastomosis has the advantage of offering definitive treatment by one operation. Its opponents maintain that anastomotic leakage is more likely when dilated obstructed proximal bowel is used. This has been countered by surgeons who advocate a subtotal colectomy with an anastomosis between the small intestine and the colon distal to the obstruction (Halevy, Levi and Orda 1989).

The traditional three-stage approach to malignant obstruction of initial stoma, second-stage resection with anastomosis and third-stage closure of the stoma is now outmoded except in patients considered too ill at

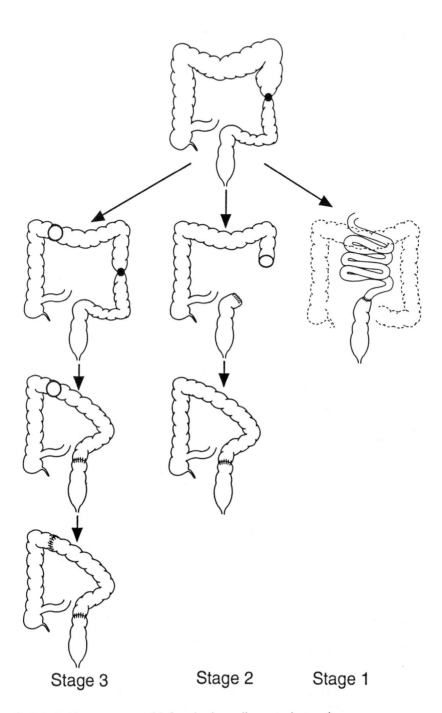

Fig. 6.7 Management of left colonic malignant obstruction.

presentation to withstand any more complex procedure than a colostomy. An initial defunctioning stoma is the preferred approach in Hirschsprung's disease and imperforate anus.

Obstructive carcinomas of the colon are usually advanced, a high proportion having regional lymphadenopathy and disseminated disease (Fielding, Stewart-Brown and Blesovsky 1979). Expeditious treatment has great advantages when considering this aspect and quality of life in general.

Perforation

Perforation is a very serious event. The mortality of faecal peritonitis is over 50% (Wood 1977). The usual causes are a perforated large bowel carcinoma, diverticular disease and trauma. Unfortunately, perforation of a carcinoma confers palliative status on the case owing to the subsequent high incidence of peritoneal involvement by tumour.

Urgent surgery is indicated. The aim includes resection of the segment bearing the perforation, lavage of the peritoneal cavity and, as discussed above, primary anastomosis or exteriorization depending on the circumstances and the surgeon's attitude.

In the case of trauma, military surgeons are now less inclined than they were to exteriorize in large bowel injury.

Pelvic floor trauma

Patients with rectal perforation and injury to the pelvic floor require a proximal defunctioning stoma with irrigation of the distal segment and debridement of the wound. Devitalized tissue should be removed. Reconstruction, if necessary, should be considered after recovery and healing.

Incontinence

Faecal incontinence may be due to diarrhoeal states (see 'Inflammatory bowel disease', above), with urgency from above, or to insufficiency of the pelvic floor. Neuromuscular weakness of the sphincters occurs in general neurological diseases; for example, disseminated sclerosis, spinal cauda equina lesions and pudendal neuropathy. This last may be due to damage to the pudendal nerve during childbirth. The sphincter becomes weaker with age and behavioural disorders (e.g. dementia) may be associated with incontinence. Other causes include fistulation from the rectum to the exterior (perineum or vagina), megarectum with relaxation of the anal sphincter and sphincter trauma.

There are several operations available to repair the sphincter muscle or to support the pelvic floor and close the anal canal. These include postanal and anterior anal repair, sphincter reconstruction and, more recently, electrically stimulated gracilis muscle sling. Their overall effectiveness in the long term ranges from 30% to 80% depending on the state of the muscle tissue. When reconstruction is unsuccessful, a stoma may be necessary. A temporary stoma forms part of management in patients having a stimulated gracilis neosphincter (Williams et al. 1991).

Functional bowel disease

This is a disease category that may involve the anal sphincter along with some form of dysfunction of the bowel above. The aetiology is not known in most cases but certain clinical groupings are evident. These include idiopathic constipation (megarectum or megacolon or both) with dilatation of the large bowel or without dilatation (severe idiopathic constipation). In these there appears to be a defect both of intestinal transit and of rectal emptying. Impairment of rectal emptying seems to be the predominant feature in the solitary ulcer syndrome and in so-called anismus.

The management of these disorders is difficult and unsatisfactory, for two main reasons: first, ignorance of their cause, and secondly the psychological component which probably plays a part in the majority of cases. Treatment involves a combination of medical management (e.g. laxatives for constipation), biofeedback, psychotherapy and surgery. In functional constipation, surgery should be a last resort. The results in the cases selected for operation are, however, reasonable with 60–70% obtaining relief over 2 or more years of follow-up.

Occasionally, a stoma is indicated when other treatment has failed to relieve intolerable constipation or difficulty in evacuation.

STOMA CONSTRUCTION

Counselling

It is the surgeon's duty to explain to the patient the nature of the disease and the treatment advised. Proper time must be allowed to do so. Diagrams help to clarify the explanation and the patient must feel free to ask questions both at the time of the consultation and on any subsequent occasion. The advantages and disadvantages of the proposed operation should be discussed.

Counselling is of course given by the stoma therapist and nurse, and surgeons recognize that points from the initial consultation will need further clarification, and technical questions concerning care of the stoma dealt with in detail. The emphasis must be on the team approach.

Siting the stoma

The stoma should be sited where it is accessible to the patient on an area of normal skin contour large enough to accommodate the flange of the appliance. Whenever possible, it should be placed below the belt line. An ileostomy or left-sided colostomy, the commonest forms of stoma, are placed in the right and left iliac fossa respectively. A transverse colostomy will lie above the belt line.

In all cases the stoma should be placed away from bony prominences (iliac crest, costal margin), the midline, previous surgical scars and skin folds (Fig. 6.8). Preoperatively it is helpful to fit an appliance at the chosen site. The patient is asked to sit, bend, stand up and walk to ascertain the suitability of the position, which is then marked with indelible ink. It may be wise to mark more than one site if the final position of the stoma is not clear preoperatively, as might obtain for one resiting procedure. Wherever possible, the stoma should be brought through the rectus abdominis muscle to minimize parastomal herniation, and the mark should therefore lie just medial to the linea semilunaris.

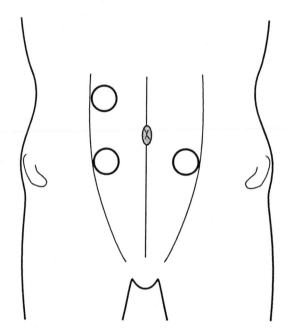

Fig. 6.8 Optimal stoma sites.

Incision

A midline incision is recommended. The skin contour on either side is left undisturbed. This is particularly important in cases of inflammatory bowel disease where there is a fair possibility of a resiting being necessary in the future. In Crohn's disease in particular, even if a resection with anastomosis is intended, a midline incision should be used to avoid creating a scar where a future stoma might be sited.

Defunctioning stoma

A stoma intended to be present for a few weeks only (e.g. to defunction an anastomosis) can be made as a loop or as an end with closure of the distal limb. While the former may not fully defunction, it does so sufficiently in most cases and it is easy to construct and to close, although it is more difficult to manage than an end stoma (Fig. 6.9a).

When the intention is to defunction for a longer period (e.g. in a case of faecal incontinence), it is better to construct an end stoma with closure of the distal bowel. No faeces can pass distally and the stoma is easier to manage than a loop (Fig. 6.9b).

Some surgeons use the stoma trephine as the only incision and bring the selected segment of bowel directly through it. This technique would apply when a laparoscopic technique is used.

It is usually quicker and safer to mobilize the loop of bowel through a short midline incision before exteriorization through the stoma trephine. Access and vision are generally more satisfactory and the trephine itself does not become distorted by the retraction that is often necessary if all the mobilization is carried out through it.

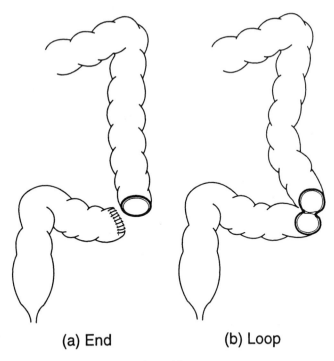

(a) End   (b) Loop

Fig. 6.9 (a, b) Defunctioning sigmoid stoma.

TYPES OF STOMA

The trephine

When a stoma has been conclusively decided upon preoperatively, the trephine should be made before opening the abdomen. The muscle layers of the anterior abdominal wall retain their anatomical relationship without sliding on each other, giving a more satisfactory stoma.

A cruciate incision 2.5 cm long is made centred on the marked stoma site. The skin is removed with curved scissors to make a circle. The subcutaneous fat, is spread with scissors to reveal the anterior rectus sheath (Fig. 6.10a). Another cruciate incision is made (Fig. 6.10b). The anterior

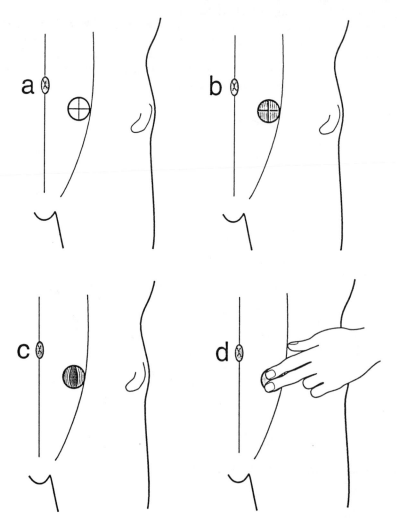

Fig. 6.10 Technique for creating a trephine stoma: (**a**) skin incision; (**b**) rectus sheath incision; (**c**) splitting of rectus muscle fibres; (**d**) ideal diameter.

rectus sheath and the fibres of the rectus abdominis muscle are spread, taking care to avoid damaging the inferior epigastric vessels (Fig. 6.10c). The transversalis fascia and peritoneum are then divided. The trephine should just accommodate two fingers (Fig. 6.10d).

End colostomy after total rectal excision

After mobilization of the rectum and while the perineal phase of the operation is proceeding, the colon is divided proximally (Fig. 6.11). The division is conveniently made at the point of the mobilized sigmoid colon level with the pubic symphysis when the bowel is held without stretch towards the legs.

The lateral space is then closed with a continuous suture. The colon is delivered through the trephine. The abdomen is closed. The colon is sutured to the skin using absorbable sutures placed through the bowel and the subcuticular portion of the skin. There must be no tension leading to retraction. The stoma should project by a few millimetres.

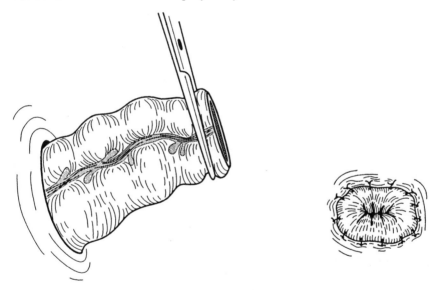

Fig. 6.11 Delivery of colon through trephine; mucocutaneous suture.

End ileostomy

The trunk of the ileocaecal artery is divided and further vessels are divided to leave the marginal artery over a distance of 6 cm. The bowel is divided just proximal to the ileocaecal junction (Fig. 6.12).

The terminal ileum is delivered through the trephine. The free edge of the mesentery is sutured to the anterior abdominal wall. The abdomen is closed. The ileostomy is everted and mucocutaneous sutures are placed to form a spout of 2.5 to 3 cm in length.

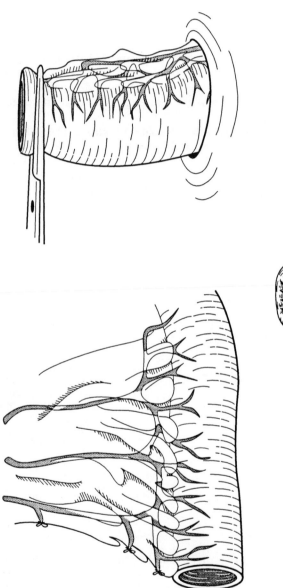
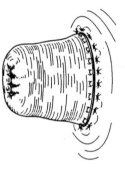

Fig. 6.12 Ileostomy construction; preparation of mesentery; everted spout.

Loop sigmoid colostomy

The sigmoid colon is mobilized. A window is made on the mesenteric border within the marginal artery arcade. A rubber catheter is passed through the window and brought out through the trephine (Fig. 6.13).

The loop is then exteriorized. The abdomen is closed. A rod is inserted through the window (some surgeons dispense with this step). The bowel is opened and the mucocutaneous sutures are inserted.

End sigmoid colostomy

After mobilization of the sigmoid, the point of the stoma is selected and branches from the marginal artery in the immediate vicinity are divided (Fig. 6.14). The bowel is then divided using a cutting stapler. The proximal end is exteriorized and the distal end is sutured to the peritoneum adjacent to the trephine. The abdomen is closed. The proximal end is opened and mucocutaneous sutures are placed.

Loop ileostomy

The technique is identical to that for a loop colostomy, except for the creation of the opening. The bowel is opened by a transverse incision on the distal limb about 1 cm above skin level. Placement of the mucocutaneous sutures should result in the formation of a spout of proximal bowel (Fig. 6.15).

Loop transverse colostomy

The technique is identical to that for a loop sigmoid colostomy except that (1) the site is in the right upper quadrant, and (2) the greater omentum is dissected from the colon before the window in the mesenteric border is made.

Kock ileostomy

A length of 45 cm of terminal ileum is measured and the distal two-thirds are folded on themselves. They are united by a seromuscular suture and the bowel is opened along a line immediately adjacent.

The distal third is invaginated to leave 5 cm projecting and the nipple created is fixed in position by the application of four lines of staples, two of which are placed as close on each side to the mesentery as possible. The reservoir is then formed by closure of the lateral sides.

The valve is tested by instillation of saline into the reservoir via a catheter inserted from the distal bowel. The distal bowel is then brought through a trephine lying just above the pubis, and seromuscular

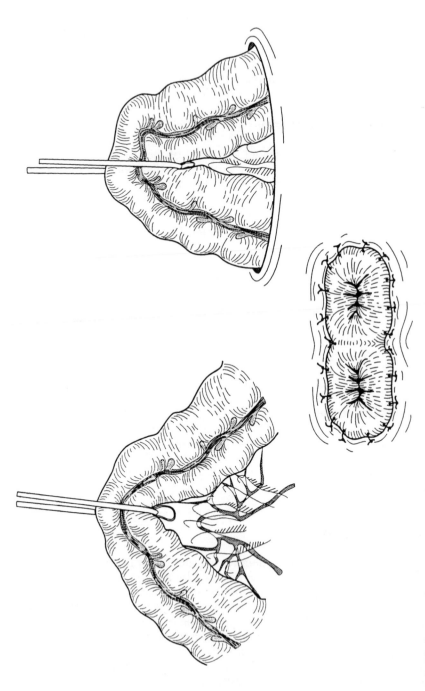

Fig. 6.13 Loop colostomy construction.

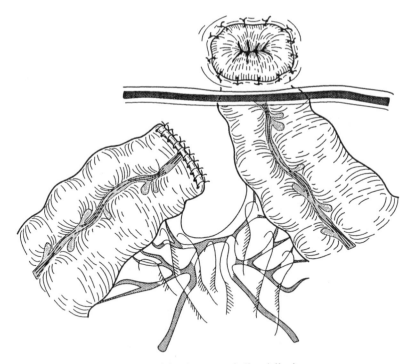

Fig. 6.14 End colostomy with closure of distal limb.

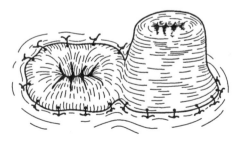

Fig. 6.15 Loop ileostomy; everted spout technique.

sutures are placed between the reservoir and the anterior abdominal wall.

A catheter is inserted into the reservoir and left in place for three weeks. An appliance is carefully placed on the stoma. The trephine in the flange should be cut to the size of the stoma and a transparent sleeve used.

POSTOPERATIVE MANAGEMENT

The stoma should be inspected regularly for signs of ischaemia in the post-operative period. The rod (if used) is removed on the fifth postoperative day.

No special management is required. The stoma will begin to act when peristalsis returns.

Output from an ileostomy may initially be considerable, and water and sodium balance (using normal (0.9%) saline i.v.) should be maintained.

The sutures are best removed on the 10th day.

COMPLICATIONS

Complications can be divided into:

- Immediate   within 12 hours
- Early   during the hospital admission
- Late   after discharge from hospital

Immediate complications

These include bleeding and ischaemia. Bleeding from the stoma can be controlled by pressure and the application of topical adrenaline solution. Occasionally, the insertion of further sutures is necessary.

Early ischaemia is rare. If it is felt that the bowel is non-viable, inspection down the stoma using a paediatric sigmoidoscope will reveal its extent. If discoloration extends by no more than 2 cm, the patient should simply be observed. If it extends much more proximally and viability is in doubt, revision will be necessary.

Early

The above complications can occur within the early postoperative course.

In addition, a loop ileostomy may be complicated by a high output or obstruction.

High output

Large volumes of effluent of up to several litres containing electrolytes may be lost over the first few days following the initial action of the stoma. The sodium concentration of ileostomy secretion is around 100–120 mmol/l and this must be replaced to prevent sodium depletion.

Obstruction

This can be caused by torsion or oedema of the stoma itself. Revisional surgery will be required if obstruction does not settle spontaneously. If this takes place at 2 or more weeks postoperatively, resection of the stoma with anastomosis should be carried out if the ileoanal anastomosis is satisfactory.

Late

Late complications are classified as either local – peristomal skin damage, stenosis, retraction, parastomal herniation and prolapse – or general – water and electrolyte loss, renal calculi and biliary calculi.

Revision procedures are frequently required for stomal complications. The cumulative incidence of reoperation ranges from 20% to 30% at 5 years.

Skin damage

Skin damage is discussed in Chapter 4.

Stenosis

Stenosis usually results from circumferential fibrosis at the mucocutaneous junction. It may respond to dilatation under anaesthesia. If recurrence follows, revision is necessary. The mucocutaneous junction is circumcised and the skin wound increased in diameter if necessary. The edge of the bowel is trimmed circumferentially for a short distance proximally and the mucocutaneous junction resutured. It may be necessary to mobilize the stoma by dissection through the subcutaneous to the anterior abdominal wall. The patient can leave hospital within one to a few days depending on recovery and home conditions.

Retraction

This complication applies to the everted ileostomy. Retraction leads to leakage under the flange of the appliance, with skin damage and lifting of the flange.

An attempt at local excision is usually successful. The stoma is circumcised and fully mobilized down to the peritoneum. It is then resutured in an everted state. Sutures placed between the terminal ileum and the anterior rectus sheath to hold it out in a projected manner should be included.

If this procedure fails, it will be necessary to carry out a more radical revision via a laparotomy.

A technique has been described in which the retracted ileostomy is elevated using tissue forceps and a line of staples applied longitudinally. This can be done as an outpatient procedure. Its effectiveness in the long term is not known. Occasionally, sepsis may result from the penetrating stapler.

Herniation

Parastomal herniation is common around an end colostomy following total rectal excision. This was particularly the case when the stoma was brought out lateral to the rectus sheath. Old people with weak musculature are particularly at risk. An incisional hernia of the main abdominal wound may also be present. Herniation around an ileostomy is less common. The complication risks the danger of strangulation. It is also disfiguring, and it may be very difficult for the patient to place the appliance. The distortion of contour may cause the appliance to become distended.

Treatment is expectant with a small asymptomatic hernia; otherwise, operation is required. There are two approaches. First the stoma itself can be mobilized and the defect in the anterior abdominal wall defined. This is then closed with interrupted non-absorbable sutures. Unfortunately, this simple approach is unlikely to succeed in the long term. The second option is resiting. This is a major undertaking, especially in an aged and obese patient. The general condition may determine whether the procedure is advisable or whether general abdominal support by a corset is preferable. The decision will depend largely on the severity of the symptoms.

Preoperatively the new site should be selected with care according to the principles described above, and then marked. The existing stoma is mobilized and closed temporarily with sutures to prevent contamination from faeces. The abdomen is reprepared and opened through the previous incision. Adhesions are divided, the stoma is completely freed and the defect in the anterior abdominal wound is closed with non-absorbable interrupted sutures. The terminal part of the bowel is then offered up to the proposed new site. Further mobilization may be necessary. The stoma trephine is then made and the bowel brought through. The base is fixed with interrupted sutures to the anterior abdominal wall including the peritoneum with posterior rectus sheath and anterior rectus sheath. The abdomen is closed after making sure that there is no torsion of the bowel in its new position within the abdomen. The stoma is then made using mucocutaneous sutures.

Prolapse

Prolapse may occur in patients with a redundant bowel. It is usually associated with a colostomy of the end or loop type. If it is mild, no action is necessary. If troublesome, surgical excision is required. The stoma is mobilized and the redundant bowel is excised. The new stoma is then formed using the proximally divided intestine.

REFERENCES

Allan, R., Steinberg, D.M., Alexander Williams, J. and Cooke, W.T. (1977) Crohn's disease involving the colon: an audit of clinical management. *Gastroenterology*, **73**: 723–32.

Bennett, R.S. (1976) The place of pull-through operations in treatment of carcinoma of the rectum. *Diseases of the Colon and Rectum*, **19**: 420–24.

Brooke, B.N. (1952) The management of an ileostomy, including its complications. *Lancet*, **2**: 102–4.

Cummings, B.J. (1986) A critical review of adjuvant preoperative radiation therapy for adenocarcinoma of the rectum. *British Journal of Surgery*, **73**: 332–8.

Dukes, C.E. and Bussey, H.J.R. (1958) The spread of cancer and its effect on prognosis. *British Journal of Cancer*, **12**: 309.

Fielding, L.P., Stewart-Brown, S. and Blesovsky, L. (1979) Large bowel obstruction caused by cancer: a prospective study. *British Medical Journal*, **1**: 575–7.

Flint, G., Strauss, R., Platt, N. and Wise, L. (1977) Ileorectal anastomosis in patients with Crohn's disease of the colon. *Gut*, **18**: 236–9.

Gerard, A., Buyse, M., Nordlinger, B., et al. (1988) Preoperative radiotherapy as adjuvant treatment in rectal cancer. Final results of a randomised study of the European Organisation for Research and Treatment of Cancer (EORTC). *Annals of Surgery*, **208**: 606–14.

Greenall, M.J., Quan, S.H.Q., Stearns, M.W., Urmacher, C. and De Cosse, J.J. (1985) Epidermoid cancer of the anal margin: pathological features, treatment and clinical results. *American Journal of Surgery*, **149**: 95–101.

Halevy, A., Levi, J. and Orda, R. (1989) Emergency subtotal colectomy: a new trend for treatment of obstructing carcinoma of the left colon. *Annals of Surgery*, **210**: 220–3.

Harper, P.H., Truelove, S.C., Lee, E.C.G., Kettlewell, M.G.W. and Jewell, D.P. (1983) Split ileostomy and ileocolostomy for Crohn's disease of the colon and ulcerative colitis: a 20 year survey. *Gut*, **24**: 106–13.

Heald, R.J. and Ryall, R.D.H. (1986) Recurrence and survival after total mesorectal excision for rectal cancer. *Lancet*, **1**: 1479–82.

Hellers, G., Bergstrand, O., Ewerth, S. and Holmstrom, B. (1980) Occurrence and outcome after primary treatment of anal fistulae in Crohn's disease. *Gut*, **21**: 525–7.

Keighley, M.R.B., Asperer, J., Grobler, S. and Hosie, K. (1991) Is a loop ileostomy desirable in restorative proctocolectomy? *Gut*, **32**: A579.

Knight, C.D. and Griffin, F.D. (1980) An improved technique for low sphincter resection of the rectum using the EEA stapler. *Surgery*, **88**: 710.

Kock, N.G. (1971) Ileostomy without external appliances: a survey of 25 patients provided with intra-abdominal intestinal reservoir. *American Journal of Surgery*, **173**: 545–50.

Mann, C.V. (1988) Total colectomy and ileorectal anastomosis for ulcerative colitis. *World Journal of Surgery*, **12**: 155–9.

McArdle, C.S. and Hole, D. (1991) Impact of variability among surgeons on postoperative morbidity and mortality and ultimate survival. *British Medical Journal*, **302**, 1501–5.

Morson, B.C., Vaughan, E.G. and Bussey, H.J.R. (1963) Pelvic recurrence after excision of rectum for carcinoma. *British Medical Journal*, **2**: 13.

Myrvold, H.E. (1987) The continent ileostomy. *World Journal of Surgery*, **11**: 720–6.

Nicholls, R.J. and Phillips, R.K.S. (1992) Surgery therapy of colorectal tumours. In: Phillips, S.F., Pemberton, J.H. and Shorter, R.G. (Eds) *The Large Intestine*, Raven Press: New York, pp. 657–86.

Papillon, J. and Berard, P. (Eds) (1992) Endocavitary irradiation in the conservative treatment of adenocarcinoma of the low rectum. *World Journal of Surgery*, **16**: 451–7.

Parks, A.G., Nicholls, R.J. and Belleveau, P. (1980) Proctocolectomy with ileal reservoir and anal anastomosis. *British Journal of Surgery*, **67**: 533–8.

Phillips, R.K.S., Hittinger, R., Blesovsky, L., Fry, J.S. and Fielding, L.P.

(1983) Local recurrence following curative surgery for large bowel cancer. 1. The overall picture. *British Journal of Surgery*, **71**: 12–16.

Pollett, W.G. and Nicholls, R.J. (1983) The relationship between the extent of distal clearance and survival and local recurrence rates after curative anterior resection for carcinoma of the rectum. *Annals of Surgery*, **70**: 159–63.

Quer, E.A., Dahlin, D.C. and Mayo, C.W. (1953) Retrograde intramural spread of carcinoma of the rectum and rectosigmoid: a microscopic study. *Surgery, Gynecology and Obstetrics*, **96**: 24–30.

Ritchie, J.K. and Lockhart-Mummery, H.E. (1973) Non-restorative surgery in the treatment of Crohn's disease of the large bowel. *Gut*, **14**: 263–9.

Williams, N.S., Price, R. and Johnston, D. (1980) The long-term effect of sphincter-preserving operations for rectal carcinoma on the function of the anal sphincters in man. *British Journal of Surgery*, **67**: 203–8.

Williams, N.S., Nasmyth, D.G., Jones, D. and Smith, A.H. (1986) Defunctioning stomas – a prospective controlled trial comparing loop ileostomy with loop transverse colostomy. *British Journal of Surgery*, **73**: 566–70.

Williams, N.S., Patel, J., George, B.D., Hallan, R.I. and Watkins, E.S. (1991) Development of an electrically stimulated neo-anal sphincter. *Lancet*, **338**: 1166–9.

Wood, C.D. (1977) Acute perforation of the colon. *Diseases of the Colon and Rectum*, **20**: 126–8.

FURTHER READING

Phillips, S.F., Pemberton, J.H. and Shorter, R.G. (Eds) (1991) *The Large Intestine: Physiology, Pathophysiology and Disease*. Raven Press: New York.

Keighley, M.R.B. and Williams, N.S. (Eds) (1993) *Surgery of the Anus, Rectum and Colon*. W.B. Saunders: London.

Nicholls, R.J., Bartolo, D.C.C. and Mortensen, N.J.McC. (Eds) (1993) *Restorative Proctocolectomy*. Blackwell Scientific: Oxford.

7 Appliance leakage

Celia Myers

INTRODUCTION

There is a multitude of reasons why appliances leak. This chapter attempts to set out and clarify problems that can be faced by both patients and stoma care nurses. Some of the problems outlined are easy to solve but others may need medical intervention. In most cases, the patient approaches the nurse first to find a solution.

There is no worse scenario than an appliance that leaks, and one of the first questions asked by the new patient is, 'Will it leak?' A leaking appliance causes embarrassment and lowering of self-esteem so the effect on lifestyle can be very dramatic. Patients lose confidence and worry that this could happen again. The fear of a possible leakage may never leave them; they are constantly checking the appliance and always carry a spare appliance and even a change of underwear. The horror of the smell and sight of bowel content on clothing in public or in private can be devastating and result in personal and professional rejection; sadly, a few of these patients can even become the butt of smutty jokes. Leakage must be avoided at all costs, for a stoma that leaks is a high price to pay for health.

SITING OF THE STOMA

Careful consideration must be given to the chosen site (Fig. 7.1). If good preoperative assessment has been undertaken, the site will have been chosen by the patient, the stoma care nurse and the surgeon, after considering the following:

- The potential site must be visible to the patient
- Avoidance of skin creases
- Avoidance of old operation and drain site scars
- Surface anatomy and avoiding bony landmarks
- Avoidance of waist or belt line
- Unobscured by pendulous breasts
- Employment factors (e.g. if a driver, the need to wear a seat belt)
- Positioning within the rectus sheath

If the patient is wheelchair bound, the siting must be assessed with the

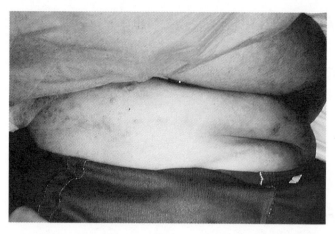

Fig. 7.1 Urostomy lost in a deep skin crease, resulting in severe skin condition.

patient in the wheelchair. If an artificial limb is worn with straps, the limb must be worn when the stoma is sited.

If the stoma is too high, the appliance can be visible through clothing. A stoma that is sited too low can make it difficult for the surgeon to mobilize the bowel, and the appliance may interfere with normal activity. A common complaint is that the appliance clamps can cause soreness to the upper thighs and also catch pubic hair. If all the preoperative factors are considered the permanent stoma should not need resiting. Unplanned stomas formed as life-saving procedures on sick patients, often with distended abdomens, can cause future management problems.

POOR DEXTERITY

Once it has been established that a stoma is necessary and the stoma care nurse is asked to see the patient for the first time, an early observation must be the patient's dexterity and degree of physical ability in practical care (e.g. to manage adhesive appliances, the ability to clean him- or herself and to use scissors). If a drainable appliance is necessary, it is of paramount importance that the patient is able to use a clamp, or, in the case of formation of an ileal conduit, to manipulate the tap and connect the appliance to an overnight drainage system. If patients are well supported at home, it may be possible to engage family help in the early stages. If problems are encountered, the most suitable and easy-to-use appliance should be selected; for example, with a single release paper and precut hole size. If easily managed equipment is not available, manufacturing companies can be consulted and the problems discussed with them. Prescription services are also very helpful as they will cut flange sizes and are always willing to prepare appliances ready for use.

Patients with poor dexterity must be given plenty of time and commitment; elderly people may need extra help, and will benefit from repeated demonstration. Talking through the procedure in the early stages is vital and the patient must not be rushed or assumed to be capable. Once the appliance is safely in place the stoma care nurse will take the time to demonstrate its use and leave in the patient's stock box a spare appliance for practice. If clips and clamps are necessary, extra supplies of these should also be available. If it is necessary for holes and shapes to be cut, a template can be prepared and scissors and card left so that this skill can also be practised.

POOR VISION

During the preoperative assessment the stoma care nurse will ensure that the patient can handle the equipment; it is vital to make time for the patient to become competent with hygiene procedures. Patients who require them should wear their glasses. On occasion it may be necessary to consult and refer to an optician.

In some cases it may be necessary to encourage a family member to help, although partially sighted and blind patients have been known to cope very well. Routine and didactic teaching on positioning of equipment in the same place each time is vital for learning stoma care by touch.

Throughout the patient's stay in hospital, the stoma care nurse will, in his or her educative role, encourage a pattern of appliance change and will emphasize the importance of establishing a routine to ensure that appliances are changed regularly before leakage occurs. When the patient is discharged home, the local stoma care nurse will be contacted and an early follow-up visit arranged to ensure continuity of care and to provide peace of mind and reassurance for the patient and family.

Many patients find it helpful to join appropriate support groups. Welfare organizations lend audio and video tapes which can reinforce teaching and are useful adjuncts to patient care.

Table 7.1 Correcting poor technique

1. Listen to the problems patiently, pick up any key points and really hear what patients are saying. Careful questioning will elicit subtle pointers for management.
2. The appliance should be changed to detect potential problems. During this procedure the appliance should be checked closely to see if it has been worn for many days.
3. Establish that all release papers have been removed.
4. If the patient is wearing a drainable appliance, the clamp and tails should be checked to ascertain that they are clean, that the clamp has been applied in the correct manner and that the appliance has not been rolled or pleated over the clamp.
5. The appliance should be checked to see if it has leaked and been left to dry.
6. The appliance should be checked to see if it has been patched.
7. If the patient has been using extra adhesive to 'picture frame' the appliance edge for security, ask why this has been done.
8. If a belt is worn, it should be checked to make sure that it is in the correct position and is tight enough to be effective.

POOR TECHNIQUE

In case a leakage occurs, it is a good idea to establish a protocol with guidelines to help establish the cause of the problem and develop a sound problem-solving strategy such as outlined in Table 7.1.

Patients should always be asked to remove the appliance so that there is an opportunity to observe their technique. Many patients remove the appliance in a fashion similar to 'stripping off wallpaper', which can lead to skin inflammation and infection, and inflammation of the hair follicles (Fig. 7.2). A more appropriate method may need to be taught, encourag-

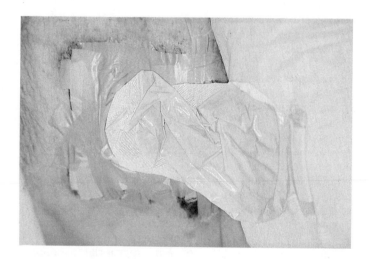

(a)

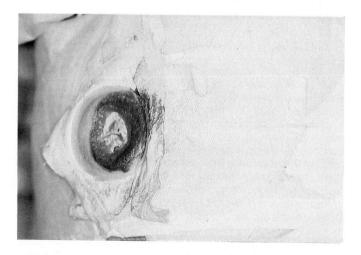

(b)

Fig. 7.2 (a) A patient whose appliance had started to leak and who has begun to patch the early leaks. **(b)** On turning the appliance over there was dry crusting stool and sore skin.

ing patients to use moistened paper (e.g. nappy liners or strong kitchen roll) and pull gently at the appliance from top to bottom. The moistened cloth can be used to wipe the stoma opening and then to cover the aperture of the used appliance to prevent odour and spillage. The reverse of the appliance should be inspected and the following questions answered:

1. Has it been placed off-target?
2. Are there any leakages?
3. Is the hole too large or too small, and is the shape correct for the stoma?
4. Has the adhesive worn away? If so, which area is involved? The peristomal skin should be checked for creases/crevices that may be responsible for the problem.

Other important factors include:

5. The skin should be checked for potential soreness seen with some appliances. 'Pseudo-redness' fades away quickly and must not be confused with inflammation.
6. If the patient has prepared a new appliance, this provides the opportunity to see it, observe the aperture size and ensure it is correct. If the aperture has been prepared by the patient, the nurse should note how well this has been done, if there are any jagged edges and that it is the correct shape and size. It may be necessary to make some suggestions for improving technique. Regular discussions about appliance changes can help to prevent bad practice. It may be necessary for a complete reassessment of the appliance worn as it may no longer be suitable and an alternative may need to be found.
7. It is good practice to check the position of the stoma in different postures (e.g. sitting before the appliance is reapplied), as this may reveal hidden creases and other factors that could be the cause of leakages. Sometimes it is necessary to introduce Dansac soft paste as a filler or perhaps the slightly stronger Stomahesive paste to the base of the stoma, or to consider the use of simple washers (Salts, Coloplast).
8. Patients should be asked to demonstrate their technique for reapplying the prepared appliance; this provides an opportunity to check that they have cleaned and dried the skin properly, avoiding excessive force, while observing the normal changing position. In some cases the use of a mirror can resolve difficulties.

It is best if patients pull gently upwards at the peristomal skin so that the appliance can be placed with the stoma in the correct position and to ensure that the shape is mirrored on the appliance. They should be encouraged to handle the appliance with its top turned back so that it can be seen more easily during its application and a secure, accurate fit achieved. Patients should be taught to 'firm down' the appliance with the fingers to facilitate adhesion; if a drainable appliance is used, a routine check of the clamp should be made at this stage.

Any of the potential problems mentioned above can cause devastating leakages. In some cases it may be necessary to admit the patient to hospital for retraining, but the stoma care nurse can usually identify faults and help the patient to make the necessary changes to solve the problems. If the skin is sticky or greasy, all that may be required is skin barrier wipes but these should be used with caution as over-frequent application can cause skin irritation.

AN OVERFULL APPLIANCE

An overfull appliance should be avoided at all costs, as the weight will pull the appliance from the skin. The presence of excessive flatus can also lead to loss of adhesion and leakage. If flatus causes severe problems, extra filters can be attached on closed appliances. Some drainable appliances (Hollister, Simcare) are also available with filters, which, provided they are not in contact with liquid faeces, can be safely applied to other drainable appliances.

When patients have excessive wind, the stoma care nurse should discuss with them the types of food and fluid they consume and dietary modifications that may have to be made. Regular meals should be encouraged and food chewed thoroughly.

PANCAKING

'Pancaking' (caused by firmer stool staying on top of the stoma, causing leakages) is not an easy problem to solve but various remedies can be tried. For example, a small amount of baby oil on the inside of the top of the appliance will help the stool to slide into the bag. All closed appliance packages contain an adhesive disc, which can be applied over the filter to prevent the appliance from 'sucking' on to the stoma. The adhesive disc can be removed to release excess flatus.

Also available on prescription is an adhesive bar (Simcare) which can be placed on the outside of the appliance close by the stoma; it can be manipulated to form a bridge that will prevent sucking and pancaking.

APPLIANCE LEFT ON FOR TOO LONG

Appliances that remain in position for longer than necessary will result in leakage and skin irritation (see Fig. 7.2). Patients must be dissuaded from 'patching up and making do' until a certain number of days elapse which sometimes happens if they are advised that a drainable appliance can remain in place for 5–7 days. If drainable appliances are left on for too long there is also the danger of odour breakthrough. Patients may not be aware that they smell, with consequent catastrophic effects on their social and private lives – which is a huge price to pay for appliances that are not changed regularly.

Another factor that can influence the patient to try to make the appliance last longer is if the information provided about appliance costs engenders a feeling of guilt and the need to economize. Cost issues are better discussed in the context of product quality, to reassure patients that appliances are well researched and safe. In the present climate of cost efficiency in the National Health Service, general practitioners in particular should be aware that patients' appliances need to be prescribed in adequately manageable amounts.

Patients who use the black rubber appliances change them weekly and rarely switch to modern equipment. It is particularly important for them to wash and care for the appliance properly between changes by hanging them up to dry and applying talcum powder to the inside to prevent the rubber from sticking together and then storing them flat in dry surroundings. This type of appliance can be used for up to 6 months.

Some patients are 'lazy ostomists' and change appliances only when they leak or smell – sometimes even patching the leakages. Clamps and drainable appliance access points become soiled and worn, resulting in staining on clothes and appliance covers. It may require persistent efforts at re-education before lasting changes are made to routines; and in some cases, the situation remains the same because the patient will not alter his or her hygiene habits.

It is important to recognize the patient who hates the stoma and leaves the appliance on for as long as possible, trying to cope by ignoring its existence. Such patients require careful and skilful handling by the stoma therapist, who may have to request the expertise of a psychotherapist.

APPLIANCES CHANGED TOO FREQUENTLY

It should always be established that the appliance the patient is using is the correct one for the type of stoma (e.g. a closed appliance for formed stool). A closed appliance is not acceptable for the patient with an ileostomy, especially if it is a one-piece type, as the repeated changes necessary (often up to five times a day) will cause skin problems and the appliance can overfill, turning the changing procedure into a messy one. This is also an expensive waste of resources.

The exception to this is the person with a colostomy who is admitted for further investigations and is receiving bowel preparation. It is imperative that a drainable appliance be supplied, as the usual closed pouch will overfill and become heavy very quickly, with devastating results. Overfrequent changes of appliance may be due to some patients' aversion to the presence of stool in the bag, which makes them feel very dirty – they feel 'clean' only when the pouch is empty. It is essential to explain carefully the ways of keeping drainable appliances clean between changes: for example, the two-piece type can be unhinged from the top and cleaned using a small plastic spray bottle. With the patient sitting well back on the toilet, the appliance can be flushed by using warm and mild soapy water. One-piece drainable appliances can also be flushed in the same way from the bottom of the appliance.

Patients with a colostomy and a closed appliance can develop the habit of changing whenever there is stool in the appliance and will require explanation that the colostomy should be allowed to function for its whole duration. If questioning elicits the information that the appliance is changed very frequently but that small amounts of stool are being passed all day long, diet, fluid intake and perhaps irrigation as a method of control should be considered.

WEIGHT GAIN

Cachectic patients who have been ill for a long time prior to surgery may find that, with long periods of rest and inactivity, they feel better and gain weight quickly. Although the stoma size has settled and they are now used to cutting or ordering a particular size, they may start to experience periods of leakage and become irritated, demoralized and desperate for help. In this situation it is important to measure the stoma size accurately, because as patients gain weight the base of the stoma gets larger and so a larger sized aperture is required.

Problems can also develop during pregnancy. The expectant mother should be informed early about what to expect as the abdomen increases in size (e.g. problems in seeing the stoma and so cleaning and changing the appliance correctly become difficult) and helped to find appropriate solutions such as the use of an angled mirror. As the abdomen enlarges, the shape of the stoma base changes, becoming larger and more awkward. Use of an appliance with a 'starter hole' (Fig. 7.3) will enable the patient to cut the correct shape and leave plenty of adhesive so that a good seal is obtained and she feels safe and reassured.

Excessive weight gain can also cause extra bulges and creases: when the patient sits up without an appliance in place, folds of fat can fall and may obstruct or obliterate the stoma. In this instance, the appliance range should be reviewed; for example, a rigid two-piece system may have to be changed to a one-piece that can be moulded into creases. The potential benefits of fillers and pastes should be considered carefully with indi-

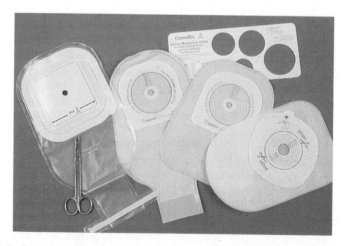

Fig. 7.3 Starter holes are very useful for new patients, who can then use a measuring guide and mirror to adapt the holes.

vidual patients, as they make the whole procedure more time consuming and alarming.

Attention should also be paid to diet and lifestyle, and appropriate advice given. Sometimes weight gain is unavoidable, as when steroids are prescribed; patients can be assisted both to adopt the right techniques for appliance changes and also to select the most appropriate appliance while taking this particular medication.

WEIGHT LOSS

It is usually unlikely that weight loss is simply the result of a desire to be trim and to feel good. With marked weight loss, the appliance hole may need to be made smaller. Any skin inflammation caused by leakage usually resolves following a single application of a secure and correctly fitting appliance. Patients in advanced stages of terminal disease may develop shrinkage or retraction of the stoma (Fig. 7.4), which makes stool evacuation difficult, especially if the patient is receiving opiates. In this situation, suitable stool softeners are needed in addition to an appliance that is large enough and fits.

The key to selecting an appliance of the correct size is careful measurement of the stoma. When patients are almost ready for discharge, it is advisable – as part of routine procedure – to demonstrate and discuss the use of the measuring guide that is in all stock boxes. Most stoma care nurses use starter hole appliances for patients at this stage, and they can size themselves down with the aid of a mirror. When their stoma size has been determined, patients can order precut hole sizes, which avoids having to cut and prepare the appliance. Also before discharge, patients should be encouraged to think about how they would change an appliance at work/school/college or when visiting friends. The facilities that can be used can be discussed in detail as well as potential problems and appropriate solutions. An example is the 'travel pack' which can ensure that the

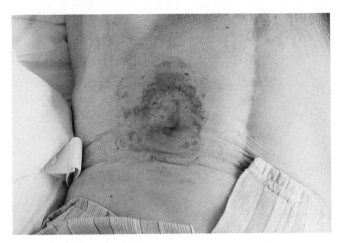

Fig. 7.4 Retraction of the stoma in a terminally ill patient.

patient will be able to cope even in the worst circumstances and that appliances can be changed and disposed of safely. A 'travel pack' should consist of (in addition to an appliance):

- A moistened nappy liner carried in a small resealable plastic bag
- A bag for a dirty appliance
- Scissors (if the circumstances are appropriate) to cut the corner of a closed appliance or to prepare a new appliance

The appliance should then be placed under the toilet flush to remove most of the bulky stool. Aluminium foil is very useful if immediate disposal of the used appliance is not possible. The carefully sealed package can be wrapped and kept out of sight until it can be conveniently disposed of.

RETRACTION OF THE STOMA

A stoma that has retracted can cause leakages; in some cases surgical revision is necessary. As part of a careful assessment, patients should sit so that skin creases, dips and folds can be identified. Patients can be questioned about their use of accessories such as seals, belts or wafers, how long the appliance changing procedure takes before a seal is achieved, and the nature and timing of leakages.

A range of appliances is available to help to minimize this problem. Convatec produce convex inserts (Fig. 7.5) that can be placed in the two-piece range of flanges. The insert makes the stoma protrude and prevents effluent from seeping under the adhesive, which is especially helpful for those patients with a retracted urostomy or ileostomy. A range of ready prepared convex appliances is manufactured by Hollister. If convex appliances are used with extra washers and seals, the convexity is diminished.

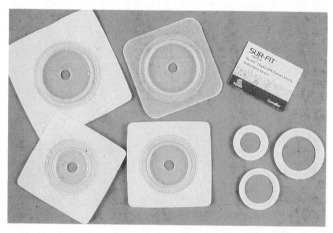

Fig. 7.5 Convex inserts.

PERISTOMAL HERNIAS

Patients can get very alarmed by the protruding swelling that is visible through the clothes and the aching sensation that suddenly develops around the stoma (Fig. 7.6). Following an initial appointment with the general practitioner, the patient is invariably referred back to the operating surgical team. In some cases it may be very difficult to correct the defect surgically, especially if the patient has already had many abdominal operations, and in this instance resiting is a legitimate consideration.

If the problem is mild to moderate, it is possible to correct leakages by increasing the size of the appliance aperture or by using a different type of appliance and accessories such as a belt or abdominal support garment.

The patient's lifestyle should also be reviewed and advice given to avoid lifting. For the rare occasions that lifting is unavoidable, correct technique should be taught; nevertheless, some patients in the building or removals trade may not be able to continue with this employment. Peristomal hernias can recur, even after surgical correction, so support garments should be worn, especially during working hours.

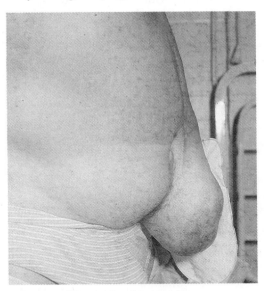

Fig. 7.6 Protruding swelling around a stoma.

PROLAPSE OF A STOMA

This is very alarming, and can occur abruptly without any apparent reason (Fig. 7.7). Lifting or periods of heavy exertion are often blamed for the prolapse of a temporary loop colostomy. Patients sometimes present in accident and emergency departments with large prolapses that have previously been reduced manually and early surgical intervention is then required; such a patient who is on a waiting list for surgery may be able to have the operation brought forward.

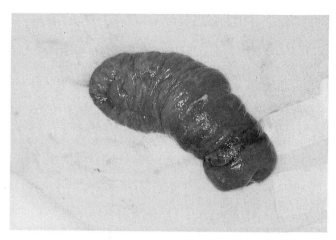

Fig. 7.7 Prolapsed stoma.

It is essential that patients with a prolapsed stoma are clean, free from any leakages and can be reassured and supported at all times. The most useful appliance is a large postoperative type that can accommodate the prolapse and the stool (CliniMed). A small ileostomy prolapse that reduces spontaneously with rest but relapses following fatigue or exertion can be prevented from further prolapse if the patient wears a Convatec Shield (available free of charge from the company). It can also be used by younger patients involved in contact sports to provide protection from trauma.

PERISTOMAL SKIN IRRITATION

During preoperative assessment the patient should always be asked about allergy to sticking plaster. In such cases the stoma care nurse must carry out a patch test, on the abdominal wall, of all common adhesives used in stoma care to see if there is a reaction. The adhesives used in the manufacture of stoma care products are claimed to be hypoallergenic, but patients can react adversely to a specific yet unknown constituent. It may be necessary to work through a range of adhesives and find the most suitable type by a process of elimination.

In patients with psoriasis, care should be taken to site the stoma away from any affected areas. Patients who use a one-piece appliance (Fig. 7.8) may experience an improvement in skin condition if it is possible to change to a two-piece appliance in the same range. Hair follicles can become infected if strict hygiene practices are not adhered to; for those who require it, shaving should be undertaken using a clean razor.

Skin irritation can best be dealt with by using a square of Comfeel or Stomahesive between the skin and the appliance; this usually permits continued use of the preferred appliance. Their effectiveness can be enhanced by the use of barrier wipes. Occasionally a patient may be sensitive to the plastic bag. If it is undesirable to change the type of appliance, a cotton pouch cover can solve the problem.

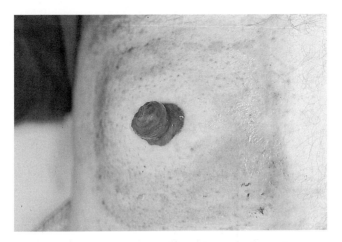

Fig. 7.8 Improvement of condition after change of use from one to two-piece appliance.

Fungal infections flourish in moist, warm and badly aerated areas. Standard anti-fungal medicines will combat the infection and improve appliance adherence. Creams are sometimes recommended for mild inflammation; if used sparingly, they can also improve appliance adherence. Caladryl lotion is a useful preparation, particularly in hot weather when patients can suffer skin irritation and have a tendency to scratch. Applied sparingly to intact skin before attaching the appliance, the lotion will soothe the skin and resolve the problem in a short time. This inexpensive preparation can be bought without prescription at dispensing chemists.

Radiotherapy to the abdominal wall causes redness and tenderness of the skin. Considerable problems with appliance adherence may be experienced by the patient and it may be necessary to change to a two-piece appliance. Patients with a colostomy who undergo radiotherapy may experience loose stools, so a drainable appliance in the same range as that usually used would be an advantage.

The nurse faced with a patient in the stressful situation of a leaking appliance needs to handle this with understanding and empathy. Many people come to surgery after living with disease and increasing debility over many years, persuaded by the promise of an improved quality of life. Those with a leaking appliance will often consider that they are no better, and feel cheated of the chance to lead a normal life. Nurses caring for this group of patients need the knowledge and expertise to assess the cause of the leakage and resolve this effectively and so restore their patients' dignity and quality of life.

8 Irrigation technique

Karen Davis

INTRODUCTION

Irrigation is a method of cleansing the bowel by instilling water via a stoma. It is used to ensure a clean bowel prior to surgery, X-rays or other investigative procedures such as colonoscopy. The method is also effective in the treatment of severe constipation. Irrigation has been in use for many years, mostly performed by nursing staff, but as the equipment has improved it has become a safe way for ostomy patients to control their stomas. It is not very popular in the UK at present but this is probably because only 4.7% of the ostomy population are aware of its existence (Wade 1989). Irrigation is not suitable for every ostomist: it has its disadvantages as well as its advantages and each patient needs careful assessment by a trained nurse before considering irrigation as a method of colostomy management. Patients must be given a full explanation of all aspects of irrigation before they can make an informed decision.

ADVANTAGES

1. The patient is continent again and requires only a small appliance or dressing over the stoma.
2. Regained confidence improves self-esteem and self-image; patients often report a better quality of life as a result,
3. Intimacy between partners can be more relaxed.
4. A more varied diet can be enjoyed and the effects of flatus, constipation and diarrhoea are reduced.
5. Patients do not have to deal with the disposal of soiled equipment.
6. The equipment is reusable, lasting for several years, is easily stored and can be packed discreetly when the patient is away from home.
7. Irrigation can help reduce skin problems, especially those associated with leaking bags and allergic reactions.

DISADVANTAGES

1. The method can be time consuming and may need to be performed

as frequently as every day. It cannot be performed periodically (e.g. just when on holiday) if the patient is to achieve any kind of success.
2. It can cause disruption to a busy household as the bathroom may be occupied for up to an hour.
3. If irrigation is practised for some time and then stopped (e.g. because of ill health or old age) the bowel will be sluggish and normal evacuation will prove difficult. Adjusting back to an ordinary appliance may create problems physically and mentally.
4. Poor technique could increase the risk of bowel perforation. The procedure must always be carried out unhurriedly and following the correct guidelines.

CRITERIA

As stated above, irrigation is not a method that can be used by all ostomists. Several criteria must be met in order to decide that a patient is a suitable candidate.

1. The patient must have an end colostomy with formed stool.
2. There should be no complications such as stenosis, herniation or prolapse around the stoma.
3. There must be no further inflammatory bowel disease.
4. Patients with a history of cardiac or renal disease will need careful monitoring as they may become overloaded with fluid.
5. The patient must be physically able to use the equipment; arthritis or other physical impairment such as poor vision may cause unnecessary anxiety and difficulty.
6. The patient must be well motivated and keen to succeed.
7. The patient's family must be supportive, patient and understanding.
8. The patient needs adequate facilities at home; a separate bathroom and toilet is especially useful because of the length of the procedure.
9. A calm, relaxed approach is needed – nervous, mentally disturbed or elderly patients may become too anxious and worried.

The consultant's approval must be obtained before teaching the patient, and the general practitioner should also be aware of the patient's intention to use the method.

TEACHING THE PATIENT

The best time to teach the patient is the subject of great debate (Allen 1984). There are those who advocate teaching immediately after surgery to form a stoma, and others who feel it is better to wait. Most of those patients taught in the first few days after surgery are outside the UK where the financial aspect of care is often forcing people to seek the cheapest option. Whilst there are some centres in the UK that advocate early learning, most stoma care nurses prefer to wait. Today we are all aware of the need to be cost conscious but to teach a particular method just to save money is the wrong way to care for patients. Irrigation is not successful for everyone and the sense of failure that may follow unsuccessful attempts can be very damaging to the patient's confidence. Patients have more than enough to cope with, coming to terms with major abdominal surgery, without complicating things further by teaching them irrigation. In 2–3 months the wounds will have healed and patients will have established a routine and a better understanding of how their stoma works. They will be confident when handling the equipment and will be more sure of what they want to do.

Suitable patients can be made aware of the irrigation technique during their preoperative counselling sessions. Once they are fit and healthy postoperatively, they can be given more counselling and explanations of the technique, and the nurse can use books, videos and successful irrigators to make sure that all aspects of irrigation management are understood.

It is useful to visit patients in their homes to advise on any adjustments that may be necessary. Usually, only the addition of a hook above the toilet is required, from which to hang the water reservoir (Fig. 8.1). The time of day the irrigation takes place also needs to be discussed. As far as bowel activity is concerned, it does not matter which time of day patients choose (Phillpots et al. 1976). What is important is what fits best with the family schedule; choosing a quieter time for the bathroom, such as the evening, may cause less disruption than first thing in the morning.

Ideally, the method should be taught at home, but it is possible at the hospital as long as private facilities are available.

The procedure needs to be taught daily for at least a week. The first few days are spent demonstrating the equipment and its use. Gradually, each aspect of the technique can be handed over to the patients so that by the end of the first week they are observed carrying out the whole procedure on their own. Written instructions, feedback and teaching videos can be used to ensure that patients have fully understood everything. The daily irrigations should continue until they are confident that the stoma will not work between irrigations. It is advisable for patients to wear their normal appliance during this time. It generally takes 2 more weeks for the bowel to become accustomed to the irrigations. The length of time between irrigations can be extended as long as no stool comes through the stoma. This is a highly individual thing and for some patients an irrigation every 24 hours will always be necessary. Constant reassurance will be needed; although patients will be managing on their own after the first week, regular follow-ups over the next few weeks are advisable to ensure they are not having any difficulty.

EQUIPMENT REQUIRED

The equipment that is needed (Fig. 8.2) comprises:

1. Irrigation kit, consisting of:
   graduated reservoir

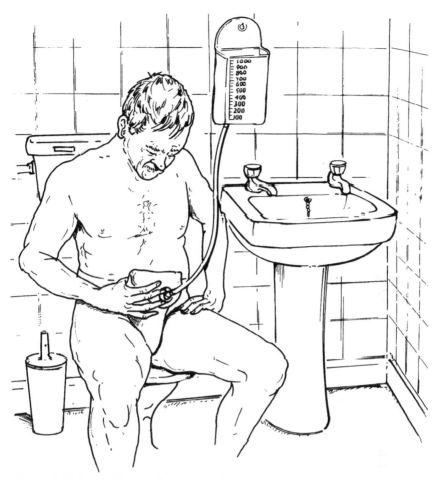

Fig. 8.1 Height of hooks for reservoir.

      cone and tubing
      clamp
      irrigation sleeve with adhesive or belt attachment
      belt if required
      pegs
      cleaning brush
      (This kit is available on prescription as a starter set.)
2. Lubricating jelly
3. Disposable gloves
4. Tissues
5. Jug
6. Clean appliance, cap or dressing

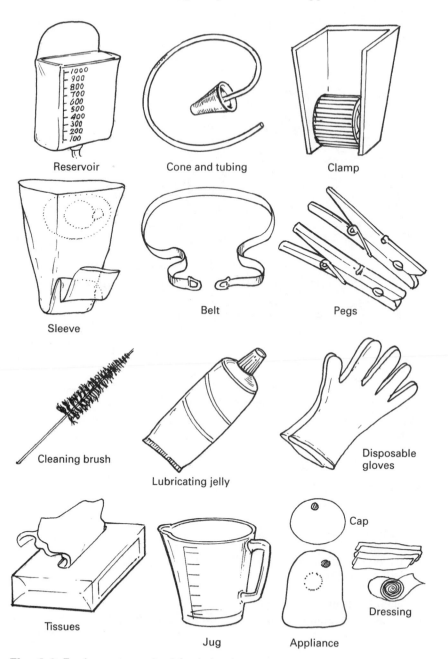

Reservoir Cone and tubing Clamp

Sleeve Belt Pegs

Cleaning brush Lubricating jelly Disposable gloves

Tissues Jug Appliance Cap Dressing

Fig. 8.2 Equipment required for irrigation.

THE IRRIGATION PROCEDURE

1. Connect the cone, tubing and reservoir together.
2. Ensuring that the clamp is closed, fill the reservoir with just over 1 litre of warm tap water.
3. Secure the reservoir on a hook positioned at head to shoulder height in reach from the toilet.
4. Open the clamp and run through some of the water until all the air is expelled from the tubing. A litre of water should be left in the reservoir and the clamp firmly closed.
5. Remove the old appliance from the stoma and cleanse the surrounding skin.
6. Securely fix the irrigation sleeve over the stoma, using the belt or adhesive backing.
7. Sit on the toilet with the irrigation sleeve between the legs and passing into the pan of the toilet. If the sleeve is too long, the bottom can be trimmed.
8. Once comfortable, place a gloved finger into the stoma to determine the direction of the bowel. This can be a little off-putting at first, but can be stopped after a few weeks if the direction of the bowel has not changed.
9. The lubricated cone can then be passed into the colostomy, in the direction of the bowel, and gently held in place with one hand.
10. The clamp is gradually opened. The water should run slowly into the bowel, over a period of 10–15 minutes.
11. Once the reservoir has emptied, the cone can be removed and the top of the sleeve folded down and secured with pegs.
12. Faecal matter, together with most of the water, will be expelled into the sleeve and down the toilet. This might be explosive at times.
13. It takes about half an hour for all the faecal matter to pass through, but once the majority of the fluid has returned the patient can use the jug to flush water through the sleeve from the top, clean the bottom and roll up the sleeve, securing both ends together with the pegs, in order to carry on other bathroom activities.
14. Once the colostomy has stopped draining the sleeve can be removed, the skin cleansed and a new appliance fitted.

The equipment can then be rinsed through and the cone cleaned using the brush, leaving it to dry ready for future use. Disposable sleeves are available that can be rinsed and thrown away clean, which is often much more acceptable than storing a used sleeve for several days.

During the first few weeks, patients may experience a few common problems. They should be made aware of these beforehand so that they can employ simple remedies as listed in Table 8.1.

Each patient is different and slight adjustments to the timing and amount of water used may be necessary for complete success. Some patients only need a few hundred millilitres to promote peristalsis, whilst others may require considerably more than a litre. Any changes made should be done gradually and under supervision.

There are occasions when, despite employing the right method,

Table 8.1 Common problems and likely remedies

Problem	Possible cause/remedy
The reservoir does not empty freely into the bowel	The direction of the cone may need to be adjusted slightly The patient may need to relax a little more The cone or tubing may be blocked by faecal matter and need cleaning The reservoir may be hung too low The patient may need to use a little less water
The patient experiences abdominal pain	The water is running too fast and causing cramping. Stop the irrigation until the cramping ceases, then slowly start it again. The patient may feel faint with this pain too The temperature of the water is too hot or too cold
Faecal matter is slow to return	Peristalsis may be sluggish – it can be encouraged by massaging the stomach, moving around the room or having a drink The colon does absorb some of the water – if the patient is dehydrated, more water may be absorbed and less expelled
Breakthrough stool between irrigations	The patient may be waiting too long between irrigations The patient may not be waiting long enough for all faecal matter to pass through the stoma before completing the irrigation The patient may need to use less water The patient's diet may need to be looked at for any foods that may be having a laxative effect
Bleeding from the stoma	Occasionally, the stoma will go into spasm and tighten, making it difficult to insert the cone, causing trauma. The patient needs to remove the cone and try to relax before starting again

irrigation is inexplicably a failure. It may be necessary to abandon the procedure altogether, giving counselling to the patient to help him or her return to using a regular appliance.

In general irrigation is a safe, effective method for achieving continence as long as the correct procedure is taught and followed.

NURSING PROCEDURES

All irrigations or washouts performed by the nurse must be ordered by the doctor first. The procedure is very similar to the irrigation technique already described, but the doctor may wish to add medication or change the type of fluid used.

End colostomy washout

The procedure is identical to that described above except that warm oil may be instilled first to soften stool in cases of obstruction.

Transverse, loop or double-barrelled colostomy washout

This is perhaps the most common stoma irrigation that the nurse will be required to perform. There are two types of washout: one in the distal loop and one in the proximal loop.

Distal loop washout (Fig. 8.3)

This irrigation should not be performed if there is any indication of an obstructing lesion in the distal end. The nurse must ensure that the patient is sitting on the toilet or commode. (The procedure can be lengthy, so patients should be kept warm and their privacy respected.) Once the

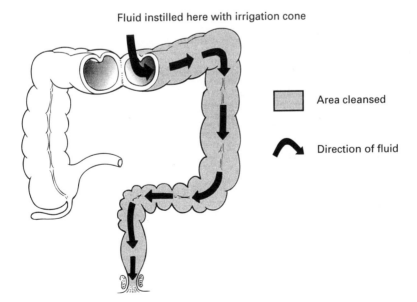

Fluid instilled here with irrigation cone

Area cleansed

Direction of fluid

Fig. 8.3 Distal loop washout.

patient is comfortable, the nurse should examine the stoma and determine by digital examination which of the openings in the stoma leads to the distal loop. In theory, it should be the left side but, to be certain, both openings need to be examined. The proximal loop will have faecal content whilst the distal loop will contain only mucus. It is worth asking the patient which opening seems to be active, but do not rely on this alone. Once you have located the distal loop, water can be instilled as for a normal irrigation; however, most of it will pass through into the toilet via the patient's rectum. In many cases, the nurse must continue the washout until the water comes through clear.

Proximal loop washout (Fig. 8.4)

Having established which opening leads to the proximal colon, the nurse

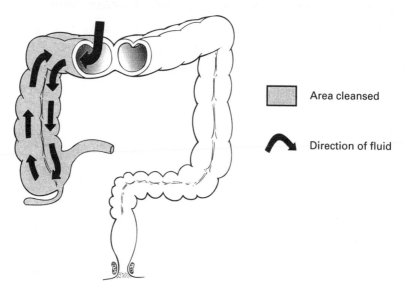

Area cleansed

Direction of fluid

Fig. 8.4 Proximal loop washout.

can irrigate the stoma in the same manner as for an end colostomy; however, it should run slightly slower in order to prevent back-flow into the sterile ileum via the ileocaecal valve.

Ileostomy washouts

This irrigation is rare and should be performed only by a nurse experienced in the procedure.

Loop ileostomy washouts

These are performed as for loop colostomy irrigations except that a fine rubber catheter should be used instead of a cone.

Ileostomy

An ileostomy irrigation is usually attempted only if the patient is obstructed and only at the doctor's wishes following abdominal X-rays. As little as 30 ml of sterile saline is introduced via a fine rubber catheter, and all 30 ml must be returned before attempting to instil further amounts.

Washouts in babies

This is a rare procedure and must initially be carried out by an experienced nurse. It is most often performed on babies with a loop colostomy following surgery for Hirschsprung's disease and only at the request of the consultant paediatrician.

The baby should be made comfortable on a waterproof sheet – a clean nappy can remain in place. A second nurse may be required to keep arms and legs still. Using a syringe (without the plunger) and a fine-bore soft catheter, 15–30 ml of sterile saline is instilled slowly into the distal loop. The saline will be passed via the rectum on to the nappy. Occasionally the consultant will request the same procedure with saline instilled via the rectum. The parents can eventually be taught to carry out the procedure if they are confident and willing.

REFERENCES

Allen, S. (1984) Stoma management. *Nursing (London)*, **2** (30): 877–81.

Phillpots, E.A., Griffiths, D.A., Eltringham, W.K. and Espiner, H.J. (1976) The continent colostomy. *Nursing Mirror, Midwives Journal*, **142** (21): 53–4.

Wade, B. (1989) *A Stoma is for Life – a study of stoma care nurses and their patients*. Scutari Press: London.

9 The electrically stimulated neo-anal sphincter

Barbara Stuchfield

INTRODUCTION

Earliest documentation of surgically fashioned stomas dates back to the early 1700s (Celestin 1987); stomas have been used increasingly to regain and maintain health. However, there are a number of patients who find a stoma so abhorrent that they seek alternative surgical options.

An advance in colorectal surgery to create a neo-anal sphincter, avoiding a permanent stoma, has been pioneered at the Royal London Hospital and in Maastricht, the Netherlands, with encouraging results.

The electrically stimulated neo-anal sphincter (ESNS) is a modification of previous operations which used the gracilis muscle from one leg to form a sling around the anal canal. Pickerell originally used the gracilis muscle for this purpose in 1952 (Pickerell et al. 1952). However, the gracilis muscle is a type 2 fast twitch muscle. At rest it has little or no tone and, when made to work, rapidly tires. Electrostimulation causes the transposed muscle to transform to a type 1 fatigue-resistant muscle capable of maintaining constant tone indefinitely. Stimulation of the muscle is powered by a totally implantable stimulator which can be switched on or off by a hand-held magnet.

When the patient has the urge to defaecate, the magnet is placed over the stimulator, switching it off. The neo-anal sphincter (NS) muscle then relaxes, allowing the patient's bowels to open. The muscle is stimulated again when the magnet is removed from the stimulator. This process is repeated each time the patient needs to defaecate.

The first operation of its kind was performed in 1988 by Professor N. Williams (Williams et al. 1991). In just 7 years, 70 patients have undergone this procedure. They and their successors fall into three groups:

1. Those with severe faecal incontinence for whom previous surgery has failed to provide continence.
2. Those whose sphincter mechanism has to be removed, i.e. in the treatment of rectal cancer.

3. Those whose sphincter mechanism is congenitally absent (rectal atresia).

ESNS FOR FAECAL INCONTINENCE (GROUP 1)

Faecal incontinence is a devastating and disabling disorder that profoundly undermines self-esteem. Sufferers may become housebound, life becoming a constant battle to stay clean. The stigma associated with incontinence and the fear of social isolation prevent people discussing their problems with their peers. Despite greater public awareness of the problem, many patients are reluctant to seek medical help. Although the causes of faecal incontinence have been well characterized, their management remains difficult and controversial. Many clinicians have relatively little interest and less understanding of the condition. As a result, most patients get little in the way of counselling and constructive management.

Therapeutic options range from simple dietary manipulation to surgery. The results achieved with surgical procedures such as post-anal repair are unreliable and disappointing (Yoshioka and Keighley 1989). Patients with disabling incontinence may eventually opt for a permanent stoma which, although not free of undesired effects, allows them to dispense with the multiplicity of pads, plastic pants and other incontinence devices on which they have previously been dependent. Most patients with a permanent stoma return to full and active lives. However, a number of patients find the stoma so abhorrent that they seek the ESNS operation to avoid a permanent colostomy.

Preoperative

Patients are initially assessed by the surgical unit team. A detailed medical history and examination are carried out, including comprehensive investigations of their anorectal function (i.e. sphincter electromyography and proctography). Neosphincter technique is major and complicated surgery, performed in three stages over a 9-month period, so patients must be fit enough to undergo this procedure. Motivation and desires are carefully assessed before the operation is offered to them and, clearly, patients with a positive and interested attitude will achieve better results than patients who are passive and negative.

Before making an informed decision, the full extent of the operation, its disadvantages and possible complications must be fully understood by the patients and several meetings may be required with the surgical unit team. The stoma care nurse is involved in the preoperative counselling to discuss all aspects of stoma care; showing an appliance and giving re-assurance of ongoing support throughout all the stages of hospitalization and after discharge may help to allay many fears. Anxiety is a major factor and a lot of time is necessary to clarify any confusing issues. Family involvement is encouraged from the beginning, as they may be helping to support the patient's needs at home.

There is a booklet available at The Royal London Hospital designed to answer queries about the neosphincter operation. The most common question asked is 'Will it work?' As with any new technique, a successful outcome cannot be guaranteed. About 50–75% of patients have been significantly improved by this operation, although long-term effects are not yet known.

Other issues raised concern the financial implications coupled with work or unemployment. It is important to highlight the time span of the whole procedure, as it may take up to 9 months. Time off work may need to be negotiated with an employer and therefore raise financial worries; this would certainly be a major consideration for the self-employed. In some situations, the surgeon may consent to patients returning to work between the stages of the operation. Travelling to and from hospital may incur cost and many commute long distances. Involvement of a social worker may be helpful to discuss some of the financial and social implications of surgery.

The subject of pregnancy may need to be discussed with women. Although the neosphincter is not a contraindication, a caesarean rather than a vaginal delivery would be indicated to prevent damage to the neosphincter.

Sport and activities may need to be discussed. Swimming, cycling and aerobics can be continued but more aggressive and contact sports such as rugby should be avoided in case the electrode is pulled away from the gracilis muscle.

The stimulator and electrode are available for patients to look at, as they find it difficult to visualize; it is similar to a cardiac pacemaker (with which many people are familiar). The batteries last about 5 years and a minor surgical procedure is necessary to replace the unit.

Many of the anxieties and concerns raised by patients can be allayed by discussion, and further alleviated by the introduction to patients who have already undergone surgery. Preoperative information promotes positive postoperative outcomes – certainly for these patients.

It is essential that patients themselves make the decision to proceed with neosphincter surgery. They can, at any time, opt out of the procedure and remain with a permanent stoma.

Operative technique

The procedure is undertaken in three stages.

Stage 1: Vascular delay – defunctioning stoma

Preoperatively Patients are admitted to hospital 1–2 days prior to surgery. The bowel is prepared in a standard fashion. Patients are prescribed free fluids only for 48 hours and clear fluids only for 24 hours, two sachets of sodium picosulphate for 24 hours before surgery and then nil by mouth for 6 hours on the day of surgery. The stoma therapist visits to site a stoma and discusses any outstanding questions. Each patient's physical, psychological and spiritual needs are identified to enhance care during the hospital stay. All visits are fully documented and consent is obtained by the medical staff.

Perioperatively Vascular delay involves the preparation of the gracilis muscle for the next stage of the operation. Through a 15 cm incision in the medial aspect of the thigh, the gracilis muscle is identified. The minor blood vessels that serve the distal two-thirds of the muscle are ligated and divided. This allows anastomotic channels to open between the main vascular pedicle and the distal part of the muscle. This procedure improves the vascularity and viability of the muscle after transposition.

A defunctioning loop stoma is fashioned, laparoscopically if possible. This diverts faecal stream from the anal canal, minimizing the risk of infection after the second stage of the procedure.

Postoperatively Vital signs are closely monitored and recorded on return from theatre; the intervals between recordings are extended as the stability of the patient improves. The wound and stoma are observed for colour and drainage. Fluid balance is accurately recorded and maintained by intravenous fluids as prescribed, progressing to oral intake once gastric function has returned. The intravenous infusion can be discontinued once oral intake is sufficient.

Pain control is an important factor and regular analgesia is given as prescribed. Early mobilization is encouraged to prevent postoperative complications such as deep vein thrombosis and chest infections, and this highlights the value of the physiotherapist as part of the multi-disciplinary team.

Participation with stoma care is encouraged as soon as possible. A clear plan of aims and objectives is introduced, and a series of goals to achieve before discharge home. Patients are encouraged to participate with care by first familiarizing themselves with the pouch and clip; the stoma care nurse and ward nurses will help in the postoperative period and, with supervision, encourage gradual independence. Looking and touching the stoma may initially be difficult for the patient but with reassurance and support this can be achieved, leading to full independence when a complete pouch change is managed unaided. Other aspects discussed include dietary advice, disposal of appliances and stoma products. Many of the questions/answers can be supported by the use of stoma care booklets.

Discharge Discharge is planned for the seventh to tenth postoperative day, with support in the community from the stoma care nurse or district nurse. A small amount of stoma products are given until further supplies have been obtained from the chemist/delivery service. Prescription details and a contact telephone number are given on discharge.

Subcutaneous sutures are removed from the thigh on the tenth postoperative day. Readmission for the second stage is booked for 4–6 weeks later.

Stage 2: Gracilis transposition and implantation of stimulator

This stage consists of wrapping the gracilis muscle round the anal canal.

Preoperatively Patients are admitted 2 days prior to surgery. They may take fluids only for 24 hours and nil by mouth 6 hours on the day of surgery. It is important to note that the same medical and nursing staff are involved in the patients care at each stage of the procedure, providing the continuity of care and support which is vital for patients undergoing such long and involved treatment. Any further questions can be answered.

Perioperatively The gracilis muscle is transposed from the thigh to the perineum. It is then wrapped round the anal canal in a 'gamma' configuration (Fig. 9.1). In order to achieve this the old thigh wound (from stage 1) is reopened and extended. Further incisions are required in the perineum in order to create a tunnel round the anal canal.

At the same time, an electrode plate is sutured over the main nerve supply to the gracilis muscle (Fig. 9.2). This is connected to the stimulator which is implanted subcutaneously over the inferior costal margin (Fig. 9.3). All components of electrical hardware are checked for faults before they are implanted. At completion of surgery the system is tested once more and the stimulator is left switched off.

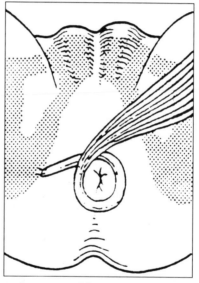

Fig. 9.1 Gracilis muscle wrapped in a gamma configuration around anal canal. (*Source*: Williams et al., 1991.)

Postoperatively Patients are confined to bed for 3 days with their ankles lightly bandaged together, in order to prevent abduction of the hips. This allows the muscle to become firmly adherent to its new attachment on the ischial tuberosity. Patients are able to lift and turn so that care can be given to pressure areas. A sheepskin can aid comfort and ease pressure areas. Although all patients return with an intravenous infusion, they are allowed to start oral fluids and diet as soon as they feel able. Temperature, pulse and blood pressure are monitored and the urinary output is recorded; a catheter remains in place until the patient is fully mobile. Intravenous antibiotics are used to prevent infection of the implanted

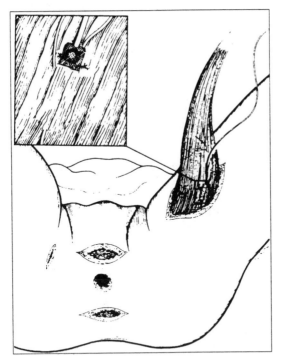

Fig. 9.2 The left gracilis muscle is fully mobilized. The electrode plate is sutured over the nerve to the muscle and the lead connected to an implanted stimulator. (*Source*: Williams et al., 1991.)

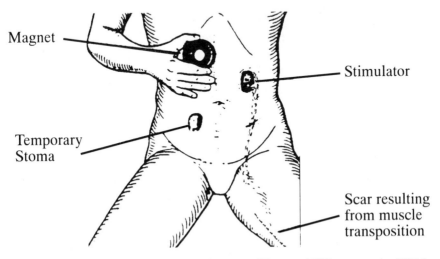

Fig. 9.3 Stage 2 prior to closure of stoma. (*Source*: Williams et al., 1991.)

electrical equipment and are usually continued for 5 days postoperatively and adequate analgesia given as prescribed. The perineum is protected by sterile pads and Netelast or elastic underpants.

Preoperative instruction and follow-up by the physiotherapist help to prevent complications such as deep vein thrombosis and chest infection. Gentle mobilization begins on the fourth day, and is gradually increased until full mobility is achieved.

The occlusive dressing seals the stimulator implantation wound until the sutures are removed.

Electrostimulation This usually starts 10–12 days postoperatively. A standard training regimen is employed to convert the gracilis muscle from type 2 (fatiguable) to type 1 (fatigue resistant). This is achieved by graduated increases in the stimulation parameters. The muscle is initially set to contract for 2 seconds in every 8. This 'daily cycle' is increased fortnightly, i.e. 4 seconds on and 4 off at 2 weeks, and 6 on and 2 off at 4 weeks, etc. Minor adjustments in the intensity and strength of stimulus delivered usually need to be made to ensure effective stimulation of the muscle. Discomfort in the thigh and anus may occur when stimulation commences but will become less obvious as patients adapt to the sensation; if the tingling persists, the strength of voltage can be adjusted.

Discharge Discharge is planned for the tenth to fourteenth postoperative day. Sutures from the stimulator implantation wound are removed on day 10 after the operation, and the perineal sutures at 10–14 days.

Drug prescription for a mild analgesic (e.g. co-proxamol) may be required. An appointment is booked for the stimulation clinic in 2 weeks and for review at the surgical clinic in 6 weeks' time. A contact telephone number is given in case problems arise at home, and a member of the surgical team is always available for advice.

Stage 3: Closure of the stoma

This is usually carried out 3 months after stage 2.

Preoperatively Admitted 1–2 days preoperatively, the patient is prepared for stoma closure with standard bowel preparation (e.g. Picolax) to facilitate anastomotic healing. Fluids only are given for 24 hours and then nil by mouth 6 hours on the day of surgery.

Consent is obtained by medical staff and any questions clarified. The last stage of the ESNS operation can be very stressful for the patient because of the uncertainty about bowel function and the overall success of the operation. At this time it may be necessary to reiterate the potential problems that may occur in the early postoperative period.

Postoperatively Once intestinal function has returned and full oral intake has been established, any intravenous infusion may be discontinued. The return of intestinal function is often heralded by a rush of diarrhoea that may result in perianal soreness, which can be very distressing and demoralizing for the patient. Perianal hygiene is encouraged with regular use of the bidet or shower; the area needs drying thoroughly by patting with soft toilet tissues or the use of a low temperature hairdryer. Excoriation is best managed by the combination of emollient cream and topical local anaesthesia (e.g. lignocaine 1% and Drapolene emulsion). However, with time and the return to a more normal diet and bowel habit, continence gradually improves and the effect of the neosphincter becomes apparent. Early mobilization is encouraged in order to minimize postoperative complications. Sutures are removed from the wound on the tenth postoperative day.

Use of the magnet Once bowel function has started, the patient is taught how to operate the stimulator using the magnet. The training period commences 4–5 days postoperatively. A small hand-held magnet is placed on the skin overlying the stimulator. This switches the stimulator off and it remains turned off while the magnet remains close to it. When the magnet is removed, the stimulator switches on again automatically. Therefore, when the patient feels the desire to defaecate it is necessary only to hold the magnet over the stimulator until defaecation is completed. Removing the magnet switches the stimulator on again.

Discharge Discharge is between day 10 and 14 after the operation. Dietary advice is provided for the patient, with the aim of improving stool volume and regularity of bowel habit. A combination of constipating drugs such as loperamide 2 mg eight times a day may be used to slow activity; laxative agents such as Mil-Par 10–20 ml b.d. increase bowel activity. It is left to the patient's discretion to titrate the medicine according to his or her specific needs.

A great deal of reassurance is needed at this time as it may take several weeks or months before a regular bowel habit is achieved. Follow-up continues on a regular basis with the surgical unit team, and a member of staff is always available for urgent consultation if the need arises.

Patients are encouraged to aim for a normal lifestyle as soon as possible. Work can be resumed 6–8 weeks after discharge; it may be possible to negotiate part-time hours with an employer to ease the transition to full-time work.

Sporting activities can commence after a few months; swimming, cycling and aerobics can be undertaken at a gradual pace but it is suggested that rugby, football and other potentially 'rough' contact sports should be avoided as the electrode may be pulled away from the gracilis muscle.

After the delicate surgery securing the electrode plate to the nerve supply, it is strongly suggested that sexual intercourse be withheld for 6 weeks to ensure that the electrode is not disturbed.

The magnet should be kept in a safe, readily accessible place (e.g. toilet) but away from children and their friends, who can have much enjoyment playing with the magnet without realizing the damage it can cause expensive computer equipment, disks, and cassette tapes. Only one magnet is given per patient but if it is lost or becomes broken it can be replaced.

If foreign travel is planned the stimulator may show up on the airport security X-ray. A letter explaining the operation is given to patients for any over-zealous customs officer. Alarm systems such as the ones in stores and libraries may also be triggered by the stimulators. It is wise to inform patients that this may occur, as it may cause embarrassment if they are apprehended by security staff!

ESNS AS A RESTORATIVE PROCEDURE (GROUP 2)

Despite recent advances in sphincter-saving operations a number of patients still require abdominoperineal excision of the rectum for low rectal cancer. The ESNS technique can be performed as a restorative procedure for patients who would normally be managed with a permanent stoma or for a small number of patients who are desperate to have their stomas closed.

A full clinical assessment is made to ensure a curative operation: this includes a full medical history and physical examination together with comprehensive investigations to exclude metastatic spread. A chest X-ray, liver function tests, abdominal ultrasound and CT scan are included.

During preoperative counselling it is essential that patients/family/carers are aware that the ESNS restorative technique is still in its infancy with no guarantee of a successful outcome. They must fully understand the nature and extent of the procedure, possible complications, time scale involved as well as the social and financial implications. Another issue highlighted is the lack of sensation to defaecate once the anal sphincter has been removed; this is due to damage of the receptors responsible for continence during surgery and an erratic bowel habit when rectum is replaced by colon. As with any surgical technique requiring rectal excision, the risk of sexual dysfunction must be discussed with patient and partner if appropriate, together with the need for a temporary ileostomy during stages 1 and 2. There are many information booklets available regarding stoma care.

Preoperative counselling is essential and most patients need several meetings with the surgical unit team and the stoma care nurse before the operative technique is fully understood by patient, family and carer. This group of patients are faced not only with the choice of ESNS versus a permanent stoma but also with the deep psychological effects of learning they are cancer victims. This news can evoke such intense feelings that some people feel they are no longer able to control their lives. A major life decision has to be made with an underlying sense of urgency owing to the implications of cancer. The anxiety about the forthcoming operation may precede the fears of cancer, which may surface at a later date.

Helping patients manage transition requires behavioural changes, coping strategies, adjustment and adaptation. Subsequently, the psychological support for patient/family/carer is very demanding for all health care professionals involved.

Surgical technique

This operation is performed in three stages over 12–18 months (minimum).

Stage 1

Stage 1 comprises abdominal perineal excision of the rectum, formation of a colonic pouch (loops of colon formed into a reservoir at the anal outlet) or simple colonic pull-through. Vascular delay and a loop stoma are performed at this stage, as described earlier. Six months later, the patient is admitted for stage 2.

Stage 2

Stage 2 involves wrapping the muscle round the terminal part of the colon and implantation of the stimulator, electrodes and plate. The stimulation programme commences on day 10 after the operation.

Stage 3

Stage 3 is closure of the stoma. The nursing care of patients is as has been described previously.

CONGENITAL ANOMALIES (GROUP 3)

A small number of patients have required stoma surgery within the first few days of life because of imperforate anus. A colonic pull-through may be performed at a later date but incontinence may result. The ESNS may be an alternative procedure for these patients to provide continence.

Preoperative counselling is essential and information should be clearly explained and fully understood. Many of the patients are adolescents and have experienced a difficult childhood, subjected to bullying and teasing at school, and have suffered deep psychological scarring; they are still coming to terms with their appearance, body image and sexuality. It is important to create an atmosphere in which they feel accepted and understood, so that they can express and share their feelings as they manage the transition into adulthood and into a new way of life which is, hopefully, an improvement in continence.

The surgical procedure and subsequent nursing care are the same as for group 1 patients.

CONCLUSION

Recently there have been changes in the surgical technique for patients in groups 1 and 3. Stage 1 (vascular delay) has been performed without a covering stoma. The stimulator is inserted at stage 2; it is connected to the implanted wires 1 week later, when the risk of infection is less. This reduces the operation to a two-stage procedure.

The electrically stimulated neo-anal sphincter is an exciting new operation. Although early results have been encouraging, there have been some technical problems and a few clinical failures. Although success is highly probable for well selected patients, a good result cannot be guaranteed. This treatment, however, affords hope for many people who would otherwise be committed to a stoma for life. This innovation has provided many patients with better anorectal function and consequently has dramatically improved their quality of life.

REFERENCES

Celestin, L.R. (1987) *Colour Atlas of Surgery and Management of Intestinal Stomas.* Wolfe Medical: London.
Pickerell, K.L., Broadbent, R., Masters, F.W. and Metzger, J.T. (1952) Construction of a rectal sphincter and restoration of anal continence by transplanting the gracilis muscle. *Annals of Surgery*, **135**: 853–62.
Williams, N.S., Patel, J., George, B.D., Hallan, R.I. and Watkins, E.S. (1991) Development of an electrically stimulated neo-anal sphincter. *Lancet*, **338**: 1166–9.
Yoshioka, K. and Keighley, M.R.B. (1989) Critical assessment of the quality of continence after post-anal repair for faecal incontinence. *British Journal of Surgery*, **76**: 1054–7.

ACKNOWLEDGEMENTS

Thanks to Elaine Macleod, CNS – Stoma Care, Royal London Hospital, for her help and support, and to John F. Abercrombie, FRCS, for his advice on the technical aspects of the procedure.

10 Restorative proctocolectomy: the nursing implications

Theresa Porrett

However managed, however we delude ourselves, a permanent potentially incontinent stoma is an affront difficult to bear, so that I marvel that we and our patients have put up with it so long.

Dudley (1978)

INTRODUCTION

It is more than 15 years since restorative proctocolectomy was pioneered at St Mark's Hospital by Sir Alan Parks and Mr John Nicholls (Parks and Nicholls 1978). In that time it has become one of the major developments in colorectal surgery and has offered many patients the opportunity to avoid a permanent ileostomy. However, it is recognized that such procedures are associated with significant complications and both physical and psychological morbidity. It is often nursing staff who detect and monitor the problems associated with pouch surgery. In this chapter the surgical aspects of restorative proctocolectomy are outlined and the nursing care and management of complications discussed in detail.

WHAT IS A RESTORATIVE PROCTOCOLECTOMY?

Restorative proctocolectomy is a procedure that involves resection of the colon and proximal rectum, mucosal stripping of the distal rectum and construction of an ileal pouch with ileoanal anastomosis. A number of terms are used to describe this type of surgery, including Park's pouch, ileoanal pouch and restorative proctocolectomy. Although the mixed terminology can be confusing, all operations involve the construction of a reservoir from distal small bowel. The procedures can differ in the technique used in the construction and final configuration of the pouch. The original Parks' pouch was constructed using three loops of ileum aligned to form an S shape. About 30–40 cm of small bowel is required. Early pouch configurations were fashioned with a relatively long segment of ileum connecting the pouch to the anus. This resulted in difficulty with spontaneous evacuation, although pouch catheterization was feasible. The pouch design was subsequently altered to overcome this problem and the modified S-shaped pouch continues to be popular.

More recently, other pouch shapes have emerged. The J-shaped pouch has proved particularly successful. It is formed from 30–40 cm of terminal ileum folded into two segments, and the J shape of the pouch is formed by a side-to-side anastomosis. The W-shaped pouch (described by Nicholls and Lubowski in 1987) provides the largest volume: 60 cm of terminal ileum is incorporated to form this pouch, which is associated with a lower frequency of defaecation.

WHO IS SUITABLE FOR THIS PROCEDURE?

When selecting patients for a restorative procedure, it is important to define the aims of such surgery and the optimal outcome that can be achieved. Disease control *per se* can be gained satisfactorily by panproctocolectomy and ileostomy, and a stoma can be avoided by ileorectal or ileoanal anastomosis. However, only the restorative proctocolectomy provides a low frequency of bowel motions and optimal disease control in the absence of a stoma. Thus the prime indication for pouch surgery is where an optimal functional result is of paramount importance to the patient.

The operation is most commonly carried out in patients with ulcerative colitis, but is also of value in familial adenomatous polyposis and constipation due to megacolon or megarectum. Occasionally, it has been used in the surgical treatment of rectal carcinoma. Restorative surgery is absolutely contraindicated in Crohn's disease because of the high risk of enterocutaneous fistula formation. Restorative proctocolectomy is a major procedure that should be undertaken only in the fit patient. Patients suffering acute exacerbation of their ulcerative colitis should be managed with restorative surgery in mind at the time of their emergency operation. Colectomy with formation of ileostomy and mucous fistula is preferred so that a pouch can be considered once the patient has made a full recovery and is no longer dependent on steroids.

Advanced age is not an absolute contraindication for restorative surgery, as patients aged btween 3 and 70 years have undergone pouch procedures, but cardiorespiratory fitness and strong motivation are very important. Thus, restorative surgery is uncommon in patients over 60 years. Good anal sphincter function is required for successful restorative procedure. Studies have revealed that resting tone in the anal sphincter deteriorates with ageing, which can lead to an increased incidence of incontinence after restorative proctocolectomy in people over 50.

Effluent from a pouch is often liquid; although it may become semi-formed as the pouch matures, good sphincter control is essential if incontinence is to be avoided. In fact, pouch incontinence is far more socially restricting than a permanent ileostomy. Anal sphincter function can be evaluated preoperatively by digital examination but many centres now measure a number of physiological parameters associated with anorectal function, which allows more accurate detection of sphincter weakness or sensory loss. Pudendal nerve integrity, anorectal manometry, anal sphincter resting tone and voluntary 'squeeze' pressures are measured.

In summary, the main contraindications to pouch surgery are Crohn's disease, low rectal carcinoma, defective anal sphincter mechanism and poor cardiac or pulmonary function.

Preoperative preparation

The pouch is not a return to normal, and great care must be taken to explain carefully the alternatives and disadvantages to any potential candidates.

Mortensen (1993)

Before a final decision is made about the surgery there is much information that must be made available to prospective patients, and they should be encouraged to take an active role in the decision to opt for restorative surgery (Coloplast Foundation 1987). Patients are frequently seen on more than one occasion in the outpatient department before operation, which allows a rapport to be established between patients, surgeon and stoma care nurse.

A great deal of information is communicated to this group of patients but in the stressful surroundings of the outpatient department it may be forgotten or become confused. The stoma care nurse is in a position to see the patient again preoperatively to reinforce information already given. This preoperative counselling is essential if the patient is to be psychologically prepared to cope with what can be a variable functional outcome to the procedure (Salter 1990a).

The operation itself may be performed in one or two stages, and patients need to be aware of the length of time that may be required off work. If the operation is performed in two stages, patients may not go back to work between the stages, which in some cases may mean a period of 5 months away from work.

The subject of pregnancy needs to be raised with young women, as there is a risk of damage to the anal sphincter during vaginal delivery. In the UK a caesarean section is recommended rather than risk any trauma to the sphincter, as sphincter damage might result in incontinence, requiring excision of the pouch. This is not a hard-and-fast rule, and each case must be assessed individually, taking into account the size of the baby in comparison with the pelvic girdle. At the Mayo Clinic there has been a series of successful vaginal deliveries.

In males, the subject of sexual dysfunction must be discussed. In any procedure that involves excision of the rectum there is a risk of damage to the pelvic autonomic nerves, which could result in impotence. However, in pouch surgery, in which a close dissection of the rectum is undertaken, the risks are low, and greatly reduced compared with the risks when undergoing an excision of rectum for carcinoma (Nicholls 1987). If there is concern about the possibility of sexual dysfunction, the facility to store semen preoperatively should be made available.

Negative as well as positive aspects of pouch surgery should be fully discussed and the risk of complications made clear. The full potential range of pouch frequency needs to be identified; at best the pouch could function twice during the day and not at all at night but equally it could function eight times daily and once at night.

Peer support is extremely useful at this stage. If potential pouch patients can be put in touch with someone of a similar age who has undergone the surgery, it will help greatly in allaying their fears.

In summary, the psychological preparation of these patients is essential if they are to cope with the varying functional outcomes. Pemberton (1993) describes informal psychological criteria for selecting patients at the Mayo Clinic: Patients should be bright, have an understanding of their underlying disease, be able to follow instructions, be compliant and compulsive about follow-up.

Preoperatively, the stoma care nurse has the opportunity to discuss with the patient the temporary loop ileostomy and its management, and the various appliances can be shown. The stoma is sited and the patient is shown the range of appliances that may be suitable for use postoperatively. A large, clear postoperative appliance is also shown to the patient and the reasons for its use explained.

When the patient is admitted to hospital for surgery, the bowel needs to be prepared for the operation. Most hospitals have their own particular method of bowel preparation, but it is commonly acknowledged that people with ulcerative colitis, with their frequent loose bowel actions, need less bowel preparation; often, 2 days of fluids only is sufficient.

The operation

The operation may be performed in one or two stages. In a two-stage procedure the ileoanal pouch is formed and anastomosed to the anal margin but a covering loop ileostomy is formed to protect the pouch anastomosis. The loop ileostomy is subsequently closed after 6–12 weeks once the anastomosis is patent. When the surgery is performed in one stage the operative procedure to form the pouch is the same, the only difference being that no loop stoma is raised. This reduces the number of hospital admissions to one and avoids the risks associated with closure of an ileostomy. To protect the pouch anastomosis a soft rectal catheter is sutured into the pouch. There may be an increased risk of leakage from the pouch anastomosis and consequent infection when performed in one stage, but research does not yet appear to show this conclusively.

The operation itself can vary greatly in length, depending on many factors such as the surgeon's experience and whether the anastomosis is hand sutured or stapled; if previous surgery has been undertaken, adhesions may take longer to divide.

Postoperative care

The care immediately after restorative proctocolectomy is that for any major abdominal surgery (Bridges 1987). Intravenous fluids are administered until bowel sounds are present and the ileostomy is passing flatus. Oral fluids are started when bowel sounds are present, gradually increasing to a light diet. A large clear postoperative appliance covers the loop stoma, enabling close observation of the stoma and rod. The rod is removed from the ileostomy at between 5 and 7 days and the patient's teaching begins. It is outside the scope of this chapter to discuss the management of a loop ileostomy but it is important to stress the fact that loop ileostomies can be extremely difficult to manage. The vast majority of patients accept and cope very well with the stoma, presumably bcause they know it is only a temporary situation.

There will be a Redivac type of drain in the pelvis. Accurate monitoring of the drainage is important. The drain can usually be removed at 3–5 days, when the drainage will have significantly reduced. A urinary catheter is placed in the bladder to drain urine continuously but can be removed as soon as the patient is mobile, often at about 4–5 days. Pain control is essential if the patient is to be able to become mobile quickly and will therefore be motivated and co-operative. Many centres use some form of continuous subcutaneous analgesia such as 120 mg of papaveretum (Omnopon) made up to 60 mm in normal (0.9%) saline and administered at a rate of between 1 and 4 mm per hour. The patient will also receive three doses of intravenous antibiotics prophylactically (e.g. metronidazole and gentamicin).

Initially following surgery there may be leakage from the pouch despite its being covered by a loop ileostomy. The output from the pouch may be blood and faecal debris from the surgery. The patient might be incontinent of this, and pads and disposable pants may be necessary. The perianal skin is at risk of becoming excoriated from this leakage, so strict perianal hygiene is required with regular use of the bidet. The skin should be thoroughly cleaned and gently patted dry, not rubbed. Nappy rash preparations are useful in preventing excoriation. The amount of leakage quickly decreases, leaving only the occasional build-up of mucus. The amount of mucus produced differs. Many patients find that sitting on the toilet once a day and passing any mucus that has collected helps to avoid the sensation of wanting to defaecate.

Patients are usually discharged home at around 10 days postoperatively, but only when they are caring for their stoma independently.

Advice at discharge

Patients are reviewed in the outpatient department in 6 weeks. They will have been advised not to return to work before then, to gradually increase exercise but not to lift heavy weights or drive for 6 weeks. If there is any increase in mucus discharge from the pouch, they are asked to contact the hospital immediately. If the output from the loop ileostomy is high (over 1.5 litres per 24 hours), patients are advised on methods to control/prevent possible dehydration and electrolyte imbalance.

STAGE 2: CLOSURE OF ILEOSTOMY

Closure of the ileostomy normally takes place 3 months later. The patient is reviewed in the outpatient department and a 'pouchogram' is performed: radio-opaque dye is inserted into the pouch to check that the pouch anastomosis is patent. Closure of the ileostomy may be delayed for up to a year if it is more convenient for the patient to go back to work first. It is important that patients know that this is an option and that no damage will occur to the pouch if the ileostomy is not closed immediately.

On admission, the only preparation necessary is 2 days of fluids only to prepare the bowel. This can be a period of great anxiety for patients and time must be taken to explain the likely erratic behaviour of the pouch immediately postoperatively.

On return to the ward from theatre, patients will be allowed nil by mouth: they will have an intravenous infusion, a small wound and dressing over the ileostomy site and be wearing disposable pads and pants. The routine postoperative care is the same as for any closure of stoma.

The pouch can begin to function 12–24 hours postoperatively. The effluent will be bile-stained and explosive in nature and patients may be incontinent at this stage. They are advised to evacuate the pouch as soon as they are aware of the sensation of wanting to defaecate. Initially, the pouch can function 10–15 times per day and perineal soreness can be a problem but conscientious perianal hygiene and the use of a nappy rash preparation or barrier cream should prevent excoriation.

Patients commence fluids and then gradually increase to a soft diet once they have good bowel sounds. It is only once they are taking an ordinary diet that the output from the pouch begins to be less liquid. It can be difficult to motivate patients to take an ordinary diet and fluids, as they sometimes think that eating will make the output from the pouch even more frequent. The opposite is true and the effluent from the pouch becomes much more porridge-like in nature, decreasing the number of times the pouch requires exacuating. Foods such as mashed potatoes and rice pudding are effective in thickening up the output. By using a stool chart, the frequency of the pouch can be monitored over a 24-hour period. A great deal of patient reassurance is needed at this time, when it is normal for the pouch to work so frequently. Loperamide capsules, 2–4 mg half an hour before meals, can be used to thicken the stool and reduce frequency.

At first the capacity of the pouch is small but over the course of 6–12 months the pouch will expand. In some cases it may have a capacity of 1 litre; this can reduce the frequency of pouch evacuation to twice daily. To aid pouch expansion, patients are encouraged not to evacuate the pouch immediately they feel the sensation to, but to wait for 10 minutes; by increasing this period by 5 minutes each successive occasion, pouch evacuation can in some cases be delayed for up to 4 hours.

The patient is usually discharged from hospital at between 7 and 10 days. At this stage, day-time frequency may be five or six times and once or twice at night.

Advice at discharge

Patients will be reviewed in the outpatient department in 4–6 weeks. They are advised on discharge from hospital not to return to work until they have been seen and cleared in the outpatient department. There are no dietary restrictions but it is advisable to introduce new foods gradually into the diet. Advice is given that, if the pouch stops working or the frequency increases, they should contact the hospital immediately. The fact that the initial pouch frequency is normal should be reinforced: it can take 6–12 months to reduce day-time frequency to three to four times and to eliminate the need for night evacuation altogether. People with ulcerative colitis who have undergone the surgery may feel that their position is no better than before with regard to frequency in the early stages, but there will not be the associated urgency that was present with their colitis (Nicholls 1993).

COMPLICATIONS

Pouchitis

Pouchitis is an acute inflammation of the pouch, and is the most common late-onset complication following restorative proctocolectomy. Patients present feeling generally unwell, and they may have a fever. The effluent from the pouch is increased and is more fluid in nature, with fresh blood.

The treatment of pouchitis tends to vary from hospital to hospital but many centres use metronidazole as their first choice. Other antibiotics (e.g. amoxycillin) have been used but not all cases of pouchitis will respond to antibiotics alone. Steroidal enemas such as hydrocortisone acetate (Colifoam) or 5-ASA have proved to be effective, but occasionally short courses of oral steroids are required.

The majority of cases can be treated on an outpatient basis but patients requiring hospital admission will often only need intravenous rehydration.

Compliance with the treatment could be a problem in some cases as the medication is very similar to that used to treat ulcerative colitis, which the patient may have taken for a number of years with little effect. Therefore, encouragement is needed if the patient is to comply with treatment.

Pouchitis can occur at any time following pouch formation, and patients may experience more than one episode (Williams and Johnson 1985). The majority of cases resolve following treatment but in some a chronic/acute inflammation may persist with symptoms that are intolerable and require excision of the pouch and a permanent ileostomy.

Outflow problems

Some patients may experience problems spontaneously evacuating the pouch. This can be caused by some degree of nerve damage or by a long ileal segment, resulting in a constant feeling of fullness associated with lower abdominal or perineal pain and abdominal distension. Once a differential diagnosis has been made by digital examination and a pouchogram, treatment can be begin. If outflow problems are caused by a stricture, the patient will require dilatation of the stricture under anaesthetic; in most cases more than one dilatation will be required. If the cause is a long ileal segment, the patient needs to be taught to intubate the pouch using a rectal catheter. This will need to be done every 6 hours but is a relatively quick procedure and the catheters can be carried discreetly in a handbag or pocket. The ileal segment can be revised but this involves major abdominal surgery which should not be undertaken or suggested lightly if the patient is managing by catheterizing the pouch. These problems can be very distressing for patients, especially until a diagnosis is made, and a great deal of support will be needed.

Night incontinence

A small number of patients experience occasional night incontinence. This may be resolved by taking their main meal at midday and just having a light snack in the evening. The use of loperamide at night has proved to be effective alongside some form of bulking agent such as Fybogel. The patient should be advised to empty the pouch completely before going to bed, and this may necessitate the use of a rectal catheter.

CONCLUSION

The demand for all types of continent and restorative procedure is increasing as an ever-greater number of patients seek an alternative to a permanent stoma (Salter 1990b). Society in general has little tolerance or understanding of bowel problems. We have formed very rigid boundaries about what is and is not socially acceptable, and are constantly reminded by the press and media of what is an attractive and beautiful figure. It is from this background of social stigma that patients hope to escape by undergoing a restorative proctocolectomy.

To support, educate and inform patients with or considering pouch surgery a Pouch Support Group has been formed as part of the Ileostomy Association and many centres now performing the surgery have their own support group networks. Support groups are useful in helping patients decide if the surgery is the best option for them; it must be stressed, though, that the objective of surgery is to allow patients to return to a normal life and so, for many, the support groups are unnecessary postoperatively. For the majority of patients the surgery will be successful in that it cures their disease and avoids the need for a permanent stoma. However, for some the adaptation to life with an ileoanal pouch is difficult and it is in this area of patient support and information that continuity of care in a team approach is essential.

REFERENCES

Bridges, J. (1987) Restorative proctocolectomy to avoid a stoma. *Nursing Times*, : 63–6.
Coloplast Foundation (1987) *The Ileo Anal Pouch.* Coloplast Foundation.
Dudley, H.A.F. (1978) If I had carcinoma of the middle third of the rectum. *British Medical Journal*, **1**: 1035–67.
Mortensen, N. (1993) Patient selection for restorative proctocolectomy. In: Nicholls, R.J., Bartolo, D., Mortensen, N. (Eds) *Restorative Proctocolectomy.* Blackwell Scientific: Oxford, chapter 2.
Nicholls, R.J. (1987) Restorative proctocolectomy with various types of reservoir. *World Journal of Surgery*, **11**: 751–62.
Nicholls, R.J. (1993) Controversies and practical problem solving. In: Nicholls, R.J., Bartolo, D., Mortensen, N. (Eds) *Restorative*

Proctocolectomy. Blackwell Scientific: Oxford, chapter 5.

Nicholls, R.J. and Lubowski, D.Z. (1987) Restorative proctocolectomy: the four loop (w) reservoir. *British Journal of Surgery*, **74**: 564–6.

Parks, A.G. and Nicholls, R.J. (1978) Proctocolectomy without ileostomy for ulcerative colitis. *British Medical Journal*, **2**: 85–8.

Pemberton, J.H. (1993) Complications, management failure and revisions. In: Nicholls, R.J., Bartolo, D., Mortensen, N. (Eds) *Restorative Proctocolectomy*. Blackwell Scientific: Oxford, chapter 4.

Salter, M. (1990a) Current trends in stoma care. *Nursing Standard*, **14** (22):. 22–5.

Salter, M. (1990b) Overcoming the stigma. *Nursing Times*, **86** (18): 67–71.

Williams, N. and Johnson, D. (1985) The current status of mucosal proctectomy and ileo anal anastomosis in the surgical treatment of ulcerative colitis and adenomatous polyposis. *British Journal of Surgery*, **72**: 151–68.

11 Continent urinary diversions – the Mitrofanoff principle

Rachel Busuttil Leaver

HISTORY OF CONTINENT URINARY DIVERSIONS

Prior to the last century, many attempts had been made to try diverting urine by attaching ureters to the non-intestinal structures of the body such as the vagina or the fallopian tubes. During the late 1800s and early 1900s much experimental and some clinical surgery was carried out in an effort to use intestine as a conduit for urinary drainage. Emptying was controlled by the anal sphincter (Bellinger 1989). Ureterosigmoidostomy became the most popular form of diversion after the turn of the century. This offered a relatively simple method and remained popular for a long time. The lack of knowledge about the metabolic side effects and the frequent deterioration of renal function also contributed to this popularity (Kock 1992). Before the advent of prefabricated collecting devices in the middle of this century, surgeons tried to develop methods for continent external diversion using a caecal reservoir and a short segment of ileum to connect the reservoir to the skin. Whether true continence was really achieved, however, especially at night is debatable (Kock 1992) and there were many complications. This led to the formation of the ileal conduit (popularized by Bricker in the 1950s) which became the most frequently used diversion.

An internal pouch was described by Gilchrist in the 1950s, and in the 1960s Nils G. Kock modified his Kock pouch for ileostomy for use as a urinary diversion.

Urinary undiversion was first described by Lome and Williams (1972) and Hendren (1973); this surgery did not become popular, however, because of its difficulties, lengthy operative time and high revision rate (Hampton and Bryant 1992). More recently, the longer survival of the patients, greater knowledge and acceptance of the psychological, social and somatic impact on patients of incontinence, and the long-term negative consequences associated with ileal conduit have resulted in renewed interest in continent diversion and bladder reconstruction.

Today a number of different types of continent diversion are performed, and these will probably continue to be developed as more is learned about the outcome for patients. Perhaps it is fair to say that the ideal diversion has not yet been found, though undiversion and continent diversion are being offered to many patients. Will this lead to the end of diversions requiring external appliances and ureterosigmoidostomies in the future? The numbers will certainly diminish, but they remain viable options for certain patients with conditions that would preclude them from having major reconstructive surgery.

WHAT IS A CONTINENT URINARY DIVERSION?

The surgeon's aim is to replace or rebuild the body's urinary system. The ideal bladder substitute should:

1. Preserve the upper urinary tract
2. Avoid metabolic disturbances
3. Give the patient total control over emptying bladder/pouch without an external appliance.

Therefore the new bladder must have the same qualities as a normal bladder:

- Low pressure
- Ability to store a large volume of urine
- No or minimal absorption of urine
- No reflux to upper tract
- Voiding controlled voluntarily by sphincter or valve.

A continent diversion consists of three main parts:

1. A reservoir for urine
2. A tunnel or channel to let the urine out
3. A continence mechanism to retain the urine until the reservoir needs to be emptied.

The reservoir can be the patient's own bladder or augmented bladder, or completely remade out of ileum, colon or a combination of the two. The tunnel can be formed of already existing tunnel-like tissues such as the appendix, fallopian tube or ureter, or a tube can be made of rolled up ileum. The continence mechanism is a valve formed during the operation by using part of the tissues already being used to form the new bladder – for example, intussuscepted or invaginated ileum or tunnelled appendix. These valves vary according to the type of diversion being formed. Though nurses should know the main differences between the valves so as to explain to patients which one they have and how it works, the nursing care of the various types of diversion is essentially the same.

THE MITROFANOFF PRINCIPLE

Many different types of continent diversion are available today that are 'psychologically and socially acceptable to the patients and clinically acceptable to the surgeon' (Kock 1992). These include the Kock, the Indiana and the Benchekroun pouch, to name but three. This variety means that there is a diversion to suit each individual patient's needs and condition or that can be adapted to suit. Some surgeons, however, prefer one type of diversion and will adapt that to their patients' needs and available body tissues. In this chapter, one type of diversion, which is arguably the one most commonly performed in the UK, will be described – the Mitrofanoff (Fig. 11.1).

In 1980, Paul Mitrofanoff, a French paediatric surgeon, described using the appendix as a tunnel. One end of the appendix is buried in a submuscular tunnel in the bladder wall, forming an obstructed flap valve. The other end is brought to the surface of the abdominal wall as an easily catheterizable continent stoma. As the bladder fills with urine, it increases the pressure on the valve, obstructing and shutting it tighter still and rendering it even more continent. Urine is drained out of the bladder by passing a catheter into the stoma, down the tunnel, through the valve and into the bladder. Once empty, the catheter is removed and the valve closes once more. The patient is therefore dry and appliance free.

This is Mitrofanoff's principle, which has been adapted by surgeons for use with tissues other than just the bladder as the reservoir and the appendix as the tunnel when forming continent diversions (Woodhouse 1991).

Patients eligible for the surgery may have any of the following:

- Neuropathic bladder
- Congenital abnormalities
- Trauma to the bladder
- Carcinoma of the bladder/pelvic organs
- Incontinence
- Fistulae

Patients with a history of multiple bowel resection, bowel disease or radiation damage may be considered by many surgeons to be unsuitable candidates for diversion.

Stage 1: Preoperative preparation

The most important part of the preoperative care begins with careful selection of a suitable candidate for such surgery. It is vital that such patients are assessed by the designated nurse specialist at this stage as well as by the surgeon.

Patients must be fully aware of the change in function that will be achieved by the surgery and, most importantly, understand every step of the procedure and how involved they will be with the recovery and care of the new diversion. There is a lot of information for patients to absorb, so, as well as a consultation with the surgeon, it is advisable for them to have a separate (and more leisurely) consultation with the nurse specialist to reinforce and fully cover all aspects of the operation and care. It is important to remember that some patients will only hear 'you will be continent' or 'you will not need a stoma bag any more' and may block out any other important details. Above all, patients must be given enough information to ensure they give truly informed consent to the operation. Their responsibility and participation in maintaining the new reservoir must be clear so that unrealistic expectations do not lead to frustration,

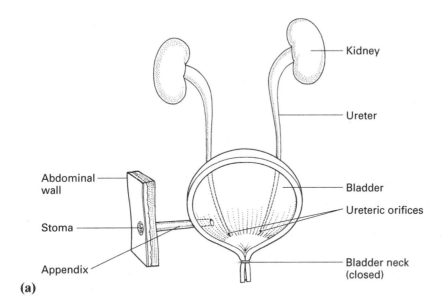

(a)

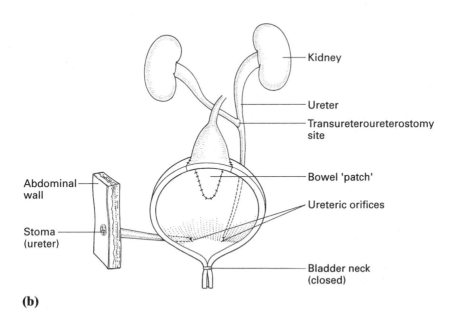

(b)

Fig. 11.1 (**a**) The 'classic' Mitrofanoff. The bladder neck is closed. The appendix is tunnelled into the bladder to form a continent catheterizable stoma. (**b**) An augmented bladder with a right-to-left transuretero-ureterostomy. The redundant right ureter is brought to the surface as a catheterizable stoma.

disappointment and non-compliance with the after-care.

This preoperative time will also give patients time to organize their work and family commitments and to arrange support and help after discharge. A well planned admission will mean fewer problems postoperatively.

The ideal patient should:

1. Be fit enough to undergo surgery (these operations are lengthy: up to 4–6 hours long)
2. Have healthy bowel
3. Be dexterous enough to manipulate a catheter
4. Be motivated
5. Be compliant.

Assessment should also take into account the patient's:

1. Intellect (and/or the carer's)
2. Understanding of the condition and how the operation is going to change this
3. Financial status
4. Lifestyle
5. Job (the patient may be off work for up to 3 months)
6. Partner
7. Disabilities
8. Previous surgery
9. Commitment to self-care
10. Learning ability.

Physical preparation

Many investigations will have been carried out during the assessment period and will have involved a short stay in hospital. These tests include:

- X-rays – kidney, ureter and bladder (KUB) and/or intravenous urogram (IVU)
- Ultrasound
- Kidney function tests – e.g. glomerular filtration rate (GFR)
- Cystoscopy*
- Bladder pressure test – video cystometrogram (VCMG)*
- Blood tests
  *cystoscopy and VCMG are performed only when the patient still has a bladder or part of one.

Stage 2: Preparation for surgery

This is similar to the preparation for any major abdominal surgery that is going to involve the bowel. The patient is admitted 2–3 days preoperatively for bowel preparation and the usual preoperative investigations. This is the ideal time to go over any points that patients feel they need to cover again. It is especially important that patients are warned of all the postoperative tubes they will return to the ward with, their function and a rough guide to when they can expect these to be removed. Patients need support and reassurance at this time as they have to endure tests, food deprivation and undignified bouts of diarrhoea as well as the natural worries of an impending major operation.

Stage 3: Postoperative care

Reconstructive surgery is lengthy (5 hours or more), and has a significant complication rate. Patients may need a 24–48 hour stay in a high dependency or intensive care unit postoperatively.

The care postoperatively should focus on:

1. Adequate analgesics such as continuous opiate infusions given via an intravenous or epidural route (patient-controlled analgesia)
2. Accurate measurement and recording of urine output
3. Ensuring that all drainage tubes are kept patent and draining (Fig. 11.2)
4. Ensuring that the reservoir is not stretched before it is properly healed.

The new reservoir must be kept empty of urine for 6–8 weeks after the operation. This allows it to heal and will ensure that urine will not leak out into the peritoneum.

The pouch is drained by:

1. One or two ureteric stents from the kidneys
2. A pouch catheter (also known as a suprapubic catheter)
3. A stoma catheter.

All are on free drainage. Most of the urine will drain via the stents for the first 5–7 days. As the bowel continues to secrete mucus there is a potential danger of the pouch and stoma catheters becoming blocked by this mucus and debris from the operation. Both catheters must be flushed twice daily using 20 ml of saline each time and commencing from day 1 postoperatively. At day 4 postoperatively the amount of saline can be increased to 100 ml and the pouch can be gently washed out using gentle suction via a bladder syringe. Once patients are able to take on some of their own care, this is the first skill they need to be taught and they should be encouraged to do their pouch washouts twice daily. Besides giving patients some responsibility for their own care, it will help them become more confident in handling the catheters, syringes, etc., and help prepare them for discharge home where this care will continue. By about 10–12 days after the operation, patients should have had their intravenous infusion, wound drain, stents and clips removed. An X-ray (a pouchogram) is sometimes taken at this point to check that the pouch has healed and to see if there are any peritoneal leaks. The pouch catheter is then removed, leaving the stoma catheter in place. Patients are discharged home for 4–6 weeks with this catheter in place on free drainage. This time at home will help patients to recover from the trauma of the surgery, allow the pouch further healing time and prepare them for the next stage.

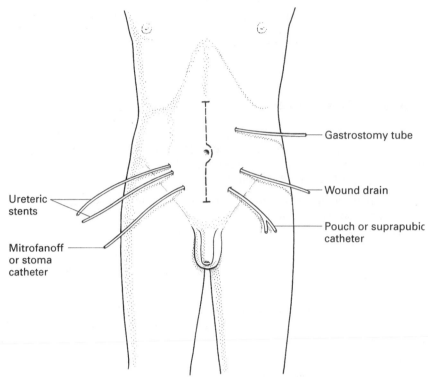

Fig. 11.2 Position of the catheters and drainage tubes postoperatively. The gastrostomy tube is used in some patients instead of a nasogastric tube. If the bladder neck has not been closed, the patient may have a urethral catheter in place as well as, or instead of, the suprapubic catheter.

Stage 4: Readmission

The patient is readmitted 6–8 weeks after the operation for the next stage in the procedure. During this admission the pouch is expanded to assess its volume. The patient:

1. Becomes used to the feeling of a full pouch
2. Starts intermittent catheterization
3. Will acquire the knowledge and skills to enable him or her to take over this care on discharge
4. Will be confident and knowledgeable enough to cope with most problems at home.

The pouch catheter is clamped and patients are encouraged to drink fluids and allow the pouch to become full. It is unclamped every 2–3 hours (sooner if painful or uncomfortable). Most pouches initially hold 200–400 ml and may reach 500–600 ml before discharge. In some cases the pouch continues to stretch and may eventually hold 800–1000 ml. Patients may experience some discomfort or pain and a feeling of fullness and/or nausea. They must be reassured that this may happen and should ease as the pouch expands further.

Once the pouch has been expanded, the stoma catheter is removed and catheterization can begin.

Catheterization

This is a clean procedure (Fig. 11.3). Catheterization is done 2–3-hourly at first and is slowly extended to 4-hourly. The process is tailored to each individual patient's needs and may take 1–3 weeks to achieve. Patients should never go longer than 4–6 hours without catheterization.

If the pouch gets overfull:

1. It may leak
2. Pressure on the valve will increase and make catheterization difficult or impossible
3. The pouch may rupture.

Patients are encouraged to set an alarm to wake them up at least once at night to empty the pouch. Once a regular pattern has been established and patients are aware of how much the pouch can hold comfortably and safely, most of them find that, by cutting back on their evening drinks and

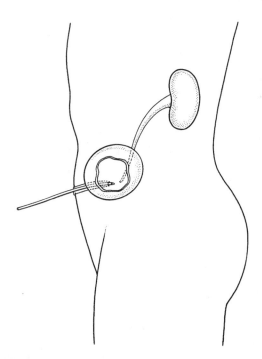

Fig. 11.3 Emptying the pouch by clean intermittent self-catheterization via the continent abdominal stoma.

by emptying before bedtime, they are able to sleep all through the night.

Catheterization, though a fairly simple skill, can be frightening and unnerving for patients (Hampton and Bryant 1992). It is unlike anything most of them have experienced, so reassurance, careful explanation and supervision are important. Patients need time to practise their new skills and to absorb all the new information they need to gain confidence when handling the pouch. Some patients may prefer to have a fixed pouch-emptying schedule rather than develop their own routine. This is perfectly acceptable as long as they realize that a fixed schedule does not take into account their lifestyles and changing situations. In time, patients become more confident and are able to modify the catheterization routine to fit in with their habits (Hampton and Bryant 1992).

Details of the procedure are given in the Appendix to this chapter.

Catheter care

Most catheters are disposable. The ones of choice are PVC, male-length Nelaton-type catheters. Female-length catheters are not long enough to reach far enough into the pouch to empty it of all the urine.

The most common size used is a 12 or 14 Ch but this depends on the size of the stoma or tunnel. After use, the catheter is rinsed out in hot soapy water, patted dry with a tissue and stored in a clean dry receptacle such as a plastic bag or make-up purse. Patients should be advised to check with the catheter manufacturer as to the recommended care for their particular appliance. Catheters should be changed weekly, and patients should make sure they have spare catheters with them at all times.

Complications

Patients may experience a number of complications postoperatively. These may be short-term teething problems while the pouch settles down and the patient gains control of it. Although the Mitrofanoff is a relatively new procedure, some long-term complications have been identified. Some patients may have to undergo additional surgery or treatment until the pouch function is acceptable.

The most common complications are:

1. Infection
2. Leaking via the stoma
3. Stenosis of the stoma
4. Loss of the tunnel
5. High-pressure bladder system
6. Stone formation
7. Acidosis
8. Renal failure
9. Rupture of the pouch.

An extensive follow-up programme ensures that any complications are discovered and treated before they become a major problem. Patients are seen in clinic at 3-monthly intervals at first, then six-monthly and eventually annually. At present they are not discharged from our clinics because the long-term complications (other than those listed above) of these procedures are not known.

Discharge advice

Patients are advised always to empty their pouches before doing any strenuous activities, to minimize the pressure put on the pouch. Pouches must be emptied every 4–6 hours, depending on fluid intake. Leaving it for longer periods may result in infection, mucus build-up, discomfort, leaking via the stoma, or leaking or rupture of the pouch.

Patients, carers and community health workers should all be given information on the procedure and its care, as well as a contact number to a hospital 'link' nurse or the ward. Patients should wear a safety chain or bracelet such as Medic Alert or SOS in case of accidents. Some of these stomas are very small, sometimes looking like a dimple in the skin, and may easily be missed by an uninformed examiner.

It is important that patients attend for their follow-up clinic appointments and investigations.

CONCLUSION

The only certain advantage to the patient undergoing this diversion is cosmetic. This is a considerable advantage, of course, but it is important to remember that it is not a good enough reason to put an unfit or unwilling patient through such lengthy operations (Woodhouse 1991).

In the zeal to try out these new operations and offer them to as many patients as possible, full consideration of their circumstances and the effect on their lifestyle may not be taken when selection is made. This may be a result of incorrect assumptions made by carers and patients regarding the outcome of these operations. There is a danger of assuming that patients will accept the changes in their bodily function more readily than if a urostomy is formed. The other common assumption is that, because they do not have 'to wear the bag' on their stomachs, patients will not suffer the same problems with change in body image and sexuality as do ostomists. Although some patients, especially those who are having their conduits undiverted, do achieve a significant improvement in their body image and quality of life, there are many who find the abdominal scars, and the fact that they had to have a diversion at all, extremely distressing: they need as much time, counselling and support as any ostomist.

Another danger is patients pinning all hope of a drastic change in their lives on the outcome of the surgery (e.g. if an ostomist feels that the inability to have a sexual relationship is due to having a stoma). It is important to counsel such patients preoperatively to ensure that no such unrealistic outcome is expected. In many cases (e.g. patients with bladder exstrophy) it is the original or underlying condition that is causing the problem and, though the diversion may improve things, it will not change the fact that the problem is there and will not go away. Cavas and Makay (1991), summarizing the nurse's role in relation to these patients, say 'Patients need constant support and continuous care to deal with the demanding changes in their lives. Though the operation may free a patient from his disease, his life is changed forever. It is the nurse who plays a key role throughout by facilitating information, providing empathy, striving to detect psychosocial problems early, listening to the patient and his family and carers, confronting problems.' The nurse will also have access to further resources the patient may need, such as additional counselling. It is clear, therefore, that the success of these operations is dependent on the ability of the nurses involved with the patients at all levels to provide not only high degrees of nursing care but also the support network they need.

Despite all possible problems, urinary reconstructive surgery and continent diversion surgery such as the Mitrofanoff diversion seem to be the way forward. They offer patients a choice that was not previously available to them and, for many, a more normal lifestyle and a better quality of life than before.

Appendix: Intermittent Clean Self-catheterization of Continent Urinary Diversions*

This procedure is performed to enable complete emptying of urine from a continent urinary diversion as there is no other route for drainage of urine. It is aimed at promoting continence and preserving renal function. The objective is to ensure that the 'bladder' is empty of its contents, thereby reducing discomfort for the patient, using a technique that reduces the risk of introducing bacteria.

This policy applies to both adults and children.

Equipment required
Catheter   size and type will depend on each individual patient
Lubricant   K-Y Jelly (optional)
Receiver   to collect urine
Sterile gloves   if procedure is to be performed by a nurse.

Action

Rationale

1. The procedure is explained and discussed with the patient prior to the first catheterization, which may be performed by the nurse or by the patient under supervision.

Understanding may relieve anxiety and distress.

2. Assemble equipment in sequence.
3. Wash hands.
   Wash the exit of the catheterizing channel with soap and water.
   This may not always be

To reduce the risk of introducing bacteria into the 'bladder'.

*Adapted from a policy document by St Peter's Hospitals (UCL Hospitals Trust), London.

required. Wipe away mucus or encrustation only if necessary.

4. Assume most comfortable position – e.g. standing, sitting on toilet/bed – ensuring that the exit site of the catheterizing channel is clearly visible.

5. Discard the first 'squeeze' of jelly.

Discarding the first 'squeeze' of jelly ensures that no contaminated jelly is introduced into the 'bladder'.

Apply lubricant in either of the following ways.

To allow for ease and comfort during passage of the catheter.

   a. Apply lubricant directly on to the tip of the catheter.

   b. Apply lubricant on to a clean piece of tissue and smear on to the tip of the catheter.

6. Place the receiver in position to collect the urine.

7. Gently introduce the catheter into the exit site of the catheterizing channel and then slowly push the catheter into the 'bladder'. if you feel some resistance this is usually at the site of the valve. Keep on pushing slowly but firmly and the valve should open. Stop introducing the catheter when urine is seen flowing out of the catheter into the receiver.

To reduce the risk of traumatizing the catheterizing channel during the insertion of the catheter.

8. Allow urine to drain into the receiver. When the flow has stopped, push the catheter in further to ensure that the 'bladder' is completely empty.

To ensure that the 'bladder' is empty before the catheter is removed.

Slowly withdraw the catheter, using a rotating action. If the flow of urine recommences, stop withdrawing, allow urine to drain into the receiver until it has stopped and then recommence withdrawing the catheter.

Rotating action reduces suction effect and pain due to friction.

9. Remove catheter completely.

10. Discard urine and wash receiver. Discard catheter and wash hands.

11. Record action in nursing documentation.

Problems that may occur

Potential problem	Possible reason for problem	Remedy/Action
Difficulty is experienced in passing the catheter.	The catheter has entered a false passage.	Remove the catheter.
	The tunnel has become tighter or stenosed.	Attempt again after a short period, using a smaller size catheter.
	The valve has tightened or stenosed.	If difficulties are experienced again, seek medical help.
		Introduce the catheter further into the 'bladder'.
No urine is draining after the catheter has been introduced.	The catheter has not entered the 'bladder'.	Rotate the catheter to dislodge any material that may be causing the blockage.
	The eyes of the catheter have become blocked.	Remove the catheter and try again with a new one.
		Flush out the catheter and/or wash out the bladder to remove debris/mucus, then retry.
		If these measures fail, seek medical help.
The urine is foul smelling or discoloured.	The urine may be infected.	Obtain a specimen for culture.

GD/URO/NEPU/NP6
Reviewed April 1995

REFERENCES

Bellinger, M.F. (1989) The history of urinary diversion and undiversion. *Journal of Enterostomal Therapy*, **16** (1): 39–41.

Cavas, M. and Makay, S. (1991) The Indiana Pouch – a continent urinary diversion system. Home Study Programme. *AORN Journal,* **54** (3): 493–517.

Hampton, B.G. and Bryant, R.A. (1992) *Ostomies and Continent Diversions – Nursing Management*. Mosby-Year Book: St Louis, pp. 145–57.

Hendren, W.H. (1973) Reconstruction of previously diverted urinary tracts in children. *Journal of Paediatric Surgery*, **8**: 135.

Kock, N.G. (1992) The evolution of the urinary bladder. In: Hohenfellner, R., Wammack, R. (Eds) *Société Internationale d'Urologie Reports – Continent Urinary Diversion*. Churchill Livingstone: Edinburgh, pp. 51–5.

Lome, L.G., Williams, D.I. (1972) Urinary reconstructions following temporary cutaneous ureterostomy diversion in children. *Journal of Urology*, **108**: 162.

Mitrofanoff, P. (1980) Cystostomies continente trans-appendiculaire dans le traitement des vessies neurologiques. *Chir Pediatr*, **21**: 297.

Woodhouse, C.R.J. (1991) The Mitrofanoff principle for continent urinary diversion. *World Council of Enterostomal Therapists Journal*, **11**: Worldwide no. 1: 12–15.

FURTHER READING

Cumming, J., Worth, P.H.L. and Woodhouse, C.R.J. (1987) The choice of supra-pubic catheterisable stoma. *British Journal of Urology*, **60**: 227–30.

Duckett, J.W. and Snyder, McC. (1986) Continent urinary diversion: variations on the Mitrofanoff principle. *Journal of Urology*, **136**: 58–62.

Licklider, D. and Mauffray, D. (1991) Conventional urostomy vs. continent urostomy: case study. *Ostomy/Wound Management Journal*, **34**: 26–9.

Woodhouse, C.R.J., Malone, P.R., Cumming, J., et al. (1989) The Mitrofanoff principle for continent urinary diversion. *British Journal of Urology*, **65**: 53–7.

12 The child with a stoma

Gail Fitzpatrick

INTRODUCTION

In the 1990s children with a stoma are still a fairly unknown entity and not a topic for discussion even within the medical and nursing professions. At present, national statistics are not available, but it is known that 80% of paediatric stoma surgery occurs in the first 6 weeks of life, 10% from 6 weeks to 1 year, and the remaining 10% is performed in older children (Webster 1985).

In 1992 one regional paediatric centre performed 30 stoma procedures, excluding gastrostomy, jejunostomy and tracheostomy. The majority of stomata were colostomies; ileostomy formation was less frequent, and there were very few urinary diversions. Most were temporary and were closed within 16 months of life.

CONDITIONS REQUIRING STOMA SURGERY

Anorectal anomalies

Anorectal anomalies occur in 1:3000 live births and result from arrest or aberration of the normal development of the cloaca into a dorsal rectal tube and a ventral urinary system. They can be divided into high or low, depending on whether the anorectal anomaly is above or below the puborectalis sling. Low anomalies such as covered anus, ectopic anus, congenital anal stenosis and congenital anorectal stricture can generally be treated with anal cutback and anal dilatations. However, high anomalies are more complex: the bowel ends as an atresia or continues as a fistulous opening (MacMahon 1991a: p. 94). A fistula presenting in boys is a rectourethral fistula, and in girls a rectovaginal fistula (Fig. 12.1).

Almost two-thirds of these infants will have one or more associated malformations, most commonly genitourinary and vertebral, although malformations of the alimentary, cardiac and central nervous systems can also occur. Major sacral abnormalities are often associated with neural abnormalities that affect the nerve supply to the bladder and bowel.

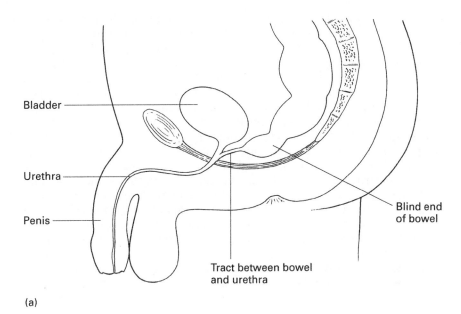

Bladder

Urethra

Penis

Blind end
of bowel

Tract between bowel
and urethra

(a)

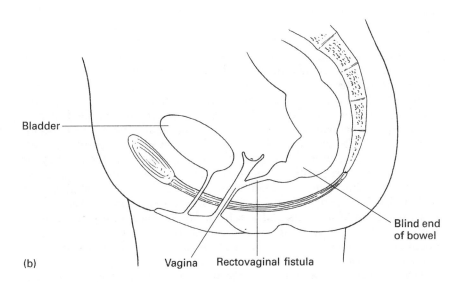

Bladder

Blind end
of bowel

(b)   Vagina   Rectovaginal fistula

Fig. 12.1 Imperforate anus with (**a**) rectourethral fistula in a boy and (**b**) rectovaginal fistula in a girl.

Anorectal anomalies are diagnosed at birth following physical examination of the baby which reveals an absent or covered anus. Other signs may be abdominal distension, constipation, intestinal obstruction and vomiting. Where there is an associated fistula, meconium will be passed from the vagina in girls and through the penis in boys.

The severity of the anomaly can be revealed by radiological tests. The infant is held upside down in front of the X-ray screen, which causes the intestinal gas to rise to the apex of the blind pouch. A marker is placed over the anal dimple, and the distance between this and the apex is measured to determine the distance between the blind-ended bowel and the perineum. Treatment for high anomalies is complex, so a temporary colostomy is performed to relieve the clinical symptoms and enable infants to thrive and grow until they are strong enough to undergo major corrective surgery, which is usually carried out between 6 and 9 months after birth. A pull-through procedure brings the pelvic colon down through the muscle sling of the pelvic floor and this enables it to be joined to an artificially constructed anus. If a fistula is present, it is ligated at the same time. The new anus has to be prepared before the colostomy can be reversed and this is achieved by performing daily anal dilatations, commencing about 7–10 days after the operation, until the anus is of an adequate size for a normal stool to be passed. It is difficult to obtain a satisfactory degree of continence owing to the total absence of a normal external sphincter. Some 50% of infants with a high anomaly would be expected to be continent, 25% to have fair continence and the remaining 25% would be incontinent.

Hirschsprung's disease

This congenital abnormality occurs in 1:5000 live births and is caused by the terminal absence of ganglion cells in the submucous and myenteric plexuses of the colon as a result of the failure, during uterine growth, of distal migration of the ganglion cells along the intestinal tract. The length of the aganglionic segment depends on the stage at which the distal migration was disrupted.

In 50% of cases the sigmoid colon and rectum are affected, in 25% the rectum only is involved, and the whole colon is affected in just 5%. Extension of the aganglionic segment into the small bowel is rare, occurring in just 1–2% of cases (MacMahon 1991a: p. 92). Hirschsprung's disease has a 7% familial incidence. Several siblings in a family may be affected and several mother–child cases have also been reported. The risk for siblings with a short segment distribution is 1 in 30 over all, with a higher risk for brothers than for sisters. In the long segment cases, there is a risk of 1:10 for sisters and 1:6 for brothers. Short segment cases are more common in boys than girls in a ratio of 5:1, whereas there is an equal sex distribution with long segment cases. The abnormality most commonly associated with Hirschsprung's disease is Down's syndrome.

The problem commonly presents with delay in passing meconium. There is often abdominal distension due to constipation, although diarrhoea may result from faecal overflow or enterocolitis. Other signs include failure to thrive, slow feeding and vomiting. The majority of cases are diagnosed in the neonatal period as the baby presents with an acute or subacute intestinal obstruction. Alternatively, infants with short segment Hirschsprung's disease may suffer from intermittent constipation and abdominal distension, and diagnosis may be delayed for months or years.

Loops of bowel distended by gas will be shown by a plain abdominal

X-ray. Diagnosis is confirmed by rectal suction biopsies which demonstrate that ganglia are absent from the submucous and myenteric plexuses together with an increase in the number of nerve fibres in the interface between the circular and longitudinal muscles. Further histological techniques stain sections for acetylcholinesterase to identify cholinergic fibres and identify adrenergic fibres using a catecholamine fluorescent technique (Jones et al. 1985c).

If a very short segment is involved, it may be possible to perform a modification of Duhamel's procedure. Otherwise, a temporary colostomy will be required to relieve the intestinal obstruction until a definitive procedure is carried out. If a long segment is affected, a temporary ileostomy will be required. The stoma needs to be created in ganglionic bowel. The location will be confirmed using frozen section histology but, if this facility is not available, it is advisable to perform a transverse, rather than a sigmoid, colostomy. Further biopsies are taken above and below the transitional zone so that, when the definitive operation is performed, the length of aganglionic bowel is accurately identified.

A definitive procedure may be undertaken at 3–6 months of age. Most commonly, a modification of Duhamel's operation is used (Fig. 12.2): the rectum is retained, ganglionic colon is joined to the posterior half of the anorectal ring and then the common wall between the rectum and colon is destroyed, forming a capacious new rectum. The stoma is reversed at the same time, wherever possible, or within the succeeding 3 months.

Necrotizing enterocolitis

This combination of ischaemia and infective gangrene affects mainly premature and low birthweight babies. The cause is unclear, but a large proportion of neonates affected have been subjected to some sort of stress such as prematurity, hyaline membrane disease, umbilical vessel catheterization, exchange transfusion or hypoglycaemia. Mesenteric vasoconstriction in a neonate subjected to stress enables pathogens to infiltrate the bowel wall and this results in ischaemia and infective gangrene, although no specific organism has been identified.

Babies present with rectal bleeding, diarrhoea, abdominal distension, bile-stained vomiting and pyrexia. Diagnosis will be confirmed by a plain abdominal X-ray, which shows intramural gas outlining the wall of the bowel (pneumatosis intestinalis) (Jones et al. 1985b). The initial treatment is to rest the intestine; the baby will receive nil by mouth, and a nasogastric tube will be inserted, then aspirated. Intravenous fluids will be commenced and broad-spectrum antibiotics administered. If the symptoms do not resolve with conservative management and the disease progresses, surgical intervention will be necessary. At laparotomy, the area most commonly affected with gangrene is the terminal ileum, and perforation and peritonitis are possible. The ischaemic bowel is resected and an ileostomy is required. Once the neonate has recovered and is thriving, the ileostomy is closed, usually within a few months.

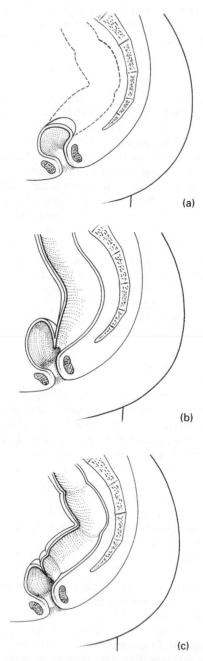

Fig. 12.2 Duhamel operation. (**a**) Aganglion sigmoid and upper rectum resected, lower half of rectum retained and closed. (**b**) Ganglion colon pulled through the posterior half of the anorectal ring. (**c**) Common wall crushed.

Meconium ileus

Fibrocystic disease is a genetically determined disease that affects the intestinal, bronchial, salivary and sweat glands and the pancreas. Meconium ileus is a condition that develops in approximately 10% of babies with fibrocystic disease (Fig. 12.3). There is a deficiency of pancreatic enzymes released into the intestinal tract. This deficiency *in utero* causes the meconium to become thick, inspissated and adherent to the intestinal mucosa, resulting in obstruction (Netter 1979). At birth, the abdomen is distended and the thick meconium is often visible and palpable. A plain abdominal X-ray will reveal various loops of bowel which range in size from smaller than normal up to gross enlargement and dilatation. In contrast to babies with intestinal obstruction due to atresia, stenosis or aganglionic megacolon, 50% of babies with meconium ileus will have an associated atresia. The bowel distal to the obstruction is normally empty and collapsed; proximally, the ileum has an appearance similar to a string of beads – the pellets of meconium. The proximal bowel is dilated and filled with gas. In severe cases, perforation and peritonitis can result.

Meconium plugs may be successfully removed from the colon and terminal ileum by administering a Gastrografin enema which makes the thick, tenacious contents of the dilated ileum more fluid, so that they can be passed rectally. If this does not succeed, formation of a loop ileostomy is necessary as a temporary measure to relieve the obstruction and enable washouts to be done via the stoma. Once the infant is thriving and there is no further evidence of the presence of meconium plugs, the ileostomy is closed, usually a few months after it is raised.

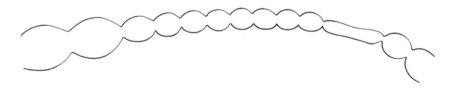

Fig. 12.3 Meconium ileus.

Trauma

Road traffic accidents are probably the most common form of childhood trauma causing puncture or crush injuries to the abdomen and necessitating emergency surgery. Depending on the injury, the child may need a colostomy, ileostomy or urostomy. On rare occasions it may be necessary to perform a double diversion of both the bowel and the urinary tract. Whenever possible corrective surgery will be performed and the stoma subsequently closed.

Inflammatory bowel disease

Both Crohn's disease and ulcerative colitis are rare in children, yet have been seen in tiny infants to teenagers. The diseases present with varying signs, including diarrhoea (which may contain mucus and blood), niggling abdominal pain, anaemia, malaise, failure to thrive and short stature. Initially, conservative medical treatment is used but, if symptoms are not arrested and the disease increases in severity, surgical intervention may be necessary. Surgery involves the formation of an ileostomy with possible partial or total colectomy. Children with ulcerative colitis may be able to have an ileoanal anastomosis with the creation of a pouch when they are in their teens.

Bladder exstrophy

This is a rare congenital condition that affects 1:1000–20000 babies. Predominating in boys (Upadhyaya 1991) at a ratio of 5:2, it is caused when the lateral mesodermal structure of the anterior abdominal wall fails to fuse together, resulting in a midline defect bounded by the rectus muscle and the pubic bone on both sides. The dorsal urethra, anterior bladder and the bladder neck fail to develop, producing an epispadias and extroversion of the exposed vesical mucosa, causing urine to constantly dribble from the ureteric orifices.

Bladder exstrophy can vary in severity. In minor defects there is epispadias with exstrophy of the bladder neck; in severe cases there is a wide separation of the pubic bones resulting in the axis of the hip joints being rotated posteriorly, which cause the child to have a waddling gait. The gap between the rectus muscle is occupied by the exposed bladder mucosa, everted due to intra-abdominal pressure.

Early detection is possible in the prenatal period if, following routine maternal serum screening, the alpha-fetoprotein is found to be elevated. Ultrasound scanning confirms the diagnosis. Following birth, usually by caesarean section, surgical repair to the abdominal wall is undertaken to achieve urinary continence without causing back-pressure from the bladder to the kidneys via the ureters and impairing renal function. Minor defects can be corrected by repairing the epispadias and reconstructing the bladder neck. The severe defects with wide bony gaps are difficult to treat and often require staged primary reconstruction. If it is not possible to achieve urinary continence even after attempting clean intermittent catheterization and renal function is impaired, urinary diversion may be necessary.

Posterior urethral valves

This condition occurs only in boys. It is the result of a developmental abnormality in the region of verumontanum which leads to the presence of obstructive valvular folds in the urethra (MacMahon 1991b). Symptoms usually arise in early infancy; they include failure to thrive, vomiting, abdominal distension, urinary tract infection, poor urinary stream, constant dribbling due to overflow from the distended bladder and a degree of renal failure.

In many cases it is possible to diagnose this condition antenatally through routine fetal ultrasound, after which various devices can be used to relieve the bladder and kidney pressure *in utero*, although these are not always completely successful. Others may be diagnosed when routine postnatal examination reveals a large palpable mass due to hydronephrotic kidneys and palpable bladder. On further investigation, serum creatinine is usually above normal levels. A thick-walled, trabeculated bladder with gross posterior urethral narrowing to an obstructive lesion at the level of the verumontanum or just below is observed at cystoscopy. A DTPA (^{99m}Tc-diethylenetriaminepentacetic acid) radioisotope scan is performed to determine renal perfusion and function. A common association with posterior urethral valves is vesicoureteric reflux or obstruction at the ureterovesical junction, causing back-pressure on the kidneys. Delay in detecting the valves is associated with increasing damage to the renal tissue.

Immediate relief of obstruction is provided by the insertion of an indwelling catheter, and this is followed by fulguration of the urethral valves. This may be required on more than one occasion to ensure their complete removal. If renal function is grossly impaired, emergency formation of bilateral ureterostomies may be necessary as a temporary measure. Once the valves are fulgurated and renal function is stabilized, ureterostomies can be reimplanted back into the bladder. Long-term management is necessary, as most have associated renal damage and abnormal bladders.

Rhabdomyosarcoma of the bladder

This is a rare childhood tumour; the main histological types are alveolar and embryonal. The embryonal type predominates in primary lesions of the genitourinary tract, often arising from the base of the bladder or prostate (Boles 1991). Children with a rhabdomyosarcoma of the bladder may present with bladder outflow obstruction or poor urinary stream, dysuria, haematuria, suprapubic mass, weight loss, malaise and anaemia.

The tumour is usually palpable on rectal examination and the diagnosis is confirmed by endoscopic bladder biopsies. Chemotherapy, radiotherapy and surgery are combined in treatment. Initially, chemotherapy is used, but if this fails to eradicate the tumour it will be followed by radiotherapy. Radical surgery is used if the combined chemotherapy and radiotherapy has failed. Surgery involves total cystectomy and the formation of permanent bilateral ureterostomies.

THE ROLE OF THE PAEDIATRIC STOMA CARE NURSE

The aim of the paediatric stoma care nurse is to work as part of a multi-disciplinary team to ensure that children with a stoma and their families receive a high standard of holistic care. The role has many challenges and can be divided into three sub-roles: counsellor, educator and adviser/liaison person.

Counsellor

From the initial contact onwards the paediatric stoma care nurse acts as a counsellor providing support to the child and the family. Counselling should include pre- and postoperative issues, future plans, treatment, and involvement of siblings and grandparents. The stoma care nurse needs to be sensitive, flexible and able to adapt to the changing needs of the growing and maturing child. There comes a time when the child may want to chat without parents present; often the first question asked is 'What do I tell my friends, boy or girl friends about the stoma?' Honesty is often the best approach, explaining to their friends what a stoma is and why it was necessary.

Educator

This aspect of the role involves formal and informal teaching sessions with the child, parents, trained and student nurses and medical staff, with the aim of passing on clinical skills and knowledge so that others acquire the competence and confidence to deliver a high standard of care.

Adviser/liaison person

The paediatric stoma care nurse liaises and advises on topics related to the care of the individual child to maintain continuity of care and to address any problems that might arise. Those with whom the nurse has a liaison role include the child, family, hospital nursing and medical staff, GP, community nurse, the child's school, community stoma nurse, patient support groups and appliance companies. The paediatric stoma nurse should be able to offer suggestions to the appliance companies to alter existing appliances or develop new ones for use in children and to increase patient choice.

PAEDIATRIC STOMA CARE

The principles and techniques of caring for children and adults with a stoma are very similar. There are, however, several important areas for consideration when planning care for individual neonates and children undergoing stoma surgery, and these aspects are considered in the sections that follow.

Family involvement and bonding

The majority of congenital abnormalities requiring stoma surgery are not apparent until after birth, giving parents no time to prepare for the consequences of giving birth to an imperfect baby. Often these babies are born in local district hospitals and need to be transferred to regional paediatric centres soon after birth, resulting in the father travelling with the infant in the ambulance and the mother remaining in hospital. The feelings of grief due to the loss of their 'perfect' baby, guilt that something they have done wrong during the pregnancy caused the defect and being separated as a family are immense. As soon as the mother is well enough to be discharged from hospital, she should be given support and encouragement either to stay with her baby or to visit regularly.

When the baby has undergone surgery and is being nursed in an incubator/baby therm, with various drains and tubing, these can act as a barrier to the parents who may feel frightened of, or prevented from, cuddling or even touching their baby. They often feel that they are no longer in control and that the doctors and nurses have taken over. It is vital that parents be involved at all times with their baby's care and in decision making. Encouragement and support should be given to mothers who wish to breast-feed, even if the baby is initially unable to feed orally. Milk can be expressed and preserved for later. It may then be given by nasogastric tube until the baby is well enough to go to the breast. Cuddling and touching the baby should be encouraged by all staff, and siblings in the family should be included and allowed to visit. Time must be set aside to explain to them why their new brother or sister needs to be in hospital.

At the appropriate time, parents will need to be taught to care for their child's stoma. Whenever possible, a grandparent, aunt or family friend should also be taught so that, once discharged, a capable babysitter can be available and the mother will be able to get out for a break. It is important that she doesn't feel isolated and that she is the only person who can look after the baby. New parenthood can be traumatic and stressful at the best of times, but for parents with a baby requiring surgery the experience can be much more difficult to deal with. The support received from staff can make all the difference (Stewart 1990).

Nutritional aspects of the child with a stoma

Neonates, children and teenagers with a stoma may have normal breast-feeds, baby formula, and a well balanced diet unless there is another medical condition that contraindicates this. As always, each child is totally different and it is a matter of trial and error to find which foods affect the individual. Weaning should be carried out at the same time and in the same way as for any infant without a stoma.

Occasionally, neonates who have undergone extensive small intestinal resection and the formation of an ileostomy develop a lactose intolerance (Blackwell 1993). This is due to mucosal damage occurring at the time of surgery, and lactase is the most susceptible enzyme to such an insult (Jones et al. 1985a), resulting in the malabsorption of lactose from the neonate's feed. The neonate presents with a high, loose stoma output, which is positive for sugar. It is usually a temporary problem and is treated by using a lactose-free baby formula (e.g Pregestimil or Pepti-Junior). When weaning commences, a milk-free diet is required. Once the ileostomy is reversed and the infant is approximately a year old, a 'cows' milk challenge' will be given and, if successful, cows' milk can be introduced into the diet. If a child with a stoma fails to thrive, urine electrolytes should be measured as it may be due to increased sodium loss. This is more common in infants with an ileostomy, and, if confirmed, oral sodium supplements may be required. These are usually required only temporarily; once begun, the infant usually begins to thrive.

Infants with a stoma can become dehydrated very quickly if they develop gastroenteritis, and it is essential that they receive an adequate fluid intake. If this is not possible by the oral route, hospital admission may be necessary for short-term intravenous fluids.

Types of appliance

Before 1988 the choice of paediatric appliances was very limited, often resulting in the use of large adult appliances on neonates and children. Fortunately, a wider selection of appliances is now being manufactured. In general, neonates and children with a colostomy or ileostomy use a one-piece paediatric drainable bag. Children's skin is thinner and more delicate than an adult's skin and can be damaged much more easily, so extra care needs to be taken to protect it.

When the appliance is changed it should be peeled off slowly and the stoma and peristomal skin washed gently and not rubbed. If necessary a mild soap can be used but this must be rinsed off thoroughly.

Babies and small children often enjoy playing and soaking in the bath so the appliance change can be timed to coincide with this routine. On the occasions when it is unnecessary to change the appliance, bathing can take place as usual but care needs to be taken afterwards to ensure that the appliance is thoroughly towelled dry. A damp appliance can cause skin soreness.

The appliance should not be changed too frequently. On average, every 2–3 days is appropriate. Tape should never be used to reinforce a leaking appliance as any leakage on to the skin will make it sore. If barrier wipes or creams are to be used, it is advisable to do a patch test on the baby's leg or arm first to check that it does not cause an allergic reaction.

Babies' stomal output is looser and more frequent, and a drainable appliance is essential to avoid frequent changing. Two-piece appliances are more rigid and can cause problems because there is a limited surface area on which to apply a base-plate and it is difficult to mould this to the shape of a neonate's abdomen.

Some parents prefer to use a two-piece appliance with a base-plate and clip-on pouch, and this is suitable for children from the age of about 4 years. Teenagers with a colostomy may opt for a two-piece system so that they are able to use a small activity pouch for 'special occasions' such as parties and swimming. Children with urinary diversions use either a one- or two-piece appliance with a non-reflux valve – as yet, there are no paediatric urinary appliances available. Parents of children under 18 months with a urinary diversion such as a ureterostomy or vesicostomy often prefer not to use an appliance, as the child would normally still be in nappies. If this option is chosen, the use of skin protective wipes on the peristomal skin is all that is necessary.

Common complications of stoma surgery in children

Diarrhoea

Children with a colostomy, and especially those with an ileostomy, can become very dehydrated and unwell if they develop gastroenteritis. Children should be encouraged to drink plenty of fluids and parents should seek medical advice if their child develops a gastrointestinal upset. On occasion, hospital admission may be necessary to rehydrate the child with intravenous fluids.

Rectal discharge

Some children with a colostomy or ileostomy may experience a rectal discharge of stale faeces or mucus. If the discharge becomes offensive or troublesome, gentle rectal washout can be effective in relieving this.

Surface bleeding

Surface bleeding may arise from a number of causes such as too vigorous cleaning of the stoma, accidental injury, an ill-fitting appliance, or granulation tissue on the stoma. The cause needs to be identified and then corrected: for example, further teaching on cleaning technique or the application of silver nitrate to remove granulation tissue. If surface bleeding is persistent the haemoglobin level should be checked and oral iron prescribed if required.

Prolapse

This occurs more frequently with a colostomy than an ileostomy. Child and parental reassurance is essential, as this can be a very frightening experience. No immediate action is required as long as the stoma remains pink, healthy and functioning and the child has no discomfort. Often when the child goes to sleep at night the prolapse will reduce. If it persists and the stoma appliance is difficult to fit, stomal revision may be necessary. The vast majority of paediatric colostomies and ileostomies are temporary, so early corrective surgery and stoma closure may be an appropriate option. If the prolapsed stoma becomes dark and dusky in colour, medical advice should be sought.

Retraction

This is more common with ureterostomies and is a major cause of leakage. A convex disc used within a two-piece appliance can prevent leakage; if this is not effective, stoma revision to create a spout may be required.

Teaching the child to manage the stoma

It is important that from an early age children are encouraged to help, even if it may seem easier and quicker for an adult to do it, so that they gain control over their stoma care and achieve confidence and independence. Children have an amazing capacity to learn to care for the stoma. From 4 years old they can begin to learn and generally start by helping their mother or the nurse to gather the equipment to change the appliance, empty the bag or peel off the soiled appliance. Children often prefer to remove the appliance than to have this done for them. It is helpful for the nurse to talk through the appliance change while it is being done, as this enables the child to get the procedure in order. If different carers slightly vary the procedure a young child will be the first to inform them that they are 'doing it wrong'. At about 7 years of age, children should be able to cut a flange base to the appropriate size with the help of a template and a small pair of nail scissors. By this stage they should also be able to learn how to change their own appliance.

Children who undergo stoma surgery from the age of 10 upwards should be taught to care for the stoma as soon as they are able to after the operation. Background support, help and encouragement must be available at all times. Each child is different and they should be assessed individually to ascertain when they are ready to start to care for the stoma. A good indication is when they start asking questions and offering to help.

Play therapy

Play is a vital part of a child's normal development and children of all ages use play as a means of expressing their feelings as well as a model to learn and come to terms with painful experiences. Toddlers and children can be prepared for surgery using play; for example, stoma dolls, hospital play, story books and colouring books. Research confirms that it is beneficial to prepare children and parents whenever possible for hospital admission and subsequent surgery. This not only reduces anxiety but also helps to establish a normal routine for a child and results in an earlier discharge home (Jolly 1981). Most paediatric hospitals run a pre-admission programme enabling the child, parents and siblings to visit the hospital ward and have the opportunity to ask questions before admission. Children are extremely sensitive and what we adults do consciously may not be as important as what we say and how we behave.

Nursery and schooling

Many parents of children requiring stoma surgery are naturally anxious about how their child will face school when the time comes. Playgroups are an ideal way to ease the toddler into the school situation as they enable the child to mix, make friends and gain confidence on their own. If difficulties are encountered in finding a suitable playgroup that is prepared to take a child with a stoma or is still in nappies, local health visitors can often help. The Pre-school Playgroups Association (PPA) believe that most handicapped children benefit from attending a playgroup.

Before children are due to transfer from playgroup to school it is advisable to approach the head of the school selected to discuss their needs. Most schools and head teachers are helpful and the transfer can occur without problems, provided careful liaison has been maintained. If, after discussion with the school, obstacles arise or school admission is refused, parents should be reminded that there is no good reason why a child with a stoma or incontinence should not go to a mainstream school. Under the 1981 Education Act there is a requirement that, whenever reasonably practicable, children with special educational needs should be educated in mainstream schools alongside other children. This means that the local education authority has the obligation to ensure that the child's needs are met as far as possible in the mainstream school. If the child's needs are still not met parents have the right to request that the local education authority undertakes a multi-disciplinary assessment of the child. It is a legal requirement that parents be involved in this. The 'assessment' consists of interviews and visits. At the end of the procedure the education authority issues a statement setting out the conclusions and, if there are special needs, what it intends to do to enable these needs to be met. The statement is maintained by the authority and is transferrable from one area to another if the child moves residence. The procedure for preparing a statement may take time and it is advisable to start this process well in advance of the time at which the child is to start school.

Children requiring stoma surgery after the age of 5 years encounter fewer problems keeping their places at school because they are already in the education system. Heads of schools and teachers know the children concerned and realize that educationally there is no reason why they should not remain in the mainstream school, minimizing the interruption in their education after the period of necessary hospitalization. Special arrangements may be needed for toilet facilities and some schools allow the children to use the staff toilets.

Teenagers and altered body image

The adolescent period is a traumatic time for any youngster. It must be remembered that the needs of teenagers differ from those of both adults and children. Three major issues of importance are independence, privacy and social needs. Teenagers need their independence and a chance to make decisions. The 1989 Children Act strongly recommends that all children should be involved in decision making and consent to medical treatment. At times, teenagers may have difficulty in communicating with parents or staff owing to the 'generation gap'. Staff must be sensitive to their needs and respect their need for privacy. Where possible, they should be given a single room in a paediatric setting and the opportunity for friends to visit.

Teenagers are self-conscious and worried about their changing body image, which is compounded by the fact that they have a stoma. Even children who have had a stoma all their lives will often say in the adolescent years, 'Why me? It's not fair.' They may cover their fears of the future by means of antisocial or brash behaviour; the opportunity to express their feelings must be provided, with appropriate support (Gillies 1992). Another major worry is about the possible reactions of friends and what they should be told about the stoma, as well as potential loss of attraction to the opposite sex. Often it is better to explain to prospective partners about the stoma rather than wait for it to be discovered.

Teenagers should be encouraged to ask questions, and to express their feelings. They, in turn, should be provided with information and advice, for instance regarding contraception. It is especially important during adolescence that the teenager with a stoma be encouraged by parents and the stoma care nurse to participate in social and school activities. There will be times of worry and anxiety when it might be easier not to join in, but swimming, sports, going to a disco, staying overnight with friends, going on school trips and on holiday are all possible. Fears should be discussed realistically as well as positive and enjoyable aspects of activities. Possible solutions to practical problems that may arise, such as the disposal of used appliances away from home, should be fully explored. It may be appropriate to change to a biodegradable appliance for short-term use such as weekends away or holidays, or to ensure that an appliance with a slightly larger capacity than usual is available for occasions when appliance emptying may be delayed because of being out all day. Helpful discussion can provide the reassurance and extra confidence that will enable the teenager to make the decision to participate.

CURRENT TRENDS IN STOMA CARE

Current trends are aimed at establishing continence in children who previously would have required a permanent colostomy or urinary diversion. The two techniques are Shandling enema continence catheter and clean intermittent catheterization.

Shandling enema continence catheter

Despite attempts to gain faecal continence, there is a small percentage of children who do not attain this. The Shandling enema continence catheter (Fig. 12.4) may prove to be a useful alternative method of achieving continence. Children born with anorectal abnormalities, Hirschsprung's disease and spina bifida can be suitable candidates. Contraindications are the presence of megacolon or inflammatory bowel disease.

Careful assessment of the children is necessary – they need to be motivated to succeed and family support is essential. The Shandling enema continence catheter works on the same principle as colonic lavage, which maintains an empty rectum and thus prevents soiling. Before commencing the programme it is essential that the child is not constipated; this may require bowel clearance by rectal washout, enema or laxatives.

Equipment required

- Shandling enema continence catheter
- Measuring jug
- Kitchen salt
- Teaspoon
- Lukewarm tap water
- Bathroom hook

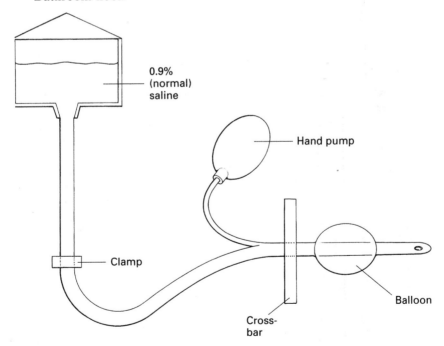

Fig. 12.4 Shandling enema continence catheter.

Enema fluid is prepared in the measuring jug using 20 ml of tap water for every kilogram of body weight and adding a teaspoon of kitchen salt for every 300 ml of water.

The enema fluid is poured into the catheter reservoir, and the clamp released to run fluid through and expel any air and then reclamped. The catheter is suspended on a hook about 1.2 metres above the child's hip level. The tip and balloon of the catheter are lubricated with water-soluble lubricating jelly and then inserted as far into the rectum as allowed by the plastic cross-piece. The balloon is inflated by squeezing the hand-pump and then the clamp is released so that the fluid flows as fast as possible into the child. If abdominal discomfort develops, the flow should be stopped for 10–20 seconds and then recommenced. The child sits on the toilet. The handpump is released to deflate the balloon and the catheter is gently removed, enabling the evacuation of the contents of the colon. This process can be assisted by rubbing the child's abdomen in a clockwise direction, commencing on the lower right-hand side. After use the catheter is cleaned with mild soapy water and left to dry.

Disadvantages of the procedure are that, for as long as it takes, children are unable to carry on with normal activities because they are confined to the toilet, and secondly, the catheter tip and balloon are fairly large and unsuitable for small children under the age of 7 years or if the anus is very tight.

Clean intermittent catheterization

Children who have persistent urinary incontinence due to congenital bladder exstrophy or neuropathic bladder as in spina bifida may be able to achieve continence during the day by using the technique of clean intermittent catheterization. Prior to 1976, children with urinary incontinence were treated with urinary diversions. In some cases 'undiversion' may now be possible (Deegan 1991).

For clean intermittent catheterization to be a viable option, the child must have a low-pressure bladder with a reasonable capacity. If the bladder is too small, especially in children with bladder exstrophy, bladder augmentation may be possible. Clean intermittent catheterization is suitable for children from the age of 18 months. It involves the child or parent performing urethral catheterization using a 'no touch' technique every 2–4 hours depending on the bladder capacity. The method works on the principle that even the abnormal bladder can contain a certain amount of urine before it leaks, so timely catheterization is essential to prevent leakage. Very young children usually adapt quickly to the technique and often from the age of 4 years upwards can be taught to catheterize themselves. Assessment of the child and family is vital for success, as it takes a substantial time commitment and needs to fit in with family life and with school (Deegan 1989). These children require long-term medical follow-up to ensure that renal function is preserved.

CURRENT DEVELOPMENTS IN PAEDIATRIC SURGERY

Mitrofanoff principle

Urinary incontinence is often successfully managed by intermittent catheterization. However, some patients have difficulty performing urethral catheterization owing to spinal deformities or urethral abnormalities. In these patients the use of the Mitrofanoff principle may be beneficial.

The Mitrofanoff technique, developed in 1986, creates a continent catheterizable channel between the abdominal wall and the bladder in order to facilitate clean intermittent catheterization. A continent cutaneous vesicostomy is achieved by detaching the appendix from the caecum, mobilizing it on its mesentery and, after amputating the distal end, implanting it via a submucosal tunnel into the bladder or neobladder. The Mitrofanoff stoma is usually situated in the right iliac fossa. If the appendix is not available, ureter or an ileal segment can be used (Dykes, Duffy and Ransley 1991).

The Mitrofanoff procedure may be suitable for children with bladder exstrophy, neuropathic bladder or cloaca. Each individual needs careful assessment for suitability because patient compliance is required, as is a low-pressure bladder, an adequate bladder capacity and bladder neck competence. Adequate bladder capacity can be made possible by bladder augmentation prior to the Mitrofanoff procedure. If bladder neck competence is poor, formal closure is required.

The Mitrofanoff catheterization procedure

Equipment required

* Jug
* LoFric Nelaton paediatric catheter (size will vary depending on the age of the child and the size of the stoma)

After the hands are washed and dried, the catheter sachet is opened by pulling the tabs at the heat-sealed end. Water is run into the catheter sachet and it is placed against a vertical surface. The LoFric catheter has a specially treated surface that becomes slippery after soaking in water for 30 seconds.

The catheter is removed from the sachet and gently inserted into the Mitrofanoff stoma. Some children may experience a slight 'pop' as the catheter enters the bladder. Once the flow of urine has stopped, light pressure is applied to the abdomen to ensure that the bladder is empty. The catheter is then removed, discarded and the hands are washed again.

A child with a Mitrofanoff should be advised to wear a Medic Alert bracelet in case of emergencies, especially if the bladder neck has been surgically closed. During the day, catheterization should be performed every 3–4 hours as overdistension may lead to bladder perforation. Weekly bladder washouts via the Mitrofanoff stoma will be necessary to prevent the build-up of mucus in the bladder if the child has previously undergone bladder augmentation.

The Mitrofanoff principle has proved invaluable in the treatment of selected children with urinary incontinence and should allow conventional urinary diversion to become a thing of the past.

The antegrade continence enema

Despite all treatment efforts, a small number of children with congenital abnormalities such as spina bifida, imperforate anus and Hirschsprung's disease remain incontinent and opt for a permanent colostomy. The antegrade continence enema (ACE) provides some of these children with an alternative. This is a technique, developed in the 1990s by Mr P. Malone, that facilitates the administration of an antegrade washout to empty the colon and thus prevent soiling. The ACE procedure is a combination of two well tried techniques – on-table colonic lavage and the Mitrofanoff principle.

One end of the appendix is reimplanted in a non-refluxing manner into the caecum and the other end is brought out on to the abdominal wall as a continent stoma. It provides a catheterizable channel through which antegrade washouts are given to produce colonic emptying (Malone, Ransley and Kiely 1990).

Equipment required

- Phosphate enema
- Measuring jug
- Kitchen salt
- Lukewarm tap water
- Lubricating jelly
- Irrigation set
- Catheter (EMS size 8–10)

Two types of enema fluid are prepared. The first consists of 50 ml of phosphate enema solution mixed with 50 ml normal (0.9%) saline. The second consists of 100–200 ml of normal saline (taken from 300 ml tap water mixed with 1 teaspoon (5 ml) of salt). The volume and dilution of the enema fluids may need adjustment to suit the individual.

The first enema solution is run into the irrigation set, and the clamp released to allow the fluid to run through and air to be expelled and then reclamped. The irrigation set is hung on a hook, suspended about 1.2 metres above the child's hip level. With the child sitting on the toilet, water-soluble lubricating jelly is applied to the tip of the catheter and this is gently inserted 5–7 cm into the stoma and then connected to the irrigation set. The clamp is released and fluid is run through, followed by the second (normal saline) enema fluid. The flow is stopped for 10–20 seconds if abdominal discomfort develops and then the flow is recommenced. The catheter is then gently removed and the contents of the entire colon can be evacuated. After use the irrigation set and catheter are cleaned with mild soapy water and left to dry.

To prevent the occurrence of stenosis of the stoma, the catheter is passed into the stoma twice a day, in the morning and evening. Initially the enema is given once a day but this can eventually be reduced to once in 48 hours for some children.

Liver and small bowel transplantation

Transplantation of the liver, kidney or heart is a well established and successful treatment for irreversible organ failure. Now in the 1990s, small bowel transplants in both adults and children have seen many advances and successes (Clark 1992), especially since the introduction of immuno-suppressant FK506 in postoperative treatment. Since 1991 Pittsburgh Hospital have performed 15 combined small bowel and liver transplants, with a 73% survival rate.

Liver and small bowel transplantation may be considered for intestinal failure due to extensive intestinal resection and motility disorders. Common causes of irreversible intestinal failure include congenital atresia, gastroschisis, necrotizing enterocolitis, 'short gut' syndrome, pseudo-obstruction and associated liver disorders. Approximately 49 children in the UK are currently receiving long-term parenteral nutrition in hospital (Booth 1992) and 20 are at home receiving parenteral nutrition.

Once a full assessment of the child's suitability is made and a suitable donor is found, the small bowel transplant is of the same magnitude as a liver transplant. During the procedure, a covering ileostomy is formed to reduce the risks of intestinal leak of the anastomosis. The main postoperative complications are related to rejection, infection and nutrition. One of the many indicators of rejection is increased stomal output, and regular bowel biopsies will be necessary via the stoma to assess the situation. Postoperative recovery is often not straightforward. Drug therapy with immunosuppressants is for life. Depending on the child's progress, the ileostomy may be reversed; this is rare before 18 months have elapsed following surgery. Throughout this time, the child and family require extensive counselling and support to survive such a traumatic period. In 1993 the first combined small bowel and liver transplant in the UK was performed; this could be the way forward for children with irreversible intestinal failure and severe hepatic complications, for whom, without a transplant, the chance of survival would be negligible.

It must always be remembered that 'All children have special needs at some time in their lives; stoma children have normal needs all of the time' (National Advisory Service for Parents of Children with a Stoma (undated)).

APPENDIX: SUPPORT GROUPS AND ASSOCIATIONS

NASPCS (National Advisory Service for Parents of Children with a Stoma)

51 Anderson Drive
Valley View Park
Darvel, Ayrshire KA1Y 0DE

Support group for parents of children with imperforate anus and associated conditions. Help and support are achieved by quarterly newsletters, local telephone contacts and local support group meetings, so that ideas and own experiences can be passed on and in turn help ease the feeling of parental isolation.

Contact a Family

16 Strutton Ground
London SW1P 2HP

Aims to promote contacts between families with physically or mentally handicapped children within the same neighbourhood to form local self-help groups.

TOFS Support Group

Tracheal Oesophageal Fistula
St George's Centre
91 Victoria Road
Netherfield
Nottingham NG4 2NN

For parents of children born with oesophageal atresia and/or oesophageal fistula.

RADAR (Royal Association for Disability and Rehabilitation)

25 Mortimer Street
London W1N 8AB

The association offers help with education, welfare, housing, aids, holidays, etc.

Network 81

1–7 Woodfield Terrace
Stansted, Essex CM24 8AJ

A national network of parents of children with special educational needs, they offer information guidance, help and advice on the workings of the 1981 Education Act and other legislation and administrative practices concerned with special educational provision.

Action for Sick Children

Argyle House
29–31 Euston Road
London NW1 2SD

Helps children in hospital and their parents. It is able to supply books and leaflets to help parents prepare their children for a stay in hospital. It also offers telephone advice and can give details about local branches.

REFERENCES

Blackwell, T.Y.D. (1993) In: *Food and Food Additives Intolerance in Childhood*. Scientific Publications: pp. 33–4.

Boles, E.T. (1991) Tumour in childhood. In: MacMahon, R.A. (Ed.) *An Aid to Paediatric Surgery*, 2nd edn. Churchill Livingstone: Edinburgh, p. 41.

Booth, I.W. (1992) Birmingham protocol for liver and bowel transplantation. Birmingham Children's Hospital, 2–3.

Clark, C.I. (1992) Recent progress in intestinal transplantation. *Archives of Disease in Childhood*, **67**: 976–9.

Deegan, S. (1989) Intermittent catheterization for children. *Nursing Times*, **81** (4): 72–4.

Deegan, S. (1991) Continence – close to normality. *Nursing Times*, **87** (44): 65, 67.

Dykes, E.H., Duffy, P.G. and Ransley, P.G. (1991) The use of the Mitrofanoff principle in achieving clean intermittent catheterisation and urinary continence in childhood. *Journal of Paediatric Surgery*, **26**: 535–8.

Gillies, M. (1992) Teenage traumas. *Nursing Times*, **88** (27): 26–7.

Jolly, J. (1981) Play. In: *The Other Side of Paediatrics*. Macmillan: London, pp. 71–79.

Jones, F.P., Brunt, P.W., Ashley, N. and Mowat, G. (1985a) Diseases of colon and rectum. In: *Gastro-enterology*. Heinemann Medical: London, p. 118.

Jones, F.P., Brunt, P.W., Ashley, N. and Mowat, G. (1985b) Inflammatory bowel disease. In: *Gastro-enterology*. Heinemann Medical: London, p. 244.

Jones, F.P., Brunt, P.W., Ashley, N. and Mowat, G. (1985c) Congenital abnormalities. In: *Gastro-enterology*. Heinemann Medical: London, p. 266.

MacMahon, R.A. (1991a) Intestinal obstruction. In: MacMahon, R.A. (Ed.) *An Aid to Paediatric Surgery*, 2nd edn. Churchill Livingstone: Edinburgh.

MacMahon, R.A. (1991b) Urinary tract infection and abnormalities of the urinary system. In: MacMahon, R.A. (Ed.) *An Aid to Paediatric Surgery*, 2nd edn. Churchill Livingstone, p. 224.

Malone, P.S., Ransley, P.G. and Kiely, E.M. (1990) Preliminary report: the antegrade continence enema. *Lancet*, **3**: 1217–18.

National Advisory Service for Parents of Children with a Stoma. (undated) *Our Special Children*. CliniMed.

Netter, F.M. (1979) Diseases of the lower digestion tract. In: Netter, F.M. *The CIBA Collection of Medical Illustrations*. vol. 1: *Digestive System*. CIBA: New York, p. 114.

Stewart, A.J. (1990) Mums and dads need care too. Supporting parents of babies in neonatal units. *Professional Nurse*, **5**: 660–5.

Upadhyaya, P. (1991) Body wall defects. In: MacMahon, R.A. (Ed.) *An Aid to Paediatric Surgery*, 2nd edn. Churchill Livingstone: Edinburgh, p. 217.

Webster, P. (1985) Special babies. *Nursing Times Community Outlook*, **81**: 19–22.

13 Sexuality and the stoma patient

Mave Salter

INTRODUCTION

Needing to have a stoma is not helped by cultural assumptions that it is essential to have a healthy, pleasing appearance. A person's looks are an important part of life, and society places enormous significance on having an attractive body (Salter 1992a). The expression of human sexuality and body image are virtually inseparable both in health and in illness (McKenzie 1988). Carolan (1983) has suggested that altered body image and sexuality are integrally linked, so in this chapter I discuss sexuality and explain its effect on patient care.

Stoma surgery has a profound effect on the mind as well as the body, and a holistic approach to care of patients with a stoma is essential because rehabilitation depends on their physical, psychological, social and sexual adjustment. Stoma surgery, whilst sometimes temporary, is mostly permanent; although some patients may have adequate time for preparation, others will present as an emergency with only a few hours' notice.

Dudley (1978) suggested that 'however managed, however we delude ourselves, a permanent, potentially incontinent stoma is an affront, difficult to bear, so that I marvel that we and our patients have put up with it for so long. It says much for the social indifference of the one (health care professions) and the social fortitude of the other (the patients)'. To this end, investigations into alternatives to conventional stomas have been underway for many years. There are now a variety of procedures being performed for bowel or bladder disease or dysfunction where the purpose is to eliminate, whenever possible, the need to wear an appliance (Church 1986).

THE PATIENT WITH A STOMA

As I reviewed the literature relating to the experiences of patients with a stoma and their subsequent adaptation to perceived body image changes, a number of common themes were revealed – for example, the difficulties experienced in coming to terms with a stoma (Dyk and Sutherland 1956; Druss et al. 1968; Devlin, Plant and Griffin 1971; Eardley et al. 1976;

Carolan 1983). Devlin and colleagues suggested that an immense price is paid for cure, and this price incorporates physical discomfort and psychological and social trauma. It is this element of patient care that we as nurses need to address.

Wade (1990a) implies that a patient facing stoma surgery also faces the prospect of a change in appearance and loss of control of elimination. The loss of control over elimination delivers a severe blow to self-esteem and gives rise to fears of rejection by friends and of being ostracized by society. There is also fear of rejection by sexual partners or of marital breakdown. Indeed, people can feel so badly about themselves that they may not want to re-initiate a sexual relationship, fearing they are no longer attractive, and may therefore give out 'vibes' to their partners that they are no longer interested.

THE PATIENT WITH A CONTINENT POUCH

The first ileal reservoir was performed in the mid 1970s. Although several hundreds of these operations have been carried out in the USA, the experience in the UK has been smaller (Everett 1989). Patients with a continent pouch feel that such a procedure has enhanced their lives over that with an ileostomy (Everett 1989; Nicholls and Pezim 1985; Pemberton et al. 1989). Rolstad and Rothenberger (undated) state that satisfaction with the pouch procedure has been high. The absence of a permanent ileostomy has eliminated many problems related to body image, and there has been no major problem with sexual function following this procedure. An ileoanal reservoir presents a unique experience, quite different from the pre-morbid state of living with a stoma, because concerns related to physical intimacy and long-term body image are minimized (Nemer and Rolstad 1985).

Bragg's (1989) study has shown that the continent ileostomy (e.g. Kock ileostomy) makes no restrictions with regard to clothing or physical activity. Social, sexual and psychological anxieties are significantly diminished compared with those of patients who have a conventional stoma. Therefore, there appear to be differences in the perceptions of body image and aspects of sexuality when comparing patients who have an ileostomy with those who have a reservoir.

SEXUALITY

According to Maslow (1970) the fulfilment of our need for love, intimacy and sexual gratification is a critical link in the mature, healthy personality. Sexuality and relationships are very closely connected – one rarely exists without the other (Carolan 1983). Carolan implies that, if people are inhibited in cultivating social relationships, they are liable to be hampered in their sexual expression. This view is supported by Nordstrom (1985), who states that the psychological aftermath of stoma surgery may be even more important than the physiological problems. These two factors are so often intertwined that they are difficult to separate. Psychological problems affect sexual function; for instance impotence and decreased libido may be a symptom of depression rather than a result of the operation.

Carolan (1983) has stated that sexuality is closely linked with body image; therefore it is important to define and discuss sexuality, both generally and with the stoma patient in mind. I believe that a person who has a conventional or continent procedure should receive instruction in the promotion of sexual health as part of their nursing care (Salter 1992a).

Nurses are often faced with a dilemma when caring for patients because of anxiety about discussing the effects of their illness on their sexuality. A common scenario is the nurse deciding that she ought to discuss sexual aspects with the patient but thinking the patient may be embarrassed, while the patient would like to ask the nurse how the illness/operation will affect him or her sexually, but feels that the nurse will be too embarrassed!

The World Health Organization's (1975) definition of sexuality states that it is the integration of the physical, emotional, intellectual and social aspects of sexual being, in ways that are positively enriching and that enhance personality, communication and love. Woods (1984) has defined human sexuality as highly complex, stating that sexuality pervades human beings, influencing their self-images, feelings and relationships with others. In addition, sexuality influences the biological basis of experiencing sexual pleasure, giving and receiving sensual pleasure and is a powerful force in a person's ability to bond to another person.

Woods' definition has affinities with nursing conceptual frameworks, which view humans as bio-psycho-social beings. Some of these frameworks include sexuality in their models of care (e.g. Roper, Logan and Tierney (1985) 'Activities of daily living'). Biological aspects include reproductive systems of male and female; for example, appearance, physical aspects of sexual activity, menstruation and contraception. Psychological aspects include body image, self-concept and self-esteem, but these are strongly influenced by social factors – which include forms and values of a specific culture, gender roles and stereotypes. Gender preferences are also important – whether people are attracted to/prefer to have sexual relationships with the same sex, different sex or both (Woods 1984).

The sexual response cycle consists of four main stages:

1. Excitement phase: initiated by whatever the individual finds sexually stimulating. If stimulation is continued, sexual tension increases.
2. Plateau phase: may be prolonged and/or decreased if stimulation is not effective or is withdrawn.
3. Organic phase: a completely involuntary response. The body responds with maximum intensity. The sexual tension is released in a total body reaction although the most intense sensation is in the pelvic area.
4. Resolution phase: characterized by decreased sexual tension as the individual returns to an unstimulated state. During the resolution phase, women are capable of having additional orgasms if stimulation continues but men experience a refractory period of varying length

when stimulation is not possible (Davis 1990).

Wells (1990) fears that nurses still appear to be experiencing difficulty in addressing the sexuality of their patients. 'People who come to us for care do not leave their sexuality at home, any more than they leave their fear behind'. Wells continues by suggesting that 'nurses mouth platitudes about activities of daily living, but how often do we mention sexuality in our care plans?' He states that, in reviewing the care of a patient with a nurse, he asked why there was no record of attention to sexuality. 'He did not mention it' was the response. 'If he had wanted to know, he would have asked' is not a worthy response from a professional nurse'. states Wells.

Webb (1987) has documented the general inadequacy of health care professionals in taking into account the sexuality of those in their care. She suggested that this is due to insufficient education and training of nurses in the sexual needs of patients – an imbalance that must be redressed if nurses are to care for patients holistically. Maguire et al. (1978) suggested that clients do not tell professionals how they feel, often because professionals don't ask. Instead, time is spent teaching patients about management without exploring their feelings. However, if sexual counselling is not seen to be part of the nurse's role, who undertakes this task?

Webb and O'Neill (1989) have suggested that, if sexuality were to become as much a regular aspect of nursing as wound care or nutrition, nurses' confidence and skill in handling such problems would improve. The personal nature of sexuality makes some people argue that this is an invasion of privacy. But it is precisely because patients may find it difficult to speak about it that the nurse should 'give permission' and indicate that sexuality is a legitimate subject for discussion.

Patients are not expected to care for a surgical wound or injury, and it is unfair to deny them help and information in adjusting and responding to changes in sexuality. This is not to imply that nurses forego their own beliefs or standards of morality, but that they are not-judgemental (Webb 1987).

Lamb and Woods (1981) suggested that assesment of sexual health brings with it a sex history, but nurses feel uneasy about this. Therefore a question could be prefaced: 'Some people have sexual intercourse every day, some a couple of times a month, others not at all'. This is a statement of fact, and a non-invasive question such as the following could then be posed: 'About how often do you have it?' However, I would question how often we as health care professionals would need to know the answer; it might be better to ask, where applicable, the following questions, as suggested by McPheteridge (1968):

1. Has your illness/treatment interfered with you being a mother/wife/husband/father?
2. Has your illness/treatment changed the way you see yourself as a man/woman?
3. Has your illness/treatment caused any change in your sexual functioning (sex life)?
4. Do you expect your sexual functioning to be changed in any way after you leave the hospital?

Patients/clients can choose how they answer such questions, which are not too intrusive about their personal relationships. It has been demonstrated (Dempsey, Buchsbaum and Morrison 1975; Lomont, De Petrillo and Sargeant 1978; Vera 1981) that, at the time of diagnosis (of cancer) and proposed surgery, sexual function is not an issue of prime consideration because initally patients are concerned with the immediate situation. However (Fisher 1979) states that neglecting to discuss the issue of patients' altered sexuality will only reinforce the fallacy that their sexual role is over.

In addition, Hogan (1980, cited in Fisher and Levin 1983) drew attention to the danger, when discussing sexuality, of placing too much emphasis on its genital aspects because it must be remembered that sexuality is more than the sex act. It is important also to dispel the myth that sex means intercourse, is incomplete without orgasm and requires an erect penis. Genital intercourse is only one way of expressing love; others include manual, digital and oral stimulation, intra-thigh or intra-mammary intercourse, and use of devices, vibrators, penile prosthesis or caverject (alprostadil, a prostaglandin E_1).

Lamb and Woods (1981) indicated that sex can be reflected in touch, smell, hearing, taste and sensual stimuli. However, a thorough exploration of a couple's values and attitudes should be undertaken before suggesting alternative methods. One must also be aware of the fact that one of the partners may want to stop sexual functioning, and illness is as good a reason as any. I can remember a patient who was accompanied by her husband when she was admitted for stoma surgery. They were in their late 50s and I had not met them before as they were referred from a fair distance away. Their first question concerned the effects of the stoma on their sexual life. In contrast, a female patient also in her 50s was admitted the same day. She had told me that she and her husband still had an active sex life, and I explained to her that there was no need for that to change. Her response was 'Please don't tell my husband that – I'm using this operation as an excuse not to have sex anymore!'

Lomont, De Petrillo and Sargeant (1978) agreed that the most important factor in total sexual rehabilitation for cancer patients is an educated and informed partner. The quality of a sexual relationship after a diagnosis of cancer has been made is related more to the previous quality of the relationship than to any other factor. Where appropriate, it is important to include a partner in teaching sessions. Frequently the focus is on the patient's sexuality and the potential effects of the illness on the well partner are overlooked. The 'well' partner can suffer from fatigue, and it is not uncommon for that partner to feel hesitant about initiating the sexual relationship with the ill partner, or either may feel guilty (Salter 1992b).

The results of a study of cancer patients with a poor prognosis (Leiber et al. 1976) suggested that, even when the desire for sexual intercourse decreased, a desire for non-sexual physical intimacy increased. Women patients seemed better able than their husbands to get their affectional needs met. In addition, when sexual rehabilitation was incorporated as a major component in the management of exenteration patients (removal of pelvic organs, often including rectum, bladder and vagina), resumption of sexual activity and satisfaction were greatly increased postoperatively.

Sexuality and the patient with a stoma

Sexuality and the stoma patient has been addressed by Bell (1989a, b). Stoma care nurses have an excellent opportunity to provide information on and direction in sexual rehabilitation for their patients (Salter 1992b).

The 'violation' of a stoma may take on sexual connotations for patients because they now have a different orifice from their previous 'normal' one. Females, especially if they have a protruding stoma, may see it as phallic (resembling a penis) whereas male patients may see theirs as having female characteristics – because a stoma may bleed when cleaned, they liken this to menstruation.

Caring for the homosexual patient with a stoma

Etnyre (1990) states that the experiences, concerns and needs of gay and lesbian ostomists parallel those of anyone who has had ostomy or related surgery. However, many gay and lesbian patients are reluctant to bring up issues and concerns that in any way reveal their sexual orientation, thus making it difficult for them to receive the help they need. The stoma care nurse is ideally placed to demonstrate sensitivity and receptiveness to people who are same-sex orientated, thus paving the way for them to reveal significant personal concerns.

When caring for a homosexual patient it is helpful to determine whether he is the recipient in the relationship. The patient should be warned against using the stoma for penetration, so great sensitivity is needed in the care of the homosexual patient who has had his rectum removed. For homosexual men who participate in anal intercourse, the loss of the anus or rectum removes a major source of pleasure and possibly sexual identity (Savage 1987).

Etnyre (1990) also states that the implication of receptive anal sex for the person who has had ileal pull-through surgery or rectal excision may not necessarily be addressed, particularly if patient or healthcare professionals are hesitant to broach the subject. He offers the following suggestions to ease the discussion of sexual orientation: 'Every patient is concerned about how their current partner or, if single, a future partner might react. Is there some special person, a woman or man, in your life?'

CARE OF THE PATIENT UNDERGOING STOMA SURGERY

Patients undergoing stoma surgery will need to make many adjustments. For example, a male patient undergoing an abdominoperineal excision of the rectum will need to take more care of his body and learn self-care of the stoma. He will undergo frequent examinations of his body by doctors and nurses; he may feel a sense of loss and also feel dependent on others. He could regard the stoma as having female characteristics: because it may bleed, he could liken this to menstruation. He may be concerned with the diagnosis of cancer and also of being impotent. How can he be helped to cope?

From the start the nurse can take steps to conceal as much as possible the extensions of his body image. For example, the patient with a catheter and urinary drainage bag should have the drainage bag concealed by, for instance, the sheet draped over the side of the bed if possible.

Patients can be complimented on their expressions of their sexuality, such as clothes, make-up and jewellery. Loss can be discussed and explained as part of the grieving process; touch is important to enable the patient to still feel 'touchable'. Giving permission after the convalescent period to try love-making and advice on what to do if things go wrong form part of the counselling process.

Sexual function may be impaired after any major stress but this should improve in time. A pan-proctocolectomy should not alter sexual function when performed for inflammatory bowel disease but patients should be given help if they experience difficulties. A stoma can influence sexual function directly because of damage to the pudendal nerve during surgery or indirectly as a result of the changed body image and its impact on sexuality. Other factors include age, gender, family status, severity of the disease, previous interpersonal relationships, beliefs, values and expectations (Cohen 1991).

Rolstad, Wilson and Volk-Tebbitt (1985) have stated that there are fears of sexual inadequacy and even marital breakdown. Therefore it is important to explain to the patient that sexual function may well improve with time.

Anxiety can be allayed by reassuring the couple that the stoma is fairly durable and that no harm can be done when gentle pressure is applied. Modern appliances are leak- and odour-proof and can stay intact during close body contact. This gives both partners confidence in re-establishing their sexual relationship.

Some ostomists will forego meals in the hope that their stoma will be less active a few hours later, during intercourse, but having regular meals is the rule to be followed. If a patient finds that his stoma acts while lying down when, previously, it was inactive while sitting, it may be of help to revert to the former position for a while, or just to wait a few minutes. It could be said that sexual intercourse is not then spontaneous, but a supportive partner is usually willing to wait while the stoma settles down. Sexual dysfunction may stem from psychological origins – fear of rejection or repulsion from the partner, accompanied by the worry that the stoma may act while making love.

If there is a risk of the patient becoming impotent after surgery, the responsibility must lie with the surgeon to discuss this with the individual before admission, thus given the patient time to talk it over with his partner. Ideally, psychosexual counselling should be available and the option to have sperm stored given to a man. It is, however, important that the patient is told there is a possibility that he may be impotent, not that he will be so (Joels 1989).

Patients should also be told that, as a result of the major surgery and possible further treatment, they will be lethargic and weak, with potential loss of libido. It is important for the nurse to spend time talking to the couple – individually if one or the other wishes to share something privately (to be agreed, in the first instance, by the patient) or together, spending time exploring their feelings before offering any advice. Reintroduction of sexual contact can be gradual (Joels 1989).

Impotence in males may be temporary or permanent. Informed consent to surgery means that the male patient who may be impotent as a result (especially when undergoing bladder removal for cancer) must have the opportunity of discussing these aspects in full. If impotence is probable, consideration should be given to penile aids, implants or papaverine injections. It is always safer to bank sperm for male patients who may want to father children in the future. For women with physical difficulty in sexual intercourse, a number of devices are available to enhance satisfaction for herself and her partner (Davis 1990).

Davis (1990) states that impotence has long been acknowledged as a common complication following major pelvic surgery. But doctors and nurses still face the dilemma of whether it is advisable to inform the patient that there is a potential for sexual problems following such surgery. Haywood (1975) and Zohar et al. (1976) suggested that it is the health care professional's duty to inform patients of all possible outcomes. If necessary, the patient and partner should be offered professional psychosexual counselling.

Topping (1990) states that impotence (the inability to have or sustain an erection firm enough for satisfactory intercourse) is one of the problems some male patients with stomas may encounter. However, it should be remembered that there can be a return of erectile function over time (Schover 1986). The less a man focuses on having hard erections, the less anxiety will impair what erectile function remains. 'Dry orgasms' means ejaculation occurring owing to damage to the parasympathetic nerves in the presacral area, or to surgical trauma to the prostate, seminal vesicles or bladder neck. Thus some men do not actually ejaculate, whereas others experience retrograde ejaculation. Although the intensity of orgasm is not disturbed, the experience is different.

Davis (1990) also states that, in men, sexual dysfunction refers to the repeated inability to achieve 'normal' sexual intercourse. In women, it is the repeated unsatisfactory quality of sexual fulfilment. By sharing this understanding and explaining to patients how their bodies work, giving clear pictures of how and why problems may occur, nurses will create a positive interaction that will help to build up an atmosphere of trust. Davis suggests that psychosexual counselling requires specific in-depth training and should be left to those who have undergone that training; however, nurses should raise awareness and recognize the needs of patients.

Joels (1989) states that sexual dysfunction occurs in 43% of male colostomy patients and in virtually all following cystectomy for cancer. In the male, the sympathetic and parasympathetic nerve supply lies in close proximity to the rectum and the bladder. Surgery may therefore cause damage to the nerves, leading to impotence.

Women undergoing abdominal perineal excision of rectum and therefore requiring a permanent colostomy may experience narrowing and shortening of the vagina. For instance, dyspareunia may be experienced by a woman on first resuming intercourse following surgery, and the perineal wound may inhibit the return of an ostomist's sex life as soon as desired. An understanding and patient partner can work wonders.

Joels (1989) postulates that, following abdominoperineal resection, women may experience loss of sensation, dyspareunia and lack of vaginal secretions. Pelvic exenteration proves to be devastating for the self-image of some women, owing to removal of reproductive organs and stoma surgery, which makes them feel incomplete.

Schover (1986) has suggested that dyspareunia can result from anatomical changes such as shortening of the vaginal vault or damage to the posterior vagina wall or from changes in the volume of vaginal secretions. Painful intercourse can be resolved by various strategies, such as adopting different positions during lovemaking, extended foreplay to encourage greater relaxation or the use of lubricants such as water-soluble gel, saliva or vaginal dilators. Practical measures, for example underwear designed to incorporate the bag, are also helpful. All these reduce the feeling of unattractiveness. A change in position when making love may help women who suffer from dyspareunia.

The World Health Organization (1975) suggested that there is increasing evidence that the problems related to human sexuality are more pervasive and more important than had been recognized. Therefore, the need for health professionals who are competent in providing sex education and counselling increases (Fisher and Levin 1983). In a study of gynaecological patients (Corpey at el. 1992) nearly one-third of the women would have liked more information on the operation's effects on sexual function. The women also mentioned that they would have liked their spouse to have received more information on sexuality.

The nurse's role

The psychological preparation and counselling of patients in the preoperative period is of great importance. Preparing patients for the outcomes of surgery makes them better able to accept a change in body image (Keighley et al. 1987). I suggest that more consideration should be given to patients' needs to learn to live with the implications of body image changes and that care should not be left unstructured. Perhaps the ideal person to co-ordinate rehabilitation in this group of patients is the stoma care nurse, in conjunction with the patients, their partner/significant others and other health care professionals (Salter, 1992c). To care for the patient holistically, the physical, mental, emotional, social, sexual and economic must be taken into consideration. When one area is disturbed, the others will be influenced (Cohen 1991).

Cohen (1991) suggests that if the loss of bodily structure and function and the creation of a stoma are planned in advance, a person may have time to anticipate the loss and adopt a more positive attitude. If the creation of a stoma is an emergency procedure, the individual is not able to anticipate the loss and work through the grief process, and may therefore have a more difficult time coping with the changed body image in the future. Some patients are able to integrate the stoma into their body image as a valued organ. This is more likely to occur if they experience good health after ostomy surgery and can compare this situation with the illness experience before operation. The meaning of the loss of an organ depends on the duration and severity of the disease.

Knowledge about actual and potential problems associated with sexuality and an alteration in body image enables nurses to assess the meaning of this for individual patients and their families, to provide counselling before and after the surgery, and to intervene so that each individual will be able to adapt to an alteration in body image and return to their previous activities of daily living and lifestyle (Cohen 1991). Kelman and Minkler (1989) suggest that the first year after surgery be classified as one of disability because of hospitalization and experimentation, learning and relief in being alive. The one-year period of adaptation is related to the duration of mourning and the loss that must be worked through.

Watson's (1983) study on the effects of short-term postoperative counselling in cancer/stoma patients found that subjects who received counselling demonstrated positive alterations in self-concept/self-esteem, as compared with subjects who were not counselled. Age, gender and type of stoma were not found to be significantly related to these body image changes. McKenzie's (1988) study of women undergoing total pelvic exenteration found that, when sexual rehabilitation was incorporated as a major component in the management, resumption of sexual activity and satisfaction were greatly increased postoperatively.

It is important, therefore, for nurses to be communicators, counsellors and patient advocates. We must take a careful history and assessment, organize (where applicable) patient conferences, encourage patient/family-centred care, and plan discharge and rehabilitation within our roles in the multi-disciplinary team.

Smith (1984) has stated that each patient has individual needs and worries that only a careful history and access to the family will reveal. The carer's reaction and acceptance of this new change will in turn affect the attitudes of the patient towards him- or herself. How people have reacted in the past will affect their present coping mechanisms.

Pre- and postoperative counselling is aimed at returning patients to the lifestyle enjoyed prior to surgery, enabling them to pick up the threads of life. Rehabilitation must include the patients and their partner (or other significant people) and should be an enabling process on the part of the nurse (Salter, 1988). Part of the rehabilitation process includes encouraging patients to view themselves as 'normal' after surgery. Nurses should encourage the patient to view the stoma as an inconvenience rather than a disability or handicap.

In Kelly's (1987) study of a non-random, self-selected volunteer sample of 50 ileostomists, the data revealed that patients face two great uncertainties: one psychological and the other technical. The hospital stay appeared to do little to resolve patients' uncertainties. Some patients reported having had little or no preoperative counselling. Sometimes this was unavoidable because the onset of the ulcerative colitis was very sudden and emergency surgery was indicated. For the majority of patients, however, there was the opportunity for counselling. Yet 21 people reported that they left hospital with a clear impression that medical and nursing staff had only the vaguest idea of what having an ileostomy involved and even less interest in discussing the matter with them. But the issue was not just lack of knowledge. Some respondents referred to an apparent relunctance by staff to confront the issues of stoma care – the patients left hospital feeling that some nurses, especially, found the whole process revolting.

Patients who have the benefit of preoperative explanation and counselling and the opportunity to ask questions and discuss their feelings will often accept a stoma more readily after surgery (Joels 1989). I have argued (Salter 1992c) that incorporating body image into patient care can be developed by using a model of care. Peplau (1969) suggested a relationship of closeness between the nurse and patient which can be a springboard for enabling health adaptation to body image changes, and Price (1989) has described a model for body image care.

Pre- and postoperative care

Gillies (1984) suggested that severe pain in any body part can create body image distortions. Because the painful part receives a disproportionate amount of the patient's attention, the part is perceived as being increased in size and so it occupies a prominent position in the body image. If severe pain persists, however, the painful part becomes progressively isolated from the rest of the body, to the point that it is eventually pushed out of body image entirely (Fisher and Cleveland 1968). Grunbaum (1985) has suggested that pain can interfere with adaptation to change. She cites the example of a patient who was in severe pain for several days following major surgery. Only after the pain subsided was she ready to start adapting to her change in body image.

Rehabilitation

Broadwell (1987) has stated that rehabilitation is the dynamic process directed towards assisting the individual to function at an optimal level within the limitation of the disease or treatment. The physical, mental, emotional, social and sexual potentials are domains of the rehabilitation process. The transition from hospital to community has been recognized as a weak link in stoma care (Keighley et al. 1987). A general practitioner's list may contain only four or five people with a stoma, and few general practitioners have detailed knowledge of their special needs. Consequently, if patients do not have continuity of treatment with the stoma care nurse, or there is no liaison with the district nurses, discharge from hospital can be a period when patients may become depressed.

Price (1989) suggests that patient education is the means by which patients resume their own health care. Social support networks (family, friends, significant others) provide the environment in which a normal body image is formed and an altered body image is integrated into society. Patients with an active social support network are likely to make better progress.

The creation of a stoma presents a physical alteration. This alteration may result in the ostomist having a poor self-concept and reduced self-esteem. In Nordstrom's (1985) study, ostomists very often perceived themselves to be less sexually attractive to their partner. A survey of ileostomists (Burnham, Lennard-Jones and Brooke 1977) suggested that this is the case in about 50% of ileostomists. Rolstad, Wilson and Volk-Tebbitt (1985) have stated that poor self-concept and lack of self-esteem may lead to the ostomist's fear of rejection which in turn can create a vicious circle as the ostomist may see himself/herself as being less sexually desirable and will, as a result, avoid intimate contact.

In their survey of ileostomists, Rolstad and colleagues (1985) revealed that 60% of females and 52% of males felt less sexually desirable after stoma surgery. However, although 36% of ostomists reported a change in the pattern in intercourse, this was a negative change for only 28%, representing a positive change for over two-thirds of the couples. I believe that a supportive, loving partner can make a tremendous difference to how well a patient accepts the alteration in body image: he or she will constantly be looking for signs of distaste and rejection. If patients are accepted by others, acceptance of themselves often follows. The partner's and the family's psychological needs must not be forgotten during this time: they may be feeling useless and inadequate, and might themselves be unable to accept the loved one's illness, especially if it is terminal (Joels 1989).

Adolescents and young adults have additional problems in deciding what to tell their boy/girl friend. If a relationship deepens and then perhaps disintegrates, are they going to blame their stoma or accept the end of the relationship? It is difficult to make hard and fast rules as to what or when people with a stoma tell significant others about their changed anatomy. On the third or fourth date one usually knows if the friendship is going to deepen, and this may well be a good time to explain. What should be avoided is continually delaying coming out into the open about stoma surgery, for then it may be discovered by accident! If the relationship disintegrates, it is important for the person to see that the stoma may not have been the reason for the break-up.

So when do people with a stoma tell a new boy/girl friend about their stoma? Or what if they are already married when they require stoma surgery – how can nurses help the partners accept the situation? What about the fear of odour and what do they do with their appliance during lovemaking? Fears of damage to the stoma or displacement of the appliance all have their effect on body image. A well-fitting, secure appliance and the interchangeable activity pouches available for sport or sexual intercourse enable the patient to be more confident during close body contact.

Partners can be helped to accept the spouse's stoma by encouraging early discussion as soon as it is known that stoma surgery is necessary. Nurses can explain (when first discussing with the couple the implications of the operation) that modern appliances are leakproof, odourproof, stay intact, and can be concealed during close body contact. Male ostomists could wear a bag cover or a money-belt type of waistband to conceal the appliance and females can wear a pretty appliance cover to match their underwear or, alternatively, crotchless pants. Some patients with an end colostomy irrigate their stoma prior to intercourse and thus do not need to wear a conventional appliance. If we can allay anxiety by reasoning with the couple that the stoma is fairly durable and that no harm can be done by gentle pressure on it, we can give both partners confidence in re-establishing their sexual relationship (Salter 1988).

As patients recover from surgery, one of their paramount concerns may well be their sexuality and their ability to make love. It may be necessary for us to point out, especially during convalescence, that sexual intercourse is not the only way of expressing love and that it is acceptable to use other means. Referral to one of the self-help groups or to agencies skilled in intervention for sexual difficulties may be appropriate, especially if sex aids are required.

As patients progress through the rehabilitation period, non-intrusive questioning in follow-up, either when attending the hospital or at home in the community, can establish how they are fitting back into their previous lifestyle. Questions such as 'Do you mind if I ask if you go out shopping (see you friends, eat out at a restaurant, go on holiday, go to work)?', 'How does your wife/husband or girl/boy friend feel about your stoma?' will help introduce the subject.

Observations of a person's voice, looks, clothes and mood can help us as nurses assess how the patient is managing. Someone who has become neglectful in appearance may well be in need of further support or help.

CONCLUSION

If we really believe that the sexual health of our patients is as important as their physical well-being, then we will demand that health professionals are educationally prepared for and professionally supported in this vital aspect of care. How well the patient functions sexually after we have finished with him will depend largely on how effective we have been. If sexuality is part of the quality of life, then we as professionals can no longer ignore these components of individual care.' (Wells 1990)

In this chapter I have discussed the issues concerning sexuality in people undergoing stoma surgery. For successful rehabilitation, the aim of the nurse caring for such patients – be it a conventional stoma or a continent procedure – is to encourage them to look in the mirror, and accept the person reflected there.

REFERENCES

Bell, N. (1989a) Promoting fulfillment. *Nursing Times*, **85**: 6.

Bell, N. (1989b) Sex and the ostomist. *Nursing Times*, **85**: 5.

Bragg, V. (1989) Continent intestinal reservoir. *Ostomy/Wound Management*, Summer: 32–41.

Broadwell, D.C. (1987) Rehabilitation needs of the patient with cancer. *Cancer*, **60**: 563–8.

Burnham, W., Lennard-Jones, J. and Brooke, B. (1977) Sexual problems amongst married ileostomists. *Gut*, **18**: 673–7.

Carolan, C. (1983) Sex and disability. *Nursing Times*, **80** (37): 26–34.

Church, J. (1986) The current status of the Kock continent ileostomy. *Ostomy/Wound Management*, Spring: 32–5.

Cohen, A. (1991) Body image in the person with a stoma. *Journal of Enterostomal Therapy*, **18** (2): 68–71.

Corpey, R., Everett, N., Howells, A. and Crowther, M. (1992) The care of patients undergoing surgery for gynaecological cancer. *Journal of Advanced Nursing*, **17**: 667–71.

Davis, K. (1990) Impotence after surgery. *Nursing*, **4** (18): 23–5.

Dempsey, G.M., Buchsbaum, H.J. and Morrison, A (1975) Psychosocial adjustment to pelvic exenteration. *Gynecologic Oncology*, **3**: 325–34.

Devlin H., Plant, J. and Griffin, M. (1971) Aftermath of surgery for ano-rectal cancer. *British Medical Journal*, **3**: 413–18.

Druss, R., O'Connor, J., Prudden, J. and Stern, L. (1968) Psychologic response to colectomy. *Archives of General Psychiatry*, **18**: 53–9.

Dudley, H.A.F. (1978) If I had carcinoma of the middle third of the rectum. *British Medical Journal*, **1**: 1035–67.

Dyk, R. and Sutherland, A. (1956) Adaptation of the spouse and other family to the colostomy patient. *Cancer*, **9**: 123–38.

Eardley, A., George, W., Davis, F., et al. (1976) Colostomy – the consequences of surgery. *Clinical Oncology*, **2**: 277–83.

Etnyre, W. (1990) Meeting the needs of gay and lesbian ostomates. *Proceedings of 8th Biennial Congress*, World Council of Enterostomal Nurses, Hollister, Canada.

Everett, W. (1989) Experience of restorative proctocolectomy with ileal reservoir. *British Journal of Surgery*, **76**: 77–81.

Fisher, S.G. (1979) Psychosocial adjustment following total pelvic exenteration. *Cancer Nursing*, **33**: 210–15.

Fisher, S. (1980) *Human Sexuality: a Nursing Perspective*. Appleton-Century-Crofts: New York.

Fisher, S. and Cleveland, B. (1968) Body image and personality. Dover Publications: New York, pp. 352–63.

Fisher, S.D. and Levin, D.L. (1983) The sexual knowledge and attitudes of professional nurses caring for oncology patients. *Cancer Nursing*, **6**: 55–61.

Gillies, D.A. (1984) Body image changes following illness and surgery. *Journal of Enterostomal Therapy*, **11**: 186–9.

Grunbaum, J. (1985) Helping your patient build a sturdier body image. *Registered Nurse*, **10**: 51–5.

Haywood, J. (1975) *Information – a Prescription against Pain*. Royal College of Nursing: London.

Joels, J. (1989) Psychological implications of having a stoma. *Surgical Nurse* (special feature on stoma care) **2** (6): x–xii.

Keighley, M., Winsler, M., Pringle, W. and Allan, R. (1987) The pouch as an alternative to an ileostomy. *British Journal of Hospital Medicine*, **12**: 1008–11.

Kelly, M. (1987) Adjusting to ileostomy. *Nursing Times*, **83** (33): 29–31.

Kelman, G. and Minkler, P. (1989) An investigation of quality of life and self esteem among individuals with ostomies. *Journal of Enterostomal Therapy*, **16**: 4–11.

Lamb, M. and Woods, N. (1981) Sexuality and the cancer patient. *Cancer Nursing*, **4**: 137–44.

Leiber, L., Plumb, M.M., Gerstenzang, M.L., et al. (1976) The communication of affection between cancer patients and their spouses. *Psychosomatic Medicine*, **38**: 379–81.

Lomont, H.A., De Petrillo, A.D. and Sargeant, E.J. (1978) Psycho-sexual rehabilitation and exenterative surgery. *Journal of Gynecological Oncology*, **6**: 236–42.

Maguire, G.P., Lee, E.G., Bevington, D.J., Kuchemann, W., Cerpetrie, R.J. and Cornell, C.E. (1978) Psychological problems in the first year after mastectomy. *British Medical Journal*, **1**: 963–5.

Maslow, A. (1970) *Hierarchy of Human Needs in Motivation and Personality*. Harper: New York.

McKenzie, F. (1988) Sexuality after total pelvic exenteration. *Nursing Times*, **84** (20): 27–30.

McPheteridge, L. (1968) Nursing history: one means to personalized care. *American Journal of Nursing*, **16**: 68–75.

Nemer, F. and Rolstad, B. (1985) The role of the ileo anal reservoir in patients with ulcerative colitis and familial polyposis. *Journal of Enterostomal Therapy*, **12** (3): 74–83.

Nicholls, R. (1983) Proctocolectomy: 1. Avoiding an ileostomy. *Nursing Mirror*, **156** (7): 46–7.

Nicholls, R., Pescatori, M., Motson, R. and Pezim, M. (1983) Restorative proctocolectomy with a 3 loop ileal reservoir for ulcerative colitis and familial adenomatous polyposis. *Annals of Surgery*, **22**: 383–8.

Nicholls, R. and Pezim, M. (1985) Restorative proctocolectomy with ileal reservoir for ulcerative colitis and familial polyposis coli. *British Journal of Surgery*, **72**: 470–4.

Nordstrom, G. (1985) Urostomy patients – a strategy for care. *Nurse Times*, **85** (18): 32–4.

Pemberton, J., Phillips, S., Ready, R., Zinsmeister, A. and Beahrs, O. (1989) Quality of life after Brooke ileostomy and ileal pouch–anal anastomosis: comparison of performance status. *Annals of Surgery*, **209** (5): 1620–8.

Peplau, H. (1969) Professional closeness. *Nursing Forum*, **8** (4): 343–60.

Price, B. (1989) *Body Image – Nursing concepts and care*. Prentice Hall: London.

Price, B. (1990) A model for body image care. *Journal of Advanced Nursing*, **15**: 585–93.

Rolstad, B., Wilson, G. and Volk-Tebbit, B. (1985) Long term sexual status concerns in the client with ileostomy. *Journal of Enterostomal Therapy*, **9** (4): 10–12.

Rolstad, B. and Rothenberger, D. (undated) *Ileal–anal Reservoir Booklet – A patient resource*. Upjohn Company: Kalamazoo MI.

Roper, N., Logan, W. and Tierney, A. (1985) *The Elements of Nursing*. Churchill Livingstone: Edinburgh.

Salter, M. (Ed.) (1988) *Altered Body Image – The Nurse's Role*. Scutari Press: London.

Salter, M. (1992a) Body image and the stoma patient. *Wound Management*, **2** (2): 8–9.

Salter, M. (1992b) Aspects of sexuality for patients with stomas and continent pouches. *Journal of Enterostomal Nursing*, **19**: 126–30.

Salter, M. (1992c) What are the differences in body image between patients with a conventional stoma compared with those who have had a conventional stoma followed by a continent pouch? *Journal of Advanced Nursing*, **17**: 841–8.

Savage, J. (1987) *Nurses, gender and sexuality*. Heinemann Nursing: London.

Schover, C.R. (1986) Sexual rehabilitation of the ostomy patient. In: Smith, D.B. and Johnson D.E. (Eds). *Ostomy Care and the Cancer Patient*. Grune & Stratton: Orlando.

Smith, R.(1984) Identity crisis. *Nursing Mirror*, **158**: ii–vi.

Topping, A. (1990) Sexual activity and the stoma patient. *Nursing Standard*, **4** (41): 24–6.

Vera, M.I. (1981) Quality of life following pelvic exenteration. *Gynecologic Oncology*, **12**: 355–66.

Wade, B. (1989) Nursing care of the stoma patient. *Surgical Nurse*, **2**: 5.

Wade, B. (1990a) Colostomy patients: psychological adjustment at 10 weeks and 1 year after surgery in districts which employed stoma care nurses and districts which did not. *Journal of Advanced Nursing*, **15** (11): 1297–304.

Wade, B. (1990b) *A Stoma is for Life*. Scutari Press: London.

Watson, P. (1983) The effects of short-term post-operative counselling on cancer/ostomy patients. *Cancer Nursing*, **6**: 21–9.

Webb, C (1987) Nurses' knowledge and attitudes about sexuality: report of a study. *Nursing Education Today*, **7**: 209–14.

Webb, C. and O'Neill, J. (1989) Nurses' attitudes about sexuality in health care. A review of the literature. *Nurse Education Today*, **7**: 75–87.

Wells, R. (1990) Sexuality: an unknown word for patients with a stoma. In Senn, H., Glaus, J. (Eds) *Results in Cancer Research*. Springer-Verlag: Berlin, pp. 115–21.

Woods, N. (1984) Human Sexuality in Health and Illness. C. V. Mosby: St Louis.

Woods, N. and Mandetta, A. (1976) Changes in student knowledge and attitudes following a course in human sexuality. *Nursing Research*, **24** (1): 10–15.

World Health Organization. (1975) Technical report series (no. 5732). *Educational and Treatment in Human Sexuality: the training of health professionals*. WHO: Geneva.

Zohar, J., Miraz, D., Macez, B., et al. (1976) Factors influencing prostatectomy – a prospective study. *Journal of Urology*, **116**: 332–4.

14 Models of care

Carol L. Cox and Maxine L.V.-T. McVey

INTRODUCTION

It has been acknowledged by Meleis (1986), a nurse theorist, that members of some sciences, such as physics, biology, sociology and psychology, have been involved in discussions about their professional existence and the nature and development of their knowledge. Knowledge is known in philosophical terms as a discipline's 'epistemology'. These sciences, unlike nursing, are well established in the development of their knowledge base. However, they are debating whether they should replace their established or mainstream 'epistemology' with new knowledge that is more congruent with the goals of their disciplines (Meleis 1986). It is from the sciences identified above, as well as others, that nursing derives some of its knowledge. Similarly, nursing is involved in debate about its own knowledge. Unique knowledge in nursing is associated with nursing theories and nursing conceptual models that underpin nursing practice (Fawcett and Downs 1992; Fawcett 1993).

This chapter will provide insight into what constitutes nursing knowledge, how nurses acquire knowledge and build on their knowledge base and gain new knowledge through research. The nature of knowledge will be examined and related to stoma care nursing. The chapter will further provide an understanding about conceptual models and how conceptual models guide nursing practice. Three types of nursing conceptual models will be explained and related to the context of nursing care.

NURSING AS A DISCIPLINE AND KNOWLEDGE

Nursing is considered to be a discipline because it is based on a particular body of knowledge. However, 'The definition of a knowledge base for a discipline begins with the separation of that knowledge which is important to the discipline and that which is not' (Visintainer 1986). Donaldson and Crowley (1978) further characterize a discipline by the unique collective way it views all phenomena, which ultimately defines its world view. The world view is the perspective and/or philosophical thought an individual or group holds within a discipline. If stoma care nurses are to define their world view and state what knowledge is important to them, they should first be able to answer the questions proposed by Manley (1991) about Visintainer's statement. These questoins are:

- What is meant by knowledge?
- Who should judge the relevance of that knowledge?
- What knowledge base is important to nursing? (Within the context of this text, specifically, stoma care nursing.)

In order to answer these questions and to discuss the knowledge important to stoma care nursing, it is necessary to reflect on the evolution of caring knowledge in nursing and the types of knowledge which have been discussed by authors such as Benner (1984), Carper (1978) and others. To begin, what is meant by knowledge will be defined.

WHAT IS MEANT BY KNOWLEDGE?

Knowledge can be defined as:

- The product of knowing (Walker and Avant 1988)
- The facts/feelings or experiences known by a person or group of people (*Collins English Dictionary* 1979)
- Theoretical or practical understanding of a subject (*Concise Oxford Dictionary* 1990)
- Familiarity gained by experience of person, thing; facts (*Concise Oxford Dictionary* 1990)

The processes of knowing are fundamental to all human activities. From birth we begin a lifelong process of learning about ourselves and our surroundings (Chinn and Kramer 1991). From this statement and the definitions cited above it can be seen that the knowledge base nurses develop encompasses experiences and understanding in addition to facts. Johnson (1968), a noted nurse theorist, has indicated she believes that knowledge differs in kind and not amount. It is the difference between 'knowing that' and 'knowing how' that is nursing's practical knowledge, and 'knowing why' and 'knowing what' that is nursing's theoretical knowledge. To conceptualize the differences, consider a nurse working on a gastroenterological ward. The nurse may 'know that' it is necessary preoperatively to determine the site of a stoma in all patients who will have a stoma formed as part of their operation. This, however, is different from 'knowing why' which is that choosing the correct site improves the quality of life for such patients once they begin to wear clothing and continue their daily lives.

WHO SHOULD JUDGE THE RELEVANCE OF THAT KNOWLEDGE?

To judge the relevance of nursing knowledge, it is important to understand the evolution of nursing. In 1985, Jean Watson discussed five epistemological categories, which Meleis (1991) has extended in her nursing text. The categories originated from research conducted by Belenky et al. (1986) associated with women's ways of knowing. These categories help to explain the perspective nursing has developed and where nursing is now in its development of knowledge. The five epistemological categories are:

- Silent knowledge
- Received knowledge
- Subjective knowledge
- Procedural knowledge
- Constructed knowledge.

Silent knowledge

Silent knowledge is the domain in which the nurse experiences self as mindless and voiceless and subject to the whims of external authority events. Formal guidelines for nurses were established by Nightingale (1859). In her seminal writings, Nightingale stressed the need for management, direction of others, teaching of both patient and family, and strict discipline. Autocratic figures of authority were evident in nursing, and remain present in some context. The Nightingale nurse was a doctor's assistant, obedient, unquestioning and subservient. This was a time when intellectual curiosity or questioning of routines was discouraged. Nursing knowledge was 'knowing that' and 'knowing how'. What mattered was the practical skills of nursing care. Oakley (1984) commented that, if Florence Nightingale had trained her lady pupils in assertiveness rather than obedience, perhaps nurses would be in a different situation now.

Silent knowing holds little benefit for the patient or the nurse in today's caring environment. On the other hand, Nightingale also stressed the need to listen carefully to patients and families before carrying out nursing care. Perhaps this was the first recognition of nursing assessment and the role of the nurse as the patient's advocate.

Received knowledge

Received knowledge is the domain in which the nurse conceives of self as capable of receiving and reproducing knowledge from external authorities, but not capable of creating his or her own knowledge. In this category, nurses have taken knowledge from others and used it in their practice. Types of knowledge described by Moody (1990) are applicable to received knowledge in nursing. The first is folklore, conventional wisdom or common knowledge. Common knowledge is transmitted from one culture or discipline to another and is available to the nurse 'merely through living' (Visintainer 1986). An example of common knowledge would be knowing that when certain foods are digested they create unpleasant wind. Using this common knowledge, nurses advise patients/clients with a stoma about foods that cause unpleasant wind. The second type of knowledge is scientific knowledge which has been generated through systematic study – quantitative and qualitative modes of enquiry. It has been acknowledged that scientific formulation of 'knowing that' has acquired a superior status for the way in which a discipline should develop knowledge (Chinn and Jacobs 1987). Why nurses received and reproduced knowledge from external authorities is best understood by examining the marxist and feminist perspectives.

The marxist viewpoint is associated with class structure, which determines modes of thought; the leading ideas are those of the dominant group in society (Cuff and Payne 1984). Within health care, doctors are the dominant group. It is medical knowledge that is approved and accepted, as opposed to nursing knowledge – which has been restricted in its development.

The feminist perspective is related to views regarding male dominance of the medical and scientific communities. This has prevented the development of knowledge in the primarily female profession of nursing. Thus, in the days of the Nightingale model, silence led nurses into the medical model of caring. The classic biomedical model focuses on correctly diagnosing disease, and the nurse's role is to accurately carry out medical prescriptions. The natural result of adherence to the medical model is the establishment of routines. An example is the taking down of dressings 'just to have a look' when there is no indication that the patient has a wound infection or that the patient will benefit from this practice. The biomedical model has given direction to nursing but it has also limited nursing's development as a profession. Received knowing is not beneficial to the further development of nursing.

Subjective knowledge

Subjective knowledge is the domain in which truth and knowledge are conceived as personal, intuitive and subjectively known and valued. Knowing in this category is not the knowledge of a discipline but more knowing of oneself. As discussed earlier, the process of learning begins at birth. In this process we become individuals within our society. As individuals we have a picture in our minds about what nursing actually is and what nurses do. This picture is based on our attitudes, ideas and values. Hence, subjective knowledge or informal models of care have always been present in nursing. This subjective knowledge remains within a nurse's personal knowing, influencing his or her own practice, and is not shared. Making such views explicit – that is, talking and writing about them – is quite new to nurses (Pearson and Vaughn 1990). It is only when subjective knowledge is made explicit by nurses that it becomes knowledge for the discipline of nursing.

Procedural knowledge

Procedural knowledge is the domain in which the nurse is invested in learning and in applying procedures for obtaining and communicating knowledge. Watson (1985) stated that in the 1970s many nurses worked and studied in other disciplines. These nurses then attempted to fit the theories of the other disciplines into nursing. Theories as a source of knowledge in nursing may be 'unique' to nursing or borrowed from other disciplines (Johnson 1968). An example of borrowed theory that has been applied to nursing practice is Maslow's psychosocial development theory.

Maslow's hierarchy of needs has been used by nurses when assessing and planning care (Minshull, Ross and Turner 1986). There is nothing wrong with borrowing theories, but it may limit nurses in producing 'unique' theories and add to the confusion about the boundaries of nursing (Cull-Wilby and Peppin 1987).

Constructed knowledge

Constructed knowledge (the highest and most integrated level) is the domain in which the nurse views all knowledge as contextual experience. The self is viewed as the creator of knowledge and the nurse values subjective and objective strategies for knowing. These different levels are evident in nursing research and are manifested as part of the evolution of nursing knowledge.

In this category, nurses create their own knowledge either inductively or deductively, or both, and generate nursing models and theories that influence nursing practice. Travelbee (1971) postulated that it is essential to build up a body of structured reliable nursing knowledge if nurses are to move from a common-sense approach to a professional level of practice. In addressing the way in which theories for practice are constructed, Travelbee (1971) defined the nursing process model as a 'disciplined intellectual approach', a logical method of approaching nursing problems to ascertain needs, validate inferences, decide who should meet the identified needs, plan the course of action and validate that course. The nursing process is a problem-solving method. In problem solving, nurses theorize about the patients' problems and the care each patient should receive. The nursing process can provide the nurse with a nursing base for research and development of new theories for practice. Through the process of constructing theories, nursing's unique body of knowledge is expanded. According to Yura and Walsh (1978), the nursing process is assessment, planning and the delivery of nursing care as well as evaluation of the care nurses deliver. Conceptual models, on the other hand, which contain theories for nursing, give guidance for nursing practice and define the boundaries of nursing.

The development of knowledge in nursing has progressed haphazardly (Cull-Wilby and Peppin 1987; Hardy 1990). It is only in nursing's recent history and research – for example, Benner's (1984) research on the role of intuition in practical knowledge – that theory construction has been recognized as a contribution to nursing's unique body of knowledge. Johnson (1968: p. 2) defined unique theory as 'that knowledge derived from the observation of phenomena and the asking of questions unlike those which characterise other disciplines'. The development of this form of scientific knowledge is seen as evolving from creative and original research. It is only by examining epistemological issues that current values attached to various aspects of knowledge can be understood (Suppe and Jacox 1985; Sarter 1988).

WHAT KNOWLEDGE BASE IS IMPORTANT TO NURSING?

Practical knowledge

Practical knowledge is 'know how' knowledge and consists of practical expertise and skills. Knowing that a patient with a stoma has or has not adapted to the change in his or her body image is an example of 'know how' knowledge in action. The nurse knows that the patient is adjusting when he or she can change the stoma bag and confirm understanding of the procedure. The nurse knowing how to change a stoma bag and how to teach this skill to others is an important aspect of practical knowledge. However, this practical knowledge must be extended into building a therapeutic relationship with patients so that the nurse can determine how well they are adjusting to their changed body image. Practical knowledge is gained through experience over time.

Benner (1984) identified six areas of knowledge that are important for a practice-based discipline, and which can be observed in 'expert' practice. First, there are 'graded qualitative distinctions'. This is when the nurse has insight into a situation. This insight is finely tuned and derived from many hours of caring for patients. An example of 'expert' practice is found in acute clinical areas: nurses can intuitively feel a change in a patient's condition even before physiological signs reflect that a change has occurred.

Secondly, 'common meanings' are developed among nurses who share common issues in practice. Here knowledge evolves from frequent exposure to an accepted meaning. At St Mark's Hospital, nurses 'digitate' fistula-in-ano wounds. This is a practice of passing a finger along the wound to ensure that it heals from the apex downwards. Digitate, according to the *Concise Oxford Dictionary*, means having separate fingers or toes. Language that addresses the anatomy of the fingers has been transposed in nursing practice to define an aspect of care.

The third area identified by Benner concerns 'assumptions, expectations and sets'. In this category, nurses have learned to predict events in a particular situation. This results from having observed many types of clinical situation. For example, the nurse has cared for a patient with a prolapsed stoma and is aware of the implications that this will have on the patient's quality of life.

The fourth area comprises 'paradigm cases and personal knowledge'. In this category, particular patients or life incidents have produced a change in a particular nurse's practice. Experience has refined 'know how' and 'know that' knowledge (Polyani 1958). For instance, an inexperienced nurse may approach teaching the skills and knowledge required for stoma care without taking into account any of the variables related to the patient. The experienced nurse, on the other hand, will be more sensitive because of his or her previous expectations that were fulfilled or not fulfilled when teaching patients about stoma care. Knowledge refinement can occur only if nurses are reflective in their own practice (Schon 1983) and also incorporate their life experiences into practice.

The fifth area identified by Benner (1984) is 'maxims' – concealed/ cryptic instructions that make sense only to those with a deep understanding of a situation. Consider, for example, the patient who has not overtly been considered unsuitable for resuscitation and subsequently suffers cardiac arrest: the maxim would be to sound the resuscitation bell but to walk slowly to the telephone to call for help.

Finally, the sixth domain is 'delegation by default'. Practice knowledge here is that of unplanned practice. Handed down practices from the medical profession have resulted in nurses becoming very skilled in certain aspects of practice. This reflects delegation by default. An illustration of this is ward nurses becoming skilled in determining stoma sites in patients. This used to be a practice performed only by doctors. Delegation by default can be viewed as a very controversial area, and its implications for the nursing profession need to be explored. Delegation by default may fragment nursing because the extension of role and newly acquired skill has not, until recently, been considered to be part of nursing practice. The UKCC (1992b) has addressed the extended role of the nurse in *The Scope of Professional Practice* guidelines. Furthermore, with the introduction of the UKCCs *Standards for Education and Practice Following Registration*, there is increased emphasis on enhanced clinical practice as nurses initiate and implement developments that contribute to the quality of care received by patients (UKCC 1994). Benner and Tanner (1987) have suggested that the sum of the six kinds of practice knowledge constitutes an expert practitioner: one who is efficient and has an intuitive grasp of the whole situation. This practical knowledge has much to offer the development of nursing theory when it is described and then studied.

Theoretical knowledge

Theoretical knowledge is 'know that' knowledge and can be related to the scientific mode of learning. In the literature, three ways of knowing that are inferior to science have been identified (Kerlinger 1973, cited in Chinn and Jacobs 1987). Tenacity is the first 'know that' domain and is based on the belief that something is as it is because it has always been that way. The second domain is authority. Here, 'know that' knowledge is knowing based on an authoritative source or person: the authority has said it is so. Third is *a priori* knowledge, which is knowing that depends on reason, and may not be consistent with experience. Meleis (1985) has identified this pattern of knowing in nursing. Here nurses hold on firmly to beliefs that have been generated from repeated experiences. Their experiences are communicated as knowledge through authoritative sources from one generation of nurses to the next. Thus knowledge is limited and restricts the progress of the development of nursing knowledge (Meleis 1985). An example of such a belief is the application of egg white to excoriated skin around a stoma. Although this was believed to be effective, it is no longer considered to be an acceptable method of treatment owing to the associated increased risk of infection. Rituals of clinical practice and organization have been discussed by Walsh and Ford (1990), who encourage nurses to question their practices and consider modifying them in the light of research evidence.

In 1978, following a review of nursing literature, Barbara Carper classified four ways of knowing that are important to the discipline of nursing. Many nurse theorists have incorporated Carper's types of theoretical knowledge into their writings. The types of knowing that Carper identified are empirical (scientific), aesthetic (art), personal and ethical (moral). Although each way of knowing is discussed separately below, they are of equal importance, and all are integrated in order for knowledge to be applied and developed (Chinn and Kramer 1991).

Empirical knowing is scientific knowledge. Its purpose is to describe, explain and predict phenomena (Moody 1990); it is regarded as superior because it is 'objective, quantifiable and verifiable' and is obtained through the senses (Leddy and Pepper 1989). This means, to the nurse, it is observable. Since the 1950s, emphasis has been placed on the development of empirical knowledge as the 'science' of nursing. Through this 'science' descriptive, explanatory and predictive theories for nursing have been developed (Chinn and Jacobs 1987).

Nursing theories lead to the generation of nursing knowledge. A theory is a 'logically interconnected set of propositions used to describe, explain and predict a part of the empirical world' (Riehl and Roy 1980: p. 3). Riehl and Roy also described theory as a 'scientifically acceptable general principle which governs practice or is proposed to explain observed facts.' Nursing science has not reached a level of development in which there is a single paradigm which governs and co-ordinates the activities of nurse theorists. There is agreement, however, that the four basic concepts of nursing, termed the metaparadigm (Fawcett 1984), are person, health, environment and nursing. These concepts are evident in nursing's conceptual models.

Aesthetic knowledge relates to the art of nursing practice. The attitude of nurses, how they approach their patients, their dexterity and expertise are expressed through aesthetic knowledge. Aesthetic knowledge is demonstrated in Benner's (1984) writings. Without this type of knowledge nurses would be unable to express creativity and style in designing and providing effective and satisfying nursing care (Orem 1991). An example of nursing care in which aesthetic knowledge is demonstrated is the fitting of an appliance to a fistula that looks clean and does not leak, coupled with the satisfaction of the patient and the nurse because the appliance has been fitted properly. Aesthetics in nursing practice inspires satisfaction and confidence on the part of both patient and nurse.

Personal knowledge is the way in which the nurse views himself or herself (Carper 1978), and is related to the relationship the nurse has with patients. It is regarded by Carper to be the most difficult type of knowledge to master and to teach as it has developed over years of life experience. Personal knowledge is gained as a lifelong process that changes as the person becomes sensitive to intuitive feelings and experiences. Benner's paradigm cases and personal knowledge are related to personal knowledge. Here, according to Benner (1984), nurses need to be able to reflect on their own practice.

Ethical knowledge is the moral component of knowing in nursing. It focuses on matters of obligation and what ought to be done (Carper 1978). Knowledge here involves being responsible for moral choices when value judgements are in conflict (Leddy and Pepper 1989). This knowledge encompasses the understanding of different philosophical positions about what is good, right and wrong. An illustration of nursing's moral code is the UKCC (1992a) *Code of Professional Conduct*. It will provide only guidance and does not offer answers to difficult moral dilemmas faced by nurses in their practice. In identifying the four patterns of knowing, Carper (1978) demonstrated the complex and diverse nature of nursing knowledge. Each pattern is necessary in the development of the expert practitioner (Benner 1984).

Theoretical knowledge ('knowing that') and practical knowledge ('knowing how') must be linked in nursing practice. Practising nurses have raised questions regarding what is perceived to be a theory–research–practice gap. Nurses must be able to give explanations for and be responsible for the nursing care they give (UKCC 1992b). This then becomes inextricably linked with accountability for actions they take. Lewis and Batey (1982) have suggested that accountability refers to a formal obligation to disclose. Therefore, in relating this back to the nursing process and the provision of nursing care, nurses should be able to state what it is they are trying to achieve (the goal of nursing care), how the care is achieved (nursing action) and why they are trying to achieve the goal (justification for nursing care). Lewis and Batey also suggested that nurses must be aware of the actions they take. Thus there must be evaluation of care.

NURSING'S EPISTEMOLOGY

Knowledge is generated from theory and, as nurses are engaged in a practice discipline, any theory of nursing must be related to practice in order that a prescription for practice may be made (McFarlane 1977). Conceptual models are considered to be nursing's unique body of knowledge. Unlike theory, they are broad and abstract and have been constructed by nurse theorists to address aspects of nursing knowledge. Thus nursing models are 'constructed knowledge'. Conceptual models may be categorized as grand theory (Fitzpatrick and Whall 1989) owing to their broad and abstract nature. However, Fawcett (1989) makes a clear distinction between theory and conceptual models based on levels of abstraction. If the purpose of the theorist's writing is to describe, explain or predict specific aspects of nursing phenomena, the work is 'most likely a theory'; if, however, the purpose is to articulate a body of distinctive nursing knowledge the work is 'most likely a conceptual model' (Fawcett 1989: p. 26). Theory, according to Walker and Avant (1988: p. 11) 'describes, explains, predicts or controls' nursing and its associated phenomena. Furthermore, conceptual models provide a comprehensive perspective of the metaparadigm of nursing. Nursing, person, health and environment are described and their relationships are explained and may be linked together.

The definitions suggest that theory may exist without conceptual models; however, the epistemological stance of conceptual models does not exist without theory. Theory may be derived from nursing's conceptual models and, at the middle range and practice levels, may be tested through research (Merton 1957). Research may also lead to the development of new theory.

Middle range theory is restricted to a limited range of nursing phenomena. It does not address the metaparadigm but is narrower in scope and encompasses a limited number of concepts and a limited aspect of nursing's world of practice. Theory at the middle range level is useful to nurses involved in stoma care. Specific problems associated with caring for the patient who has a newly formed stoma may be diagnosed by the nurse, and subsequent plans or 'theories' on how to care for the patient and the stoma are developed. At the practice level, these plans or 'theories' may be put into action. As the care is implemented, nurses evaluate the care and determine whether the outcome for the patient has been effective based on the 'theory'/plan of care. In a sense, research is conducted each time care is planned, implemented and evaluated. In action research the researcher plans a course of action, implements the action and reflects on the action (Chapman 1991). The nursing process incorporates the element of evaluation. Here the nurse reflects back on the care provided and makes decisions regarding the effectiveness of the plan. The plan may subsequently be revised, just as action research is revised or taken forward following reflection.

As already stated in this chapter, theories describe, explain, predict and control. A premise within the St Mark's model (Cox and McVey 1994) is that nursing is dynamic, reflective, responsive and progressive in its approach to caring. Therefore a theory that is explanatory and predictive in nature is one that explains the relationship of responsive and progressive nurses who promote health through education that leads to the patients/clients being able to care for their own stoma.

Conceptual models are generally categorized as developmental, systems or interactive in nature. Each type of model reflects a unique perspective regarding the nature of nursing and influences how nurses practice. Each category reflects a particular philosophical perspective or 'world view' about nursing.

Developmental conceptual models of nursing address the processes of growth, development and maturation. In this category the identification of actual or potential problems and the delineation of nursing intervention strategies become the key features of the model. The Roper, Logan and Tierney (1983) *Activities of Daily Living Model* is developmental. A major component is change and how the person adjusts. Stages are noticeable and, as in the Roper and colleagues' model, these may be identified along a dependence/independence continuum. A direction of change can be seen, and a goal or end-state that evolves through the process of becoming, developing and maturing is established with the patient by the nurse.

In stoma care nursing, if the nurse uses a developmental model as the frame of reference providing nursing care, the degree of achievement towards the goal of adjusting to and being able to care for one's own stoma would be addressed in an incremental manner. Nurses would not assume that patients could care for their stoma immediately after surgery. Nurses would expect that, over time, through their teaching and the patients' practising, the patients would come to perform their own stoma care. By the same token, nurses would know that children would care for a stoma differently from adults. Older adults may or may not be able to care for their own stoma, depending on age and ability. The plan of care is developed to take into the account the changing needs and abilities of the individual patients over time. Nurses adjust their care based on the developmental stage of the patient.

Systems models address nursing phenomena 'as if there existed organisation, interaction, interdependency, and integration of parts and elements' (Chin 1980: p. 24). As in developmental models, actual and potential problems are considered. Here, however, these problems are orientated to the whole system and nursing intervention is directed towards efficient and effective system functioning. Nurses who prefer a systems approach to nursing care would examine the patient system, its parts and the relationship of the parts within the system at a given period in time. Change is of secondary importance in systems models (Fawcett 1989). The system, which may be open or closed, considers relationships and activities within the environment. Thus, when viewing the phenomena of a person who has a newly formed stoma, the nurse would consider the stoma as a part of the intestine that has been brought to the surface of the patient's abdomen. The environment may be the patient's family, and adjustment to the stoma and how to care for the stoma includes the patient and his or her family.

The *Roy Adaptation Model* (Roy and Andrews 1986) is an example of a systems model. In this model the stoma care nurse considers adaptation as a function of the stimulus to which the patient is exposed. The adaptation level comprises a zone indicating the range of stimulation that will lead to a positive response by the patient. The patient is regarded by the nurse as having four modes of adaptation which the nurse must consider when planning and providing nursing care. In order for the system to adapt effectively, the physiological mode, self-concept mode, role function mode and interdependence mode must be addressed. The nurse considers how a patient's role in the family may change as a result of the stoma. The nurse helps the patient and the family to identify mechanisms that will lead to effective role functioning. Interdependence in the family may become a key issue in the adaptation or mal-adaptation of the patient and family to the stoma. The nurse plays an important part in helping the family and patient come to terms with the demands placed upon them by the new stoma.

Interaction or 'interpersonal' nursing models address relationships between people and social acts. Within this framework, the identification of actual and potential problems again becomes the focus; however, these are within the confines of interpersonal relationships and delineation of nursing care strategies that promote optimal socialization. A nurse who chooses to use an interaction model will be concerned with the patient's self-concept and how he or she is relating to the new stoma and the world. Aspects such as odour and privacy take on new meaning and have serious implications when a patient chooses whether to socialize with others. The patient's ability to perform roles according to self-imposed and societal standards becomes critically important in an interaction model of nursing. The patient becomes central as an active participant in interactions. Nursing care plans include elements of evaluating how the patient communicates, and measures to promote active rather than passive participation by the patient. In an interaction model, the patient actively sets goals based on his or her perceptions of relevant factors in a given situation (Fawcett 1989).

Imogene King's (1981) theory – which is an interacting systems framework – emphasizes interpersonal relationships. Nursing judgement varies relative to each nursing action, and the effectiveness of nursing action varies to the extent to which it is communicated to those responsible for providing care. Perceptions influence the interaction process of the patient and the nurse. Goals, needs and values of both the nurse and the patient also influence the interaction process. A nurse who chose to use King's (1981) interaction model would be concerned with how the patient was perceiving care and whether the patient was making informed decisions about his or her health care.

CHANGING TERMINOLOGY – REFLECTING ON NURSING'S EPISTEMOLOGY

The terms theory, theoretical framework, conceptual model, conceptual framework and model are used synonymously in nursing literature. Among some nursing theorists there is little agreement as to what the differences are between the terms. However, at practice level there is agreement that practice theories are prescriptive. Conceptual frameworks or models represent a less formal and less well developed attempt at expressing nursing phenomena than theories. Conceptual models are a broad and abstract body of knowledge that deals with concepts and propositions assembled by virtue of their relevance to a particular theme or 'world view' of nursing. Nursing models may be classified as developmental, systems and interaction. Conceptual models and theories use concepts as building blocks. However, conceptual models are more global than theories (Fawcett 1984) and contain linking statements that describe nursing, person, health and the environment in distinctive ways in order to influence nursing.

Nursing shares knowledge of the sciences and humanities with other disciplines. Conceptual models or frameworks are considered to be nursing's unique body of knowledge. Theories borrowed from other disciplines must be challenged in nursing before they can be viewed as acceptable for nurses to use in their practice.

Theory testing is an important concern in nursing. Research is stimulated through the use of theory in nursing practice. New ideas about care derived from assumptions and propositions within conceptual models, frameworks and theories serve as a point of departure for testing the adequacy of a particular theory. In testing theory, the nurse researcher deduces implications and then develops a research hypothesis. The hypothesis is a prediction about the manner in which variables would be related if the theory were correct and useful for nursing practice. Hypotheses are subjected to testing through systematic enquiry. The theory is never tested directly. It is the hypothesis deduced from the theory that is subjected to scientific investigation. The outcomes of the research and the relationships predicted by the hypothesis are compared in the research process. In this way the theory is continually subjected to potential disconfirmation. Repeated failures of the research to disconfirm the theory result in increasing support for acceptance of the theory. This then becomes knowledge for use in nursing practice.

Conceptual models of nursing may be constructed inductively. Nurse theorists who have a particular perspective related to nursing may take a specific aspect of experience, or 'phenomenon' as it is termed, and generalize it to a broader population. Once constructed, the model, which contains theory, is subjected to further research. As described above, the assumptions and propositions inherent within the model are developed into hypotheses and subjected to testing.

CONCLUSION

The members of some sciences such as physics, biology, sociology and psychology are involved in debate regarding the replacement of their established or mainstream epistemology with new assumptions and methods more congruent with their disciplines. Members within these disciplines argue that theories relating to human beings developed within their disciplines should be applied to nursing problems. However, nurse theorists advocate the development of unique nursing theories. Theories borrowed from other disciplines should be subjected to reconstruction within nursing and nursing research before being applied in nursing practice (Meleis 1991).

Nursing, like the sciences listed above, is involved in debate about its own knowledge. Within this chapter knowledge and aspects of nursing's epistemology in the form of conceptual models have been discussed. The nature of knowledge and conceptual models was examined and related to stoma care nursing.

An implication within this chapter is that stoma care nurses could examine their knowledge and make explicit their subjective knowing. Subjective knowing that has been made explicit can be developed into a theory which can then become knowledge for the discipline.

REFERENCES

Belenky, M., Clinchy, B., Goldberger, N. and Tarule, J. (1986) *Women's Ways of Knowing: The Development of Self, Voice, and Mind*. Basic Books: New York.

Benner, P. (1984) *From Novice to Expert: Excellence and Power in Clinical Nursing Practice*. Addison Wesley: Menlo Park CA.

Benner, P. and Tanner, C. (1987) Clinical judgment: how expert nurses use intuition. *American Journal of Nursing*, **87** (1): 23–31.

Carper, B. (1978) Fundamental patterns of knowing in nursing. *Advances in Nursing Science*, **1** (1): 13–23.

Chapman, J. (1991) Research – What it is and what it is not. In: Perry, A. and Jolley, M. (Eds) *Nursing: A Knowledge Base for Practice*. Edward Arnold: London.

Chin, R. (1980) The utility of systems models and developmental models for practitioners. In: Riehl, J. and Roy, C. (Eds) *Conceptual Models for Nursing Practice*, 2nd edn. Appleton-Century-Crofts: New York.

Chinn, P. and Jacobs, M. (1987) *Theory and Nursing: A Systematic Approach*, 2nd edn. C. V. Mosby: St Louis.

Chinn, P. and Kramer, M. (1991) *Theory and Nursing: A Systematic Approach*, 3rd edn. Mosby-Year Book: London.

Cox, C. and McVey, M. (1994) *The Saint Mark's Model of Nursing: Communication–Care–Consideration. Unpublished paper. St Mark's Hospital: London.*

Cuff, E. and Payne, G. (1984) *Perspectives in Sociology*, 2nd edn. Allen & Unwin: Hemel Hempstead.

Cull-Wilby, B. and Peppin, J. (1987) Towards a co-existence of paradigms in nursing knowledge development. *Journal of Advanced Nursing*, **12** (4): 515–21.

Donaldson, S. and Crowley, P. (1978) The discipline of nursing. *Nursing Outlook*, **26** (2): 113–20.

Fawcett, J. (1984) *Analysis and Evaluation of Conceptual Models of Nursing*. F. A. Davis: Philadelphia.

Fawcett, J. (1989) *Analysis and Evaluation of Conceptual Models of Nursing*, 2nd edn. F. A. Davis: Philadelphia.

Fawcett, J. (1993) *Analysis and Evaluation of Nursing Theories*. F. A. Davis: Philadelphia.

Fawcett, J. and Downs, F. (1992) *The Relationship of Theory and Research*, 2nd edn. F. A. Davis: Philadelphia.

Fitzpatrick, J. and Whall, A. (1989) *Conceptual Models of Nursing: Analysis and Application*, 2nd edn. Appleton and Lange: San Mateo CA.

Hardy, L. (1990) The path to nursing knowledge – personal reflection. *Nurse Education Today*, **10** (5): 352–32.

Johnson, D. (1968) Professional practice and specialization in nursing. *IMAGE: The Journal of Nursing Scholarship*, **2** (3): 2–7.

King, I. (1981) *A Theory for Nursing: Systems, Concepts, Process*. Delmar: New York.

Leddy, S. and Pepper, J. (1989) Patterns of knowing and nursing science. In: Leddy, S. and Pepper, J. (Eds) *Conceptual Bases of Professional*

Nursing, 2nd edn. J. B. Lippincott: Philadelphia and London.

Lewis, F. and Batey, M. (1982) Clarifying autonomy and accountability in nursing service, Part II. *Journal of Nursing Administration*, **12** (10): 10–15.

Manley, K. (1991) Knowledge for nursing practice. In: Perry, A. and Jolley, M. (Eds) *Nursing: A Knowledge Base for Practice*. Edward Arnold: London.

McFarlane, J. (1977) Developing a theory of nursing: the relation of theory to practice, education and research. *Journal of Advanced Nursing*, **2** (3): 261–70.

Meleis, A. (1985) *Theoretical Nursing: Development and Progress*. J. B. Lippincott: Philadelphia and London.

Meleis, A. (1986) Theory development and domain concepts. In: Moccia, P. (Ed.) *New Approaches to Theory Development*. National League for Nursing: New York.

Meleis, A. (1991) *Theoretical Nursing: Development and Progress*, 2nd edn. J. B. Lippincott: Philadelphia and London.

Merton, R. (1957) *Social Theory and Social Structure*, revised edition. Free Press: New York.

Minshull, J., Ross, K. and Turner, J. (1986) The human needs model of nursing. *Journal of Advanced Nursing*, **11** (6): 643–9.

Moody, L. (1990) *Advancing Nursing Science Through Research*, vol. 1. Sage Publications: Newbury Park CA.

Nightingale, F. (1859) *Notes on Nursing: What it is and what it is not*. Reprinted 1970. Duckworth: London.

Oakley, A. (1984) The importance of being a nurse. *Nursing Times*, **80** (50): 24–7.

Orem, D. (1991) *Nursing: Concepts of Practice*, 4th edn. Mosby-Year Book: London.

Pearson, A. and Vaughn, B. (1990) *Nursing Models for Practice*. Butterworth-Heinemann: Oxford.

Polyani, M. (1958) *Personal Knowledge*. University of Chicago Press: Chicago.

Riehl, J. and Roy, C. (1980) Theory and models. In: Riehl, J. and Roy, C. (Eds) *Conceptual Models for Nursing Practice*, 2nd edn. Appleton-Century-Crofts: New York.

Roper, N., Logan, W. and Tierney, A. (1983) *Using a Model for Nursing*. Churchill Livingstone: Edinburgh.

Roy, C. and Andrews, H. (1986) *The Roy Adaptation Model*. Appleton and Lange: San Mateo CA.

Sarter, B. (1988) Philosophical sources of nursing theory. *Nursing Science Quarterly*, **1** (2): 52–9.

Schon, D. (1983) *The Reflective Practitioner*. Basic Books: New York.

Suppe, F. and Jacox, A. (1985) Philosophy of science and the development of nursing theory. *Annual Review of Nursing Research*, **3**: 241–67.

Travelbee, J. (1971) *Interpersonal Aspects of Nursing*, 2nd edn. F. A. Davis: Philadelphia.

UKCC (1992a) *Code of Professional Conduct*. United Kingdom Central Council for Nursing, Midwifery and Health Visiting: London.

UKCC (1992b) *The Scope of Professional Practice*. United Kingdom

Central Council for Nursing, Midwifery and Health Visiting: London.

UKCC (1994) *Standards for Education and Practice Following Registration*. United Kingdom Central Council for Nursing, Midwifery and Health Visiting: London.

Visintainer, M. (1986) The nature of knowledge and theory in nursing. *Image*, **18**, (2): 32–8.

Walker, L. and Avant, K. (1988) *Strategies for Theory Construction in Nursing*, 2nd edn. Appleton and Lange: Norwalk.

Walsh, M. and Ford, D. (1990) *Nursing Rituals. Research and Research Actions*. Butterworth-Heinemann: Oxford.

Watson, J. (1985) *Nursing: Human Science and Human Care*. Appleton-Century-Crofts: Norwalk.

Yura, H. and Walsh, M. (1978) *The Nursing Process*, 3rd edn. Appleton-Century-Crofts: New York.

15 The St Mark's Model of Nursing: communication–care– consideration

Carol L. Cox and Maxine L.V.-T. McVey

INTRODUCTION

This chapter introduces the stoma care nurse to the definitive text on the St Mark's Model for clinical nursing practice. The model is interactive in nature because of its emphasis on social acts and relationships, perception, communication, role and self-concept. It is consistent with current perspectives in stoma care nursing. Key concepts within the model are described and substantive nursing knowledge for clinical practice is identified. Although nursing models have proliferated in the past 30 years, a model for stoma care nursing has not been developed that addresses current practice. Within the St Mark's Model, the philosophical, theoretical and conceptual bases for stoma care nursing are articulated, with the aim of influencing practice, education and research.

Within the model, a nursing process approach forms the basis for clinical judgements, the advantage being a unifying presentation of knowledge within the model which is congruent with current nursing approaches to care. This chapter begins by addressing the roots of models and theories and the research that was undertaken to develop the model. The chapter then outlines the model and gives a reflective example of how the model may be used in stoma care nursing.

Conceptual models and theories of nursing have their roots in the writings of nurse theorists from the 1950s and 1960s. Since then, conceptual models and their inherent theories have formed the foundation for nursing practice, education and research. Nursing models are conceptual descriptions of nursing based on scientific and philosophical assumptions about nursing (Andrews and Roy 1991). Generally, nursing models derive their roots from the writings of philosophers and historians and incorporate the nurse theorist's view of the nature of nursing and nursing's relation to the patient, health and the environment. Nurse theorists identify the beliefs, values and knowledge on which they base the perspective of their models. In the St Mark's Model the assumptions are based on nursing research conducted at the St Mark's Hospital, which was initiated in July 1991 by nurses at the hospital and a nurse teacher from the St Bartholomew and Princess Alexandra and Newham College of Nursing and Midwifery. Subsequently the philosophy is based on the humanistic perspectives of the nurses.

BACKGROUND

The St Mark's Conceptual Model of Nursing is a formal written representation of the staff nurses' image of nursing. It is an approximation of reality as nursing is practised and therefore includes only those concepts that are considered to be relevant to act as an aid to understanding. A conceptual model is a unique combination of concepts and presents a distinctive perspective for the phenomena of interest to a discipline (Fawcett 1989; Lippitt 1973; Reilly 1975). Nurse scholars such as Fawcett (1989, 1993), Meleis (1991) and Stevens-Barnum (1990) have postulated that it is not unusual for more than one discipline to be interested in the same or similar concepts as nursing. It is possible for a conceptual model to be developed in such a way as to reflect a multi-disciplinary view (Neuman 1989). In view of the changing face of health care into the twenty-first century the St Mark's Model has been developed to reflect a multi-disciplinary perspective to enable a team approach to the provision of care.

A conceptual model is defined by its set of concepts and assumptions, which integrate them into a meaningful whole (Fawcett 1995; Lippitt 1973; Nye and Bernardo 1981). Concepts and assumptions addressed within a conceptual model are broad, abstract and general (Fawcett 1989). Through breadth and abstraction the model can be used in a variety of nursing care settings (Fitzpatrick and Whall 1989). Unlike middle range theory which can be tested through research, or practice theory which prescribes how nursing care is provided, a conceptual model describes beliefs about nursing, the person, health and environment, and broadly lays the foundation for the implementation of the nursing process.

The perspective unique to the St Mark's Model is how the metaparadigm of nursing, person, health and environment has been specified. By describing the model, the values and beliefs underpinning nursing care are expressed. At conceptual model level, the foundation for a shared view of nursing is articulated, as well as methods of integrating its philosophical perspective into practice theories that delineate the provision of care.

The model is underpinned by the values and beliefs given in the Patient's Charter (1993) and the assumption that health care, and most specifically nursing care, is the right of all people. The model is classified as interactional because of its emphasis on communication and on the provision of care that involves some form of interaction between individuals. Also included is the social context in which care is provided, how it is provided and the relationship of the nurse to the patient and his or her family and others. How patients and their families and others perceive themselves is an outcome of the experience at St Mark's Hospital. Nurses play a major role in this experience.

DEVELOPMENT OF THE MODEL

A nursing model for guiding care at St Mark's Hospital had been in use for almost a decade. A problem-solving exercise identified that the model was not substantially influencing practice. In order to identify a conceptual model that would influence nursing practice, a working party, consisting of nursing staff and colleagues involved in direct contact with patients and their families, was formed. The remit of the working party was to review models of nursing care used to guide practice and to make informed decisions about a nursing model that would be appropriate for the requirements of nursing patients at St Mark's. Because expert advice was needed, a nurse teacher from the College of Nursing and Midwifery was invited to guide the working party as it began the difficult task of examining nursing models of care, in order to find one that would enhance patient care and would include a collaborative approach to caring. It was necessary to state the characteristics and specific needs of patients and to identify what nurses valued and believed about nursing care. A philosophy of nursing required articulation.

The working party recognized that all nurses would have to be involved so that the philosophy would be an accurate representation of the nursing staff's values and beliefs. Over several months the working party met and examined their values and beliefs about nursing. Staff nurse participation in the working party was rotated so that as many nurses as possible were involved in this process. After the philosophy had been determined, the process of examining conceptual models of nursing began. Eleven conceptual models and theories were examined, and it became clear that they did not completely fulfil the philosophy of nursing articulated by the nurses. The working party realized that extensive resocialization of nurses' views, their language and nursing practice would be required to use some of the models. It also felt that some nurses would not support the models because of their complex language and philosophical perspectives. Acknowledging the considerable commitment and time required, the working party decided to develop a model specifically for practice at St Mark's Hospital. The rationale was that the model:

1. Would be developed by and used by practising nurses;
2. Would be rooted in and determined by nursing practice;
3. Would be articulated in language that would be accessible to all those who chose to have it influence their practice;
4. Would focus on the patient and nurse as well as health, culture, society and environment.

Once the decision was made to develop a nursing conceptual model for St Mark's, the working party recognized that patients should be involved in the development of the model in order to determine whether nursing practice reflected the nursing philosophy from the patients' point of view. Patients selected to participate had to have at least two previous admissions to the hospital and should not have undergone major surgery within the last four weeks. The patients needed to be drawn from similar demographic backgrounds and be geographically bound to the London area. From a review of patient records, 41 patients were invited to participate in the project. Six patients replied and four became involved in the early stages of the model's development.

A pilot questionnaire was devised from the philosophy and given to the four patients who agreed to be part of the working party. Analysis of their written responses was undertaken by staff nurses, and then the patients were interviewed to obtain clarification of their views. Following a review of the questionnaire and redevelopment, an open-ended format of the questionnaire was posted to the remaining 35 patients; 15 patients replied, a response rate of 42%.

Postal questionnaires tend to have a low completion and return rate (Polit and Hungler 1991). When only a small number of questionnaires are returned from the overall number posted, it may be inappropriate to assume that the responses obtained represent the perspective of the entire population. To guard against this situation, the precaution was taken to ensure that the population who received the postal questionnaire were similar in terms of basic demographics. According to Polit and Hungler (1991), taking this precaution can lead to the conclusion that the respondents and non-respondents are similar enough in their views to be considered homogeneous. This precludes bias in the findings. Content analysis, as described by Burnard (1991), was completed on the returned questionnaires. The involvement of patients gave insight into nursing care and confirmed the philosophical perspective that would form the foundation of the model.

The findings from the patients' questionnaire were circulated to the nursing staff. Ward staff meetings were held to discuss the findings and to clarify issues that were raised. Notes of the discussions were taken and then content analysis of the notes, as described by Burnard (1991), was performed by the working party. Emerging themes were grouped into six categories: compassion, comforting, responsiveness, supportiveness, attentiveness and competence. Further analysis and classification yielded three key constructs: communication, care and consideration (Table 15.1).

After the constructs had been identified, another questionnaire was developed and circulated to nursing staff. Its purpose was to determine how the nurses defined nursing, person, health and environment, and whether the key constructs would be reflected in their responses. The responses, in which communication, care and consideration were evident, were analysed using Burnard's (1991) process. From the analysis, assumptions about nursing care were identified and definitions for nursing, person, health and environment were developed. The definitions were sent to all nursing staff and discussed in staff meetings. Agreement on definitions was obtained in the autumn of 1993.

In the final stages of developing the model, the definitions, written by the nursing staff, were compared with the philosophy and the responses initially obtained from the patients. The similarities were remarkable. From this comparative process, final definitions and assumptions were developed that reflect the three key constructs and the underlying characteristics of nursing care at St Mark's Hospital. In the model, the constructs form the foundation for relational statements that are used in describing the nursing process.

As already mentioned in this chapter, conceptual models are broad, abstract and general (Fawcett 1989). Inherent within conceptual models are a philosophy, definitions for the metaparadigm of nursing, person, health and environment, linking statements which incorporate aspects of the metaparadigm, the nursing process and assumptions. The philo-

Table 15.1 The three main constructs in the model and their characteristics

COMMUNICATION–CARE–CONSIDERATION

Responsive	**Supportive**	**Competence**
Amenable	Reassuring	Professional
Friendly	Encouragement	Experienced
Co-operative	Comfort	Expert
Warm	Helpfulness	Learned/Knowledge
Welcoming	Well-being	Specialist
Open	Considerate	Skilled
Manageable	Familiarity	Capable
	Sympathetic	Trust
	Understanding	Information giving
	Sensitive	Education (advocacy); how we do it
	Intimacy	
	Knowledge	
	Awareness	
	Assisting	

Comforting	**Compassion**	**Attentive**
Calm	Understanding	Considerate
Solace	Empathy	Courteous
Peace	Sympathy	Listening
Quiet	Warmth	Respectful (privacy/dignity)
Tranquillity		Guidance
Touch		

sophical perspective is underpinned by a theoretical perspective about health and health promotion. The three constructs of communication, care and consideration are underpinned by further concepts which are responsiveness, supportiveness, competence, comforting, compassion and attentiveness. The six concepts reflect characteristics of the nurse and the nurse's practice. Assumptions upon which theories can be developed and tested and upon which nursing standards for care are based are also articulated in the model.

The St Mark's Model

Philosophy

Three care constructs underpin nursing at St Mark's: communication, care and consideration (Fig. 15.1). Nurses consider each patient holistically and regard the patient as an individual who has a set of unique relationships and coping strategies. St Mark's nursing care involves a continuing partnership with the patient that often extends beyond a single admission. Nursing is dynamic; it is reflective, responsive and progressive in its approach to caring. Communication with and on behalf of patients is an integral part of nursing at St Mark's. Nursing is not practised in isolation but in collaboration with colleagues from other disciplines for the benefit of the patients. Nursing acknowledges environmental factors and appreciates the customs, values and beliefs of the individual in achieving health. St Mark's nurses, within the caring environment, enable patients to achieve their full potential of health and well-being.

Theoretical perspective

Nurses promote health through prevention, protection and education measures to help patients develop the ability, where possible, to manage their own health. Health promotion is central to nursing care. As such, health promotion activity managed under the direction of the nurse facilitates the development of coping strategies in response to changes in health experienced by patients.

The metaparadigm

Nursing is an art, compassionate, responsive and comforting. It is also a science of caring through the nursing process. It is a profession that combines art and science in the process of health recovery and promotion. Health promotion is directed towards patients and their families. Through prevention, protection and educational measures, nurses help patients develop an understanding of their health and the ability to manage their health. Nurses facilitate the formal and informal decision making process by acting as a resource, encouraging patients to look after their health.

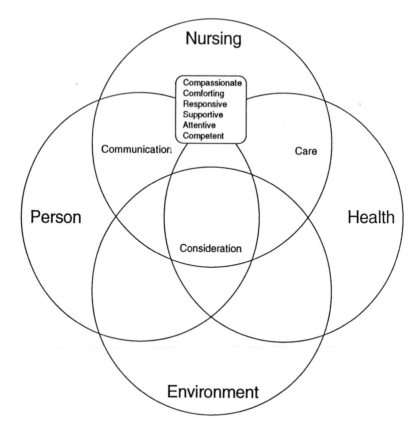

Fig. 15.1 St Mark's model of nursing.

This may or may not involve the family. Nurses create a safe and thera-peutic environment, caring for patients while they adapt to changes in their health. Nurses are considerate and competent, as demonstrated in their caring activities through use and application of knowledge derived from education, research and experience. Nurses facilitate communication between the various disciplines and act as advocates for the patients.

The person is an individual with a unique set of traits and characteris-tics, subscribing to a personal set of customs, values and beliefs. People have the right to take responsibility for their own lives. People are social beings who experience different degrees of social interaction and contact. Feelings are personal to each individual. In various states of health peo-ple adopt different roles and at times may feel vulnerable. It is within the context of various states of health that people require nursing care.

Health is dynamic, a balance of physical, psychological, environmental and social aspects. It is a perception of relative well-being defined by the person, generated or modified by social and personal perceptions. Health is the individual belief of a person's physiological and psychosocial state. People may experience a sense of well-being when they are content with their social and psychological functions, and may or may not be healthy.

Environment is all factors that influence people in their thinking and behaviour. Nursing care is provided in an environment that is responsive to a person's health requirements. Environmental factors have an impact on health, and on a person's perception of his or her health, and requirements for supportive nursing care.

Assumptions

1. Nursing is compassionate, comforting, responsive, supportive, attentive and competent. These attributes of nursing are demonstrated through communication, caring actions and consideration.
2. Nurses promote health through prevention, protection and education measures to help patients develop the ability, where possible, to manage their own health.
3. Nurses create a safe and therapeutic caring environment to facilitate the development of coping strategies by the patient.
4. The patient has a unique set of traits and characteristics and subscribes to a personal set of customs, beliefs and values, which influence the patient's health.
5. The patient is a social being with feelings unique to the individual. These feelings influence social interaction and contact with others.
6. In different states of health, patients adopt different roles and at times may feel vulnerable.
7. Health is dynamic and is defined by the patient in terms of well-being or illness based on that patient's perceptions.
8. Health is a balance of physical, psychological, environmental and social aspects.
9. The environment encompasses all factors that influence the patient in his or her thinking and behaviour. Therefore factors in the environment influence a patient's health and can be manipulated by the nurse for the purpose of achieving health.

THE NURSING PROCESS

The nursing process, which forms an integral component of the St Mark's Nursing Conceptual Model, comprises five phases which centre on communication, care and consideration. The phases, which are ongoing, include a holistic assessment of the patient's condition and concerns expressed by the patient about his or her health, formulation of a nursing opinion regarding the patient's condition and concerns (actual or potential), determination of the care required (including who will carry it out), provision of care and evaluation of the outcome of care. Evaluation of the outcome of care is evident in the patient's actual condition as well as in the patient's subjective comments regarding his or her perceptions about the outcome of care. Nurses show aspects of caring and consideration in how the nursing process is used in practice and communicated through documentation of the provision of care. The nursing process phases are:

1. Assessment
2. Formulation of a nursing opinion
3. The planning of nursing care delivery
4. The provision of nursing care
5. Evaluation of the outcome of care.

The nursing process forms the basis for clinical judgements which culminate in the provision and evaluation of care.

Communication forms the linchpin for assessment. Communication may be verbal, non-verbal or written and is evident through a system of symbols, signs and behaviour. The nurse formulates a nursing opinion based on how the patient communicates, through verbal, non-verbal and written language, his or her health care abilities and difficulties. Non-verbal communication is evident in the patient's social acts and how the patient relates to others. The focus in communication is on the identification of actual and potential problems perceived by the patient as well as objective findings obtained in collaboration with members of the health care team. The patient's relationships with others may influence the patient's perception of health and self. These relationships are identified through conversation with the patient and others as well as observation. By identifying actual and potential problems, a plan of care can be developed and care given that promotes health and the patient's perception of well-being.

Communication is important in conveying knowledge to the patients about how to care for themselves. It is important in learning roles that shape behaviour and the ability to care for oneself. Patients' perceptions of their ability to care for themselves are derived from social interations with the nurse and others. Patients may adopt appropriate health care behaviours according to how caring behaviour is communicated.

Caring takes place in the action of nursing. Nurses show interest in the individual and concern through individualized care that addresses each patient outcome. Nursing is centred on the premise that a concerted effort on the part of the nurse must be taken to help the patient. Care is given with the intent of facilitating recovery and/or the development of the patient's coping mechanisms, based on the patient's health care situation. The provision of care is substantial and requires the collaborative efforts of all members of the health care team. Caring activities are based on the status of the patient's health, the health care plan developed for the patient and the patient's present abilities to engage in care or to fully care for himself or herself.

Consideration evolves from the caring nature of nursing. Nurses give continuous careful thought about the process of care that is delivered to patients. The special interests of the patient, the family and others are considered by the nurse while continuous therapeutic actions are provided. Within this construct, the nurse considers the social context of the situation and the patient's cultural background. Therefore, through consideration, the nursing process becomes ongoing, the basis for action and research and the inducement for evaluation of care that has been given.

COMMUNICATION–CARE–CONSIDERATION

This section reflects on patient care that incorporates the St Mark's Model of Nursing. If the nurse chooses to use the St Mark's Model as the frame of reference for the provision of nursing care, the approach will be humanistic. The nurse will consider the patient holistically as a unique individual who subscribes to a personal set of customs, values and beliefs. The influence of the St Mark's Model is reflected in the following narrative.

Having worked within gastroenterological nursing for the majority of my qualified life it never ceases to amaze me how patients with drastic changes in their body image, such as formation of a stoma, develop coping strategies. Each patient requires nursing support tailored to his or her individual perceptions and health care situation.

I received the following information from midday handover. Mrs Patel was a 56-year-old lady who was seven days postoperative following formation of a colostomy for cancer of the rectum and sigmoid colon. Apparently Mrs Patel was making a 'good' postoperative recovery. She was coping well with her stoma and was virtually self-caring within this role. Her output from the stoma was liquid and she was using drainable bags. Mrs Patel had a very large extended family and, from report, it seemed that her family was very supportive. Mrs Patel was a vegetarian and the family was bringing in food to supplement her Halal diet.

After the report, as I was caring for Mrs Patel, I approached the bed area with the staff nurse from the early shift to meet Mrs Patel and assess her nursing care requirements with her. Mrs Patel introduced herself as 'Kamil' and appeared very much in control. Her bed area was surrounded by flowers and cards. I asked Kamil how she was coping. Kamil replied 'fine'. Her family was 'very grateful for all her care ... the doctors ... the nurses' – she was 'all right'. Somehow Kamil's words did not ring true to me, and although I hardly knew Kamil I knew she required my support.

Later in the shift I noticed that Kamil had gone to the bathroom with her stoma supplies. I deliberately followed and knocked on the bathroom door to offer assistance. I asked if she would like me to help her in any way. When Kamil opened the bathroom door I could see from the expression on her face she was starting to cry. I moved toward her and held her as she cried. Kamil started to apologize saying that she could not face the future. She hated the stoma. Her family had been so good, but what good was she? Kamil 'could no longer prepare the family meals'. She was 'unclean'. Kamil had always been the one who coped within the family. The sight and smell of the stoma sickened her. I listened as she poured out her feelings. Eventually the tears stopped and I emptied the bag for her and reassured her that these feelings are often experienced by people after a stoma is formed. Kamil was not 'unclean'.

We discussed ways in which Kamil could care for herself and what the change meant to her. We talked about foods that cause smells and I promised to get her some information about foods that do and do not cause wind and unpleasant smells. Kamil thanked me and said she did not realize how much she needed to express her feelings. This situation alerted me to inform the team so that they could also help Kamil during this difficult time. The team could plan to spend time with Kamil setting goals and planning strategies that would help Kamil to care for herself satisfactorily following discharge home to her family environment.

This reflection illustrates a nurse's concern regarding a patient's perception of herself and her health. Through effective communication, caring and consideration, aspects of being responsive, supportive, attentive, comforting, compassionate and competent were made evident as characteristics of the nurse and nursing. Attention to the patient's behaviour provided the nurse with an opportunity to assess and identify actual problems requiring intervention so that the patient could develop new health care behaviours and perceptions of self prior to discharge.

SUMMARY

There is a relation between a nursing conceptual model and theory that influences practice. Middle range theory, which can be tested through research, evolves from the broad, abstract and general nature of a conceptual model. Practice theory, which is prescribed by the nurse, evolves from middle range theory. A conceptual model lays the foundations for nursing care delivery. It does not prescribe how nurses will provide care. The St Mark's model provides the philosophical underpinning for care by describing the values and beliefs of St Mark's nurses. From the values, beliefs and assumptions within the model, St Mark's nurses plan and deliver nursing care. By all nurses sharing the values and beliefs described in the model, and testing the assumptions that underpin nursing practice, outcomes of care can be more clearly identified and measured, and consequently nursing care can improve. Through continual deliberative application and testing, standards are developed and revised for the benefit of the patients, their families and others.

KEY POINTS

- A conceptual model is a unique combination of concepts that presents a distinct perspective about nursing.
- The St Mark's model of nursing includes a philosophy that acts as a frame of reference for guiding nursing practice.
- Three care constructs underpin the model: communication, care and consideration.
- Nursing is not practised in isolation but in collaboration with colleagues from other disciplines for the benefit of the patient.
- Nursing acknowledges environmental factors and appreciates the customs, values and beliefs of the individual in achieving health.
- Nurses promote health through prevention, protection and education measures to help patients develop the ability, where possible, to manage their own health.
- Nurses create a safe and therapeutic caring environment to facilitate the development of coping strategies by the patient.

REFERENCES

Andrews, H. and Roy, C. (1991) *The Roy Adaptation Model: The Definitive Statement.* Appleton and Lange: Norwalk.

Burnard, P. (1991) A method of analysing interview transcripts in qualitative research. *Nurse Education Today*, **11**: 461–6.

Fawcett, J. (1989) *Analysis and Evaluation of Conceptual Models of Nursing*, 2nd edn. F.A. Davis: Philadelphia.

Fawcett, J. (1993) *Analysis and Evaluation of Nursing Theories.* F.A. Davis: Philadelphia.

Fawcett, J. (1995) *Analysis and Evaluation of Conceptual Models of Nursing*, 3rd edn. F.A. Davis: Philadelphia.

Fitzpatrick, J. and Whall, A. (1989) *Conceptual Models of Nursing Analysis and Application*, 2nd edn. Appleton and Lange: San Mateo CA.

Lippitt, G. (1973) *Visualizing Change. Model Building and the Change Process.* NTL Learning Resources: Fairfax.

Meleis, A. (1991) *Theoretical Nursing: Development and Progress.* J. B. Lippincott: Philadelphia and London.

Neuman, B. (1989) *The Neuman Systems Model*, 2nd edn. Appleton and Lange: San Mateo CA.

Nye, F. and Bernardo, F. (1981) *Emerging Conceptual Frameworks in Family Analysis.* Macmillan: New York.

Patient's Charter (1993) HMSO: London.

Polit, D. and Hungler, B. (1991) *Nursing Research Principles and Methods*, 4th edn. J. B. Lippincott: Philadelphia and London.

Reilly, D. (1975) Why a conceptual framework? *Nursing Outlook*, **23**: 566–9.

Stevens-Barnum, B. (1990) *Nursing Theory: Analysis, Application Evaluation,* 3rd edn. Little, Brown: Boston.

16 The work of the Family Cancer Clinic

Christina Harocopos

INTRODUCTION

The lifetime risk of death from colorectal cancer in England and Wales is about 1 : 50, rapidly increasing with age from 50 years (Fig. 16.1). It is the second commonest cause of death from malignant disease in western Europe, but the general public remain relatively unaware of the effect the disease has on morbidity and mortality in the community. It has been observed for many years that certain individuals with a family history of colorectal cancer may be at higher risk than others. Familial adenomatous polyposis has been recognized as an autosomal dominant condition characterized by the occurrence of multiple adenomas in the gastrointestinal tract. These polyps have considerable potential for malignant transformation: the gene responsible (*APC*) has recently been identified and other families with family aggregate of colorectal cancer have been recognized.

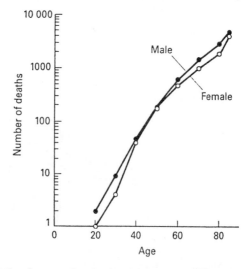

Fig. 16.1 Deaths from colorectal cancer per million population. (OPCS, England and Wales; reproduced by permission of the Controller, HMSO)

There is considerable evidence to support a contribution of genetic factors in the aetiology of colorectal cancer. Family studies in colorectal cancer have demonstrated an increased risk of colorectal cancer in first-degree relatives of between two and four times compared with the general population (Woolfe 1958; Mecklin 1960; Lynch et al. 1988). In 1974 Dr E. Lovett reported on studies carried out at St Mark's Hospital. Family histories were investigated on all patients admitted to the hospital with a diagnosis relating to the colon or rectum, and it was observed that, over all, the incidence of colorectal cancer in first-degree relatives exceeded the expected incidence in the population by a factor of three. The paper concluded: 'If we are to identify the individuals liable to develop carcinoma of the large bowel and examine them regularly, the mortality and morbidity of the disease will be reduced' (Lovett 1974). However, it was not until 1986 that a Family Cancer Clinic opened in the UK.

The Imperial Cancer Research Fund had long wanted to make a contribution towards cancer prevention. Dr Joan Slack, a clinical geneticist from the NE Thames Regional Genetics Service, in consultation with Mr John Northover, director of the ICRF Colorectal Cancer Unit at St Mark's Hospital, suggested setting up a clinic at St Mark's. The purpose of the clinic was to identify patients known through the family history to be at an increased risk of developing colon cancer and other dominantly inherited syndromes associated with colorectal cancer and to offer appropriate screening.

It is now well established that a colorectal carcinoma is commonly preceded by an adenoma (Fig. 16.2). The hypothesis of the adenoma–carcinoma sequence (Morson 1974) offers an opportunity for early diagnosis and treatment if polyps can be identified (Houlston et al. 1990).

Benign polyp   Malignant polyp   Carcinoma

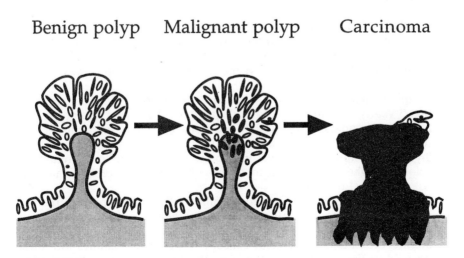

Fig. 16.2 The adenoma–carcinoma sequence.

METHODS

Risks to relatives of patients developing colorectal cancer at different ages were estimated from Lovett's pedigrees of families, ascertained through a consecutive series of patients with colorectal cancer, by life table methods (Table 16.1) (Houlston et al. 1990).

Practical policies were devised for screening individuals (Murday 1989). Patients with a risk of less than 1 in 10 would be screened by annual faecal occult blood testing, and patients with a higher risk would be offered colonoscopy. Mecklin and Jarvinen (1986) had shown that the large bowel lesions in high-risk families were mainly right sided, only 26% being within the reach of the rigid sigmoidoscope (Lynch et al. 1985). Colonoscopy allowed inspection of the proximal bowel: adenomas found at the time of screening were removed.

Table 16.1 Lifetime risks of colorectal cancer in first-degree relatives based on the Lovett series

Population risk	1 in 50
One relative affected	1 in 17
One first-degree relative and one second-degree relative	1 in 12
One relative < 45 years	1 in 10
Two first-degree relatives	1 in 6
Dominant pedigree	1 in 2

From Houlston et al. (1990), with permission.

AGE AT SCREENING

Familial colon cancer occurs earlier than in the general population (Mecklin and Jarvinen 1986) and the decision was made to start screening at 25 years. Because most of the at-risk individuals will have developed polyps by the age of 65 years, colonoscopy screening was stopped at this age (Fig. 16.3).

Follow-up adenoma studies (Williams and Macrae 1986) had suggested that 3-yearly examinations were adequate for those who had polyps and 5-yearly examinations for those found to have a 'clean' colon on the first screening. Patients already affected with colon cancers would be offered 3-yearly screening by whatever method was appropriate to the remaining colon. A higher incidence of metachronous tumours is reported in high-risk families (Lovett 1974).

It was also noted that, in some families with Lynch type II hereditary non-polyposis colorectal cancer (HNPCC), there is a high risk of certain cancers other than colon cancer. There seemed to be an increased risk of uterine, breast and extracolonic cancers. Women from families with these types of pedigree would be offered additional screening for breast, uterine and ovarian cancers (Houlston et al. 1990).

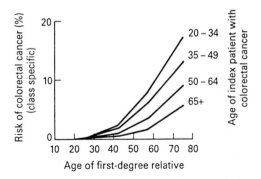

Fig. 16.3 Actual risk of colorectal cancer with increasing age in first-degree relatives of patients with colorectal cancer. (From R. Houlston, 1992, PhD thesis)

THE FAMILY CANCER CLINIC

The Family Cancer Clinic was opened in 1986 with an announcement in the press by the Imperial Cancer Research Fund. Guidance was given that screening was available for first-degree relatives of patients who had developed colorectal cancer before the age of 45 and members of families in which multiple cancers had occurred (Houlston et al. 1990). Patients attending the clinic either referred themselves because of information they received from the media, relatives or friends or were referred by GPs or hospital consultants (Table 16.2).

The purpose of the clinic was to identify patients at an increased risk of developing colon cancer and other dominantly inherited syndromes associated with it, and to offer screening appropriate to the recognized risks. Although it is possible, for research purposes, to identify individuals with germline mutations of colon cancer, diagnosis in the clinic must currently be achieved on the basis of family history alone.

There had been awareness that further anxiety and distress might be aroused in the families by discussing numerical risks and confronting the possibilities of malignancy. However, reactions have been assessed

Table 16.2 Source of referrals to the family cancer clinic

Referral	No.
Self	362
Patient via general practitioner	64
General practitioner	159
Hospital consultant	120
Other (screening programmes)	10
Total	715

From Houlston et al. (1990), with permission.

following consultations, while organizing appointments for screening, after colonoscopy and in home visits. Although no statistical analysis has been attempted, there has been a clear impression that this group of patients has been relieved to discuss the family risks of which they have usually been aware, and have derived support by undertaking a screening programme for which they have taken a personal responsibility.

Pedigree information

The first and probably the most important aspect of genetic counselling in the Family Cancer Clinic is constructing the family tree or pedigree. Symbols are used as shown in Fig. 16.4. The consultand is the individual through which the family is ascertained.

Because the family pedigree may be the only way of assessing risks and the need for screening, it is very important that the information obtained is accurate:

1. Record the date when the pedigree was taken.
2. Record dates of birth where possible as well as ages.
3. Record age and date of the onset of the cancer.
4. Take details of both sides of the family; not only does this include the whole family but may also produce findings that will add to the offspring's risk.

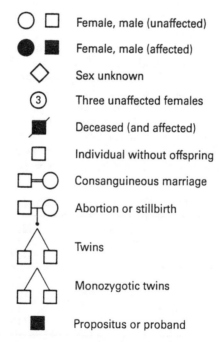

Fig. 16.4 Symbols used in drawing a pedigree.

5. Consanguinity should be asked about directly and recorded as well as miscarriages, stillbirths and early infant deaths. Documentary evidence of any significant diagnosis should be obtained wherever possible; this may come from hospital records or from death certificates, which patients are often able to supply.

Often, relatives are not sure in which site a cancer was diagnosed, and death certificates may not have recorded the fact, especially if the cancer had been removed many years previously. As much information should be obtained as possible – i.e the year of death, the address at which they were living, the hospital where they were treated – so that further information can be obtained from hospital records, if necessary.

The staff in the clinic should be aware of the possible psychological factors associated with attending for consultation, and the first contact may affect subsequent discussions and attendances. The site of the clinic is important: a non-clinical environment is ideal, in a pleasant room where, if necessary, many family members may be seen at the same time. Privacy is vital, with no distractions, both for family discussions and for examination of the individual; a properly screened couch should be available for a full clinical examination.

The patient at risk may recently have lost a family member from cancer or have a close relative who has recently had cancer diagnosed. Many of the patients may still be grieving or anxious about their own health. When discussing family events, unpleasant memories may arise and for many it may be the first time these have been discussed. Generous time should be allowed for each appointment: it is the experience of the clinic staff that patients appreciate an opportunity to express their fears and should be allowed to express their grief as well.

Genetic counselling

'It is not the duty of a doctor to order the lives of others, but to ensure that individuals have the facts to enable them to make their own decisions' (Harper 1992). This has been the principle on which the Family Cancer Clinic has been conducted.

Information, understanding and choice

The Family Cancer Clinic at St Mark's Hospital was set up as part of the Regional Genetic Service and adopted the format of a regional genetic counselling clinic. The subject of cancer in families can be difficult and worrying, yet it is important that the subject should be approached openly by patients, relatives and professionals alike. For this reason, it was decided to call the clinic 'The Family Cancer Clinic' in order to avoid any ambiguity or inhibitions about the diagnosis and the use of euphemisms among the participants in the clinic.

Patients came to the clinic by referrals from GPs and hospital consultants, but initially the majority of patients referred themselves because they had read or heard about the facilities in the media or through friends and relatives. This group of patients was exceptionally well motivated and seemed pleased to allow expression of their anxieties about their own risks and those of other family members. Many surviving relatives brought teenage children of the index patients, and their understanding of the problem impressed the counsellors and reassured us that free discussion was acceptable.

As in all genetic clinics, the diagnosis of the condition under discussion is of the greatest importance so attempts were made to verify the diagnosis of all family members. Families themselves are often able to gather important information from the extended families and the task gives them a helpful introduction to the subject among their most distant relatives. For example, see Pedigree 1.

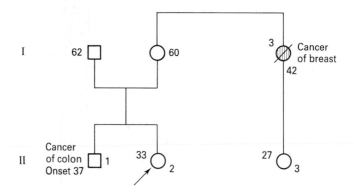

If Index Patient (IP) II.02 knows only about her brother II.01, her risk of colon cancer is 1 in 10 and screening would be offered; however, after discussion with her mother, who could also be offered screening, the information of premenopausal breast cancer in I.03 suggests the possibility of a diagnosis of Lynch type II and would indicate that breast and pelvic screening be offered to the female relatives at risk as well as colonoscopy. If I.02 is found to have colon cancer on screening, the international criteria for HNPCC are fulfilled and the family become an informative family for research with a chance of making an important contribution to DNA studies.

In the clinic's experience, patients are usually pleased to collaborate in genetic studies. Their contribution either can be by providing accurate information about the extent of the family and the diagnosis in relatives or can extend to allowing blood sampling from as many family members as possible. In this situation it is essential that all family members understand that it is unlikely that they themselves will benefit from this research in the immediate future. However, they will, as it were, fit a piece into the jigsaw puzzle and there is a real chance that they will contribute to the well-being of the next generation. It has been found that many families feel relieved and comforted by this.

After the pedigree has been examined, it is usually possible for the geneticist to assess the risk of cancer in the consultand. This can, and should, be explained in various ways: it is essential to make sure that the consultand understands the risks and how they have been estimated.

Risks

State in understandable form

The risks may be 10% for an event – and hence 90% chance against. This may be easily understood by '9 to 1 against' the event happening or '1 in 10' chance of the event happening. The converse risks often seem different to patients and these should be explained. Another way is to explain that the chance in the general population is 1 in 50 so that, if the chance is 1 in 10, there is five times the risk that everyone takes.

Answering the uninformed question

'Are my children likely to be affected?' is a common question. Discussion is often instigated concerning how to tell the children. Children like to be able to talk – to be given permission to talk. Adults also like to be 'allowed' to express their anxieties.

Model for a family cancer clinic (see Fig. 16.5)

This clinic was the first one of its kind to be set up in the UK and much has been learned over the last few years.

The general trend in community medicine is prevention rather than cure, and the population as a whole is now more aware of their health. This approach is particularly appropriate for cancer when the cure rate is not always satisfactory. Screening programmes have been set up to encourage people to protect their own health. A remarkable feature of the patients who referred themselves to the family cancer clinic was the accuracy with which they had estimated their risk (Houlston et al. 1990), but there are still many examples of health care where information is lacking and referrals are not being made.

Clinical assessment

When appointments are made, it is helpful to inform the patient of what is likely to take place and the type of information required. For this reason, the whole clinic team, including the receptionist and appointments clerk, should be knowledgeable about the clinic procedure.

In the clinic a pedigree will be compiled; if there is not enough information requests will be made for diagnosis in affected relatives to be verified before appropriate screening is recommended. A general clinical assessment will be made, including any skin abnormalities, and referrals made to specialist departments where necessary. In some cases the breasts,

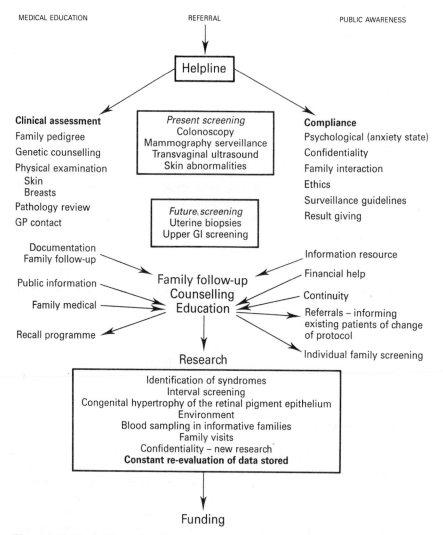

Fig. 16.5 Model for a family cancer clinic. (From Imperial Cancer Research Fund, Christina Harocopos, RGN)

thyroid and abdomen will also be examined. If any other worrying clinical feature is discussed not associated with the Family Cancer Clinic, a comment will be included in the letter to the GP. At the end of the initial interview, it is usually possible to give an estimate of the patient's risk of cancer, and time is given to explain the risk and to discuss the practicalities of a screening programme. Patients who are at relatively low risk or within the age limit are encouraged to take advantage of the national screening programmes. Further time is allowed for discussion of anxieties and the relevance of the information received to other members of the family.

Documentation following a patient's visit comprises:

- Letters to GP and patient
- Referral letters as necessary
- Pedigree categorization
- Pathology review
- Verification of diagnosis.

Risk estimate

Note that this can change as other information about the family becomes available.

Compliance

Of 606 patients, 545 (90%) took up the offer of screening, including examinations by colonoscopy, which involved time and discomfort (Houlston et al. 1990). Screening for population risk has reported much lower rates. Population compliance with Haemoccult screening is still a problem in the UK (Hardcastle and Pye 1989). Compliance among high-risk individuals is usually higher than among average-risk subjects because they may have greater insight regarding their risk and chances of benefit. It is possible that the excellent compliance rate achieved by the patients in the Family Cancer Clinic is due to the responsibility the patients themselves take for their own health care. It is therefore important that this group of patients is kept informed of any changes in screening, predictive tests and DNA diagnosis so that they may continue to take this responsibility for themselves and their families.

A helpline has evolved, as it became obvious from the beginning that patients wanted more information. Follow-up of patients and their families and encouragement in the long-term commitment to screening are essential. It has been stated that a badly informed patient is more likely to be an anxious patient. Ignorance, bad advice and neglect are more to be feared than the defective gene that patients carry (HNPCC newsletter 1992). The most frequent complaint among patients is that professional staff providing their care fail to give sufficient information about their condition or treatment (Marteau 1993).

One of the criticisms directed at the clinic was that discussing risks of cancer would cause psychological problems, cancer phobia and heightened anxiety in patients at risk. However, discussions with patients following genetic counselling and subsequent use of the helpline resulted in the majority of patients feeling reassured and more in control of the situation. They were pleased they had been taken seriously and been able to talk about their fears openly. One of their previous complaints had been the feeling of being dismissed and concern about disinformation from the media, relatives and medical staff.

The helpline as an information resource

Some patients may contact the clinic having had cancer or other problems but whose families are at no greater risk than the general population. These people are given contact numbers of other units who can offer the appropriate advice. Information is given about eating habits, the effects of smoking and sunlight; many of the women callers ask about the effect of HRT and the contraceptive pill in the higher risk families, and those staffing the helpline should be knowledgeable about these questions. If the answer is not known, a simple acknowledgement of 'I don't know but I will find out for you' is much more reassuring to an anxious patient than hedging about.

Criteria for a successful family cancer clinic

1. An ability to listen
2. An ability to impart honest, accurate information
3. Maintaining confidentiality
4. Excellent screening facilities
5. Prompt and efficient reporting of all results – positive or negative
6. Reliable recall system and follow-up
7. Long-term commitment

Family history offers an opportunity to identify those placed at high risk of colorectal, breast or ovarian cancer and to determine screening requirements. Furthermore, controlled screening in high-risk individuals may be more effective than population screening in ensuring the efficacy of screening programmes for the early detection of cancer (Houlston 1992).

Research and the clinic

At the present time there are no diagnositic genetic markers for HNPCC though linked gene markers may be available for informative familes. Patients should therefore be aware that screening of those at risk is the best that is available with the present information. Most patients are very pleased to make a contribution to research – indeed, this may be their best way of overcoming their own fears and anxieties – but it is important that they are told the relevant facts and the limitations of the screening procedure.

Constant re-evaluation of data stored is essential so that vital information is not overlooked, especially when families are geographically separated or perhaps attending different clinics. The information should not be looked at in isolation but with a team input of health professionals and scientists meeting regularly and pooling information. Collaborative studies have enabled important progress to be made in locating a single gene for breast cancer – the same success could come with collaboration between family cancer clinics in the field of colorectal cancer.

Funding

It would be unrealistic in the present state of the National Health Service not to mention finance. In the 'Health of the Nation' document published in 1991, cancer screening was given as one of the top priorities but as yet there is no extra funding available for screening the high-risk groups. Therefore the question of financing of the clinic and the screening facilities must be addressed before patients are promised a lifetime commitment: it is unethical to offer a goal that cannot be met.

APPENDIX I

Genetics and the Family Cancer Clinic

Some understanding of basic genetic principles is important for anyone involved in family cancer clinics.

Family cancer: genes and the environment

It could be said that most cancer is 'familial' in that most people with cancer will know someone else in their family who has cancer. This could be due to the fact that cancer affects 1 in 3 of the population and the shared environmental risk factors such as smoking or diet. Within families, however, it is becoming clear that shared genes are also important. In this situation, the environment may also be important, as exposure to a cancer-promoting agent may increase the risk in those inheriting an increased liability to cancer. In some families the inheritance of genes that predispose to cancer seems to be more important than any environmental exposure. In familial adenomatous polyposis (FAP), inheritance of a single abnormal gene among 100 000 results in a colon and rectum carpeted by thousands of benign polyps, one or more of which almost inevitably turns malignant (cancerous). Therefore FAP is said to be directly caused by the mutation in the one gene, now known as *APC*. In other familial cancer syndromes the causative gene has not yet been identified, though the gene for HNPCC has recently been located. However, it is known that the risk to members of families with several other syndromes is high and can be estimated fairly accurately (Marx 1993).

An introduction to the genetics of human diseases

Mendelian inheritance

Modern genetics began with the work of Gregor Mendel (1822–1884), an Augustinian monk in a monastery in what is now Brno, in the Czech Republic. Mendel was taken in at the monastery by the Abbot in order to study plant breeding. Mendel's work on peas showed that characteristics of peas (colour of petals, height of stems, smoothness of seeds, etc.) could be separated by breeding, and were therefore independent. These character variants are referred to as phenotypes and are determined by genes. Genes come in pairs, or versions, one derived from each parent. Mendel also showed that the two versions of the gene could be distinguished. This is because one may dominate the other in terms of which gene has its character expressed when they are both present in the pea. For example, when Mendel crossed pure-bred purple-petaled peas with white ones, only purple petals resulted in the next generation. Purple is therefore dominant to white and, conversely, white is recessive to purple.

Although human genetic traits cannot usually be observed as crosses as clearly as the way that Mendel saw the inheritance of plant characteristics, an analysis of matings that have already occurred can sometimes provide similar information. Pedigree analysis allows the identification of recessive and dominant phenotypes and lies at the centre of the work carried out in a family cancer clinic. Recessive conditions typically appear in the progeny of unaffected parents, and two affected individuals cannot have an unaffected child. Consanguineous matings (e.g. cousins) tend to reveal recessive conditions, for example cystic fibrosis. As shown in Tables 16.3 and 16.4, dominant disorders characteristically occur in every generation, showing 'vertical transmission'. Unaffected individuals cannot transmit except where 'penetrance' is incomplete (individuals have an abnormal gene but do not express it) and two affected parents can have unaffected offspring. However, new cases can appear as new mutations without any apparent family history. Diseases can be transmitted either by autosomal or sex chromosomes.

In both tables, the parental generation is shown in bold type. In Table 16.3 the gene version A is dominant to a, and one parent, **Aa**, has the disease. The other parent, **aa**, does not. Of four children, on average, two would be affected and two unaffected. There are no unaffected carriers,

Table 16.3 The inheritance pattern for a dominant condition (e.g. FAP)

Dominant	a	a
A	Aa	Aa
a	aa	aa

Table 16.4 The inheritance pattern for a recessive condition (e.g. cystic fibrosis)

Recessive	B	b
B	BB	Bb
b	bB	bb

as inheriting the gene gives you the disease. In Table 16.4, the abnormal version is b, and it is recessive to B. Both parents are **Bb** and therefore they do not have the disease as one of their two versions is normal. However, they both carry the disease and can pass it on to their children. On average, of four children, one will have the disease (bb), one will be completely free of the disease (BB) and two will be carriers (Bb), like their parents. It should be emphasized that these are only average figures – one could have five affected children with a recessive condition out of five born. This outcome is statistically unlikely but certainly possible.

For X-linked recessive conditions, such as haemophilia, boys have the disease and girls carry it. This is because boys do not have another X chromosome to balance the one with the abnormal gene. If a girl were to inherit an abnormal gene on her X chromosome from both parents, she would of course also have the disease, but this is unusual.

It is often possible to recognize the autosomal dominant, autosomal recessive or X-linked mode of inheritance from the family tree but it must be recognized that small families and incomplete penetrance may cause some problems.

Chromosomal disorders

Mendel could not know that genes, residing on chromosomes, were the units of inheritance that he was studying. However, chromosomal disorders are not often inherited. They can be divided into abnormalities of number and structure. Many chromosomal abnormalities result in spontaneous abortion. The phenotype of clinical disorders in liveborn babies is complex as a large number of genes are often involved. An example of a chromosomal abnormality is Down's syndrome, in which there are three copies (trisomy) of chromosome 21 – usually two from the mother and one from the father.

Structural abnormalities result from chromosomal breakage. This can result in shortened chromosomes or chromosomes that break and form unusual structures, such as rings. These can be seen in normal individuals, but if the breaks are large or in a critical place they can cause a wide range of disease. They may not be inherited if they affect fertility, but otherwise can be passed on to the next generation.

Polygenic and multifactorial diseases

In many adult diseases there is no suggestion of simple mendelian inheritance; nevertheless, there may be reasons to suspect a genetic component. Different ethnic groups within the same population can have very different frequencies of particular diseases, and migration studies have shown that an individual's risk of a particular disease may depend critically on the age at which the migration took place. In multiple sclerosis it has been shown that migration from a high to a low incidence area after adolescence does not result in a lower risk of suffering multiple sclerosis, implying a genetic and environmental interaction that is limited in time.

Analysis of families shows that there is a familial component to many human diseases. Although families have a common environment as well as common genes, a number of diseases are thought to be due to inheritance of particular mixes of genes whose products influence the response of the body to various environmental insults such as viruses, bacteria and chemicals. However, it has been extremely difficult to discover which particular genes are interacting and are thus responsible for these conditions. Coronary heart disease is an example of the interaction of environment and genetic susceptibility causing family aggregation of the condition.

The relevance of basic human genetics to the family cancer clinic

The importance of the description above is that in the family cancer clinic one may be faced by families where the cancers seen could be explained by a single dominant or recessive gene. If the gene is known, it is possible, using modern laboratory techniques, to look for defects in the chromosome or the gene structure or location. If the person has inherited the defect, he or she will be at an increased risk (possibly very much increased risk) of developing cancer in a particular organ or organs. If a particular susceptibility is recognized, appropriate action can be taken. If the gene is not known, but its approximate position in the human gene map has been established, there are other techniques that can be used to give an estimate of the likelihood that that person has inherited an abnormal copy of the gene. Again action can be taken.

If neither the gene nor its position is known, empirical estimates of risk must be made based on large studies of the type of inheritance, the number of cancers in the family in proportion to its size, the age of onset of the cancers and other factors. In this situation, determining the correct course of action is more difficult, but can be based on the individual's perception of the risk and the screening programmes that can be offered. When the empirical risk is low, it is not feasible to screen family members but reassurance can be given and sensible adjustment of environmental hazards (e.g. smoking) can be made. Finally, there may be chromosomal disorders in the family which may result in loss of genetic material that suppresses cancer. Some high-risk family members could therefore be identified by chromosomal analysis.

APPENDIX II

Familial cancer syndromes – dominant or recessive?

It is important to establish whether a particular disease is dominantly or recessively inherited. In the case of the familial cancer syndromes, most of them are dominantly inherited (see Table 16.3). This enables genetic diagnosis and/or screening to be carried out as discussed above. There are some recessively inherited syndromes such as ataxia telangiectasia and Fanconi anaemia, but affected family members are not commonly seen in adult family cancer clinics. The question of cancer susceptibility in the carriers is of considerable interest. In these syndromes, there may be abnormal sensitivity to a particular agent, such as sunlight or X-rays. Reducing exposure to the agent may have some effect on the incidence of cancer, including the apparently unaffected carrier. The typical syndromes seen in the clinic are discussed below.

Dominant pedigrees and syndromes associated with family cancer

Site-specific colon cancer and family cancer syndrome

Site-specific colon cancer (SSCC) is more often referred to as Lynch I; family cancer syndrome (FCS) is more often referred to as Lynch II. These disorders are the most common causes of hereditary non-polyposis colon cancer. The colorectal features are similar. Florid polyposis does not usually occur, but colonic adenomas (particularly right sided) are more common. Lynch II is defined by an additional predisposition to extracolonic cancers; endometrial cancer is the most common followed by breast, stomach and pancreatic cancer (Hodgson and Mahr 1992).

Muir Torre syndrome

This syndrome comprises autosomal dominant inheritance of carcinomas of the colon, duodenum and larynx in association with keratoacanthomas and sebaceous cysts (Muir, Yates Bell and Barlow 1967).

Cowden's syndrome

Adenomas and fibromas of the thyroid, gastrointestinal tract and skeletal system are found in association with lipomas, sebaceous cysts and angiomas. The greater risk is for benign and malignant disease of the breast and thyroid (Gentry, Eskritt and Gorlin 1974).

Gorlin's syndrome

This is a dominantly inherited cancer disorder characterized by multiple basal cell naevi of varying degrees of malignancy. Other features include rib abnormalities and cysts of the mandible or maxilla. Other malignancies occur, including medulloblastoma and, more rarely, colorectal cancer (Murday and Slack 1989).

Examples of dominant pedigrees seen in the clinic and screening offered

Pedigree 2

II.02   Cancer of the hepatic flexure age 63; cancer of the sigmoid colon age 66.

II.05   Cancer of the ascending colon, age 43; cancer of the rectum, age 61.

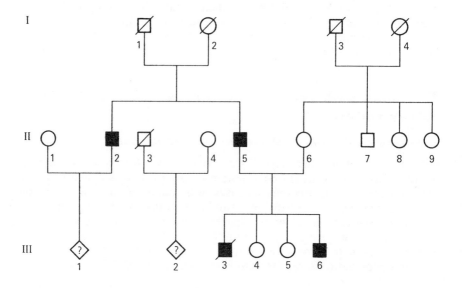

III.03   Cancer of the sigmoid colon, age 41; cancer of the stomach, age
43.
III.06   Cancer of the ascending colon, age 29 (24 polyps in specimen)

Appropriate screening offered to III.01, III.02, III.04, III.05 and follow-
up screening to III.06.

Pedigree 3

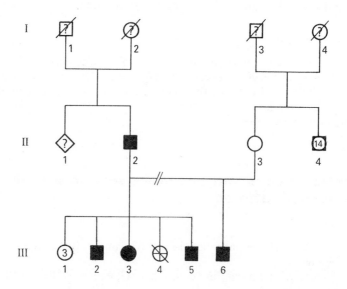

III.06 Presented with cancer of the rectum, age 38 years, June 1987
III.04 Sister died previously: carcinomatosis, aged 27 years
III.03 Sister diagnosed previously: cancer of the colon, aged 36 years
III.05 Brother diagnosed with cancer of the colon, aged 41 years, September 1991
III.02 Brother diagnosed with cancer (original site unknown), aged 37 years, September 1990

Proband III.06: not referred to the Family Cancer Clinic until 1991. If referred in 1987, III.05, III.02 and II.02 as well as III.03 would have been recommended screening.

REFERENCES

Gentry, W.C., Eskritt, N.R. and Gorlin, R.J. (1974) Multiple hamartoma syndrome (Cowden's disease). *Archives of Dermatology*, **109**: 521–5.

Hardcastle, J.D. and Pye, G. (1989) Screening for colorectal cancer: a critical review. *World Journal of Surgery*, **13**: 38–44.

Harper, P. (1992) *Practical Genetic Counselling*. Butterworth-Heinemann: Oxford.

HNPCC (1992) *Newsletter*, May: 2.

Hodgson, S. and Mahr, E. (1992) *A Practical Guide to Human Cancer Genetics*. Cambridge University Press: Cambridge.

Houlston, R. (1992) Genetic epidemiology colorectal, breast and ovarian cancer: use in clinical practice. PhD thesis, University of London.

Houlston, R.S., Murday, V., Harocopos, C., Williams, C.B. and Slack, J. (1990) Screening and genetic counselling for relatives of patients with colorectal cancer in a family cancer clinic. *British Medical Journal*, **301**: 366–8.

Lovett, E. (1974) Familial factors in the aetiology of cancer of the bowel. *Proceedings of the Royal Society of Medicine*, **67**: 751–5.

Lynch, H.T., Schuelke, G.S., Kimberling, W.J. et al. (1985) Hereditary non-polyposis colorectal cancer (Lynch syndromes I and II). Biomarker studies. *Cancer*, **56**: 939–51.

Lynch, H.T., Lanspa, S.J., Bowman, B.M. et al. (1988) Hereditary non-polyposis colorectal cancer – Lynch syndromes I and II. *Gastroenterology Clinics of North America*, **17**: 679–712.

Marteau, T. (1993) Psychological consequences of screening for Down's syndrome. *British Medical Journal*, **307**: 146.

Marx, J. (1993) New colon cancer gene discovered. *Science*, **260**: 751–2.

Mecklin, M.T. (1960) Inheritance of cancer of the stomach and large intestine in man. *Journal of the National Cancer Institute*, **24**: 55–71.

Mecklin, J.P. and Jarvinen, J. (1986) Clinical features of colorectal carcinoma in cancer family syndrome. *Diseases of the colon and rectum*, **29**: 160–4.

Morson, B.C. (1974) The polyp–cancer sequence in the large bowel. *Proceedings of the Royal Society of Medicine*, **67**: 451–7.

Muir, E.G., Yates Bell, A.J. and Barlow, K.A. (1967) Multiple primary carcinomata of the colon, duodenum and larynx associated with keratoacanthomata of the face. *British Journal of Surgery*, **54**: 191–5.

Murday, V. (1989). Family cancer screening. In: *Screening for Colorectal Cancer*. Proceedings of an international meeting (UKCCCR). Royal College of Physicians, May 1989.

Murday, V. and Slack, J. (1989) Cancer surveys. *Colorectal Cancer*, **8** (1): 139–57.

Office of Population Censuses and Surveys (1985) *Mortality Statistics in England and Wales*. HMSO: London.

Williams, C.B. and Macrae, F.A. (1986) The St Mark's neoplastic polyp follow-up study. *Frontiers of Gastrointestinal Research*, **10**: 226–42.

Woolfe, C.M. (1958) A genetic study of carcinoma of the large intestine. *American Journal of Human Genetics*, **10**: 42–7.

FURTHER READING

Connor, J.M. and Ferguson-Smith, M.A. (1992) *Essential Medical Genetics*. Blackwell Scientific: Oxford.

Harper, P.S. (1992) *Practical Genetic Counselling*. Butterworth-Heinemann: Oxford.

King, R. and Stansfield, W. (1990) *A Dictionary of Genetics*. Oxford University Press: Oxford.

Acknowledgements

I sincerely thank Dr Joan Slack for her infectious enthusiasm for the Family Cancer Clinic and her comments on this chapter, also Dr W. Foulkes and Dr R. Houlston for their contribution.

17 Discharge planning for the person with a stoma

Marion Allison

INTRODUCTION

The majority of people with a newly formed stoma will look forward to the day when they are discharged from hospital. This event signifies for many that they have made a successful recovery from the trauma of surgery and are ready to leave the protected surroundings of the hospital for their own familiar environment where they can begin to resume a normal life.

However, discharge planning for the person with a stoma involves much more than the single event of transferring the patient from hospital into the community. It is an ongoing process in which each person's individual needs in adapting to and managing the stoma are identified. A systematic plan is then developed, implemented and evaluated to ensure that these needs are met and the patient can achieve an optimum level of independence and receive appropriate continuing care at home.

The length of stay in hospital following stoma-forming surgery, and thus the time available for discharge planning, is not determined only by the patient's rate of recovery. Part of the present political agenda is aimed at improving the National Health Service. Strategies for achieving this goal include the reduction of waiting lists and providing cost effectiveness (Malby 1992). New surgical techniques for stoma formation such as laparoscopic assisted surgery, which reduce the trauma of operation, are becoming more widely used. Moves towards increasingly early discharge may therefore arise from political, managerial or medical sources; nurses need to ensure that the quality of discharge planning, patients' ability to manage at home and arrangements for continuity of care are not compromised as a result.

GOALS OF DISCHARGE PLANNING

It is important for nurses involved in the process of discharge planning to have a good understanding of the goals to be met. These focus on:

- Enabling patients to return home with the practical daily care of the stoma and appliance managed safely and effectively, through their own abilities or those of a relative or care giver.
- Enabling patients to receive continued and co-ordinated care of a practical and/or supportive nature, according to individual needs, in the community setting.
- Enabling patients to maintain progress towards physical, psychological and social rehabilitation and either resume a normal lifestyle or, where this is not possible, to maintain the optimum quality of life that can be achieved.

These goals should be considered by the nurse in relation to the unique circumstances of each patient who has stoma-forming surgery. It is essential to involve the patient, their relatives and any care givers at all stages of planning and decision making if a successful outcome is to be achieved. Such participation will help to reassure them that their needs will be met in the community and reduce the anxiety that often emerges as they begin to contemplate the reality of life at home with a stoma.

A clear idea of individual needs, which includes assessment of factors influencing the time required for development of self-care, together with accurate documentation of the patient's progress towards competence, will provide essential information to support the nurse's judgement that discharge should, on particular occasions, be deferred.

Learning needs and the teaching process

Recovery from the physical effects of surgery and the development of practical skills in stoma and appliance management are the two criteria generally used to determine the patient's readiness for discharge home (Donaldson 1989; Wade 1989). Therefore, much of the teaching that is undertaken in the postoperative period is directed towards enabling the patient to regain independence by acquiring practical stoma management skills. This focus on practical issues is entirely appropriate since it reflects patients' expressed priorities for learning (Kelly and Henry 1992). In this descriptive study by Kelly and Henry, information about equipment and appliances, management of leakage and odour, and practical ways of living a normal life with a stoma were identified as areas of most concern and the ostomists wanted to acquire the appropriate skills to cope in their new situation. In addition, as Mead (1994) points out, it is unlikely that patients will successfully adapt psychologically and emotionally to the body image changes related to stoma formation if they have not achieved confidence and competence in practical stoma care.

It is essential to assess each person's needs, concerns and unique circumstances, and then implement a planned programme of teaching in which realistic short-term goals are set (Curry 1991; Donaldson 1989) and the patient's progress is evaluated systematically. Practical self-care, or psychomotor learning, needs to be supported with sufficient understanding if patients are to become capable of initiating actions and carrying out procedures effectively when they return home. Teaching will be more effective if thought is given to the quantity and type of information the particular patient requires, which should include the principles and rationale underlying the practical aspects of the procedure, communicated in a clear and simple way that avoids the use of unnecessary jargon.

Postoperative teaching for many patients is part of a continuing process initiated and co-ordinated by the stoma care nurse; it begins with an initial assessment in their own home or the outpatient department and is developed in the preoperative period. Initial teaching will provide opportunities to discuss the construction and position of the stoma, what it will look like and how it will function, and to address any questions that the patient may have. Patients who have been able to reduce their fears and anxieties relating to stoma formation through preparation and appropriate teaching should be able to undertake new learning in the postoperative period that builds on the knowledge they have already acquired. However, when emergency surgery is performed for acute illness or trauma, the nature and focus of preoperative preparation is different owing to the patient's poor condition and the need for early surgical intervention; the shock related to the stoma, changes in the appearance of the body and the prospect of uncontrolled elimination can lead to further distress as their implications become apparent. Compassionate care and unconditional support are required, and the development of a positive outlook and successful coping can be much harder to achieve, with continuing psychological difficulties after surgery (Wade 1989). These patients will often require more time to work through their sense of loss and feelings of abnormality in the postoperative period; their readiness to retain new information and learn new skills may also be impaired, such that effective teaching commences later and proceeds at a slower pace. In common with all other patients with newly formed stomas, their ability to carry out stoma care may also vary from day to day (Dudas 1986).

Any formal teaching that is planned should progress from a comprehensive, individualized assessment that addresses the following questions:

1. What can the patient already do?
2. What does the patient already know?
3. How confident/effective is the patient in carrying out the specific aspects of care he/she has learned?
4. Does the patient need to consolidate previous learning?
5. Does the patient have specific concerns/learning needs that need to be addressed?
6. Is the patient ready to undertake new learning?
7. Is the patient willing and able to undertake new learning?

This will help to ensure that the teaching which is undertaken addresses the patient's particular needs, is paced and sequenced appropriately and, by avoiding needless overteaching (Wilson and Desrisseaux 1983), promotes effective use of the available time. Planning proceeds logically by considering the information gained during assessment and should be individualized by considering:

1. What is the next appropriate aspect of continued learning?

2. What specific goals/learning outcomes should be set?
   a. what will the patient be able to do?
   b. what essential information does the patient require?
3. Does the patient agree that the goals set are appropriate?
4. What teaching activities can be used appropriately, through which this patient can achieve the stated goals?
5. How can a suitable environment be developed to facilitate this patient's learning (e.g. time required, minimizing interruptions, providing privacy, provision of aids to learning).

Decisions about methods to be used depend on the patient's preferred ways of learning, the specific nature of the learning to be achieved, and the desired degree of patient participation. Within any particular episode of teaching, the roles of the nurse and the patient may vary according to the particular learning outcome and the patient's abilities, confidence and previous learning.

Evaluation will focus on the extent to which the patient reaches the intended goal, and it is essential that the patient is involved at this stage of the process. Besides determining the extent of the patient's understanding and practical skills, this will also provide useful feedback on his or her emotions and feelings during the learning experience. This will help the nurse in determining whether the patient is ready to progress, requires further practice to increase self-confidence, or needs to explore and resolve negative feelings or anxieties which arise.

PROGRESSION TOWARDS SELF-CARE

There is a limited amount of research-based information about the extent to which nurses caring for stoma patients are successful in helping them to achieve self-care. Collins (1988) investigated the work of 20 nurses, who each undertook an appliance change, by dividing the procedure into seven stages and observing the nurses' role during each stage, based on the helping methods identified by Orem (1980) (Table 17.1). The postoperative stage reached by the patients ranged from 2 to 33 days after surgery; 14 patients had reached at least 7 days after surgery but nurses either acted for or taught the patient throughout the procedure. In only five appliance changes were patients guided or supported to carry out patient care, and this greater involvement bore no relation to the period of time since surgery. Patients were involved to some extent in the preparation of equipment on just three occasions, and disposal on all observed changes was undertaken entirely by the nurse. Only one appliance change was carried out in the bathroom, where reasonable privacy could be expected, 16 occurred in the ward, two in the sluice area, and one in the treatment room, where a sterile technique was attempted. None of the nurses measured the stoma before fitting the clean appliance, although it is known that the size of the stoma decreases in the early weeks after surgery. The researcher also noted that nurses varied in their manner of completing written records of appliance changes in the patients' notes, which contained 'duplication, deficits and discrepancies' (Collins 1988: p. 30).

Table 17.1 Self-care and the patient with a newly formed stoma

Helping method	Roles of the nurse and patient
Acting for another	The nurse *demonstrates* skilled and dexterous stomal cleansing and change of the appliance
Teaching	The nurse *demonstrates* component subskills in an appropriate sequence that can be learned by the patient. *Verbal teaching and explanation* of how each is done
Guiding	The patient participates in guided practice *of each subskill*, learning to prepare and manipulate the appliance. The nurse provides appropriate *verbal cues, encouragement* and *feedback on performance*
Supporting	The patient continues to *practise* stoma care and appliance changing. The nurse provides *reassurance* by his or her *presence, encouragement* and *feedback*
Providing a developmental environment	Should be created with all helping methods – privacy is ensured, individual differences recognized and allowed for. Patient develops *mastery* by having sufficient opportunities to initiate and carry out appliance changes and stoma care alone in the bathroom. Nurse *discusses* adapting daily routine to home environment

Based on helping methods identified by Orem (1980).

Published in the following year, Ewing's (1989) study collected data on the extent of self-care preparation of 12 patients over time, by observing a total of 53 appliance changes. Nine aspects of physical care were identified, comprising elements of appliance management, and Orem's (1980) helping methods were again used as the basis for categorizing the nurse's role in self-care preparation. It was found that little attention was given to the preparation and disposal of equipment, and patients were not actively involved in these aspects of care. In the majority of appliance changes, the nurse provided the care for the patient. Lack of co-ordination resulted in patients developing some self-caring skills but during later appliance changes they reverted to non-participation. By the time of discharge no patient had been observed to be self-caring in all nine aspects of care. Nurses acknowledged in some cases that patients had been discharged while unable to fully manage the practical care of the stoma and appliance. In addition, they also wrongly assumed that patients had developed self-care abilities and withdrew assistance prematurely. Lack of privacy emerged as an additional problem – in 44 of the appliance changes, privacy was not assured, mainly because of interruption by other nurses.

Taken together, the results of these studies indicate:

1. Patients were insufficiently prepared to be self caring in stoma and appliance management.
2. Lack of appropriate, accurate and detailed written information contributed to the problem of insufficient preparation.
3. The approach to teaching was uncoordinated and unsystematic.
4. Teaching was not tailored to an assessment of individual patients' needs.
5. The environment in which teaching took place was usually not conducive to learning.
6. Some nurses involved in postoperative appliance changes demonstrated inappropriate care.

It would not be appropriate to attempt to generalize the findings of these studies, mainly because of small sample size and non-random selection. However, Wade (1989) interviewed 263 subjects from 21 health districts and established that 10% had not practised an appliance change before discharge and a further 10% stated that they had had insufficient practice. A significant number of people may leave hospital without sufficient skills, or lacking confidence in their ability, to carry out practical stoma management. These findings should prompt nurses who bear responsibility for helping patients to achieve self-care before discharge to question whether their own practices could be improved, and also to involve the patient in evaluating the outcomes and effectiveness of plans devised for teaching stoma and appliance management in the postoperative period.

Specific aspects of stomal and appliance management which should be included in the teaching plan before discharge are summarized in Table 17.2. The procedure that patients are taught to enable them to undertake effective practical stoma and appliance management should be as simple as possible. An uncomplicated routine will facilitate learning, lessen the time that has to be spent each day carrying out stoma care, ease the process of adapting a procedure learned in hospital to the home environment and decrease the potential for developing ritualistic and obsessive management habits which can interfere with the resumption of normal living and decrease self-esteem.

Gentle peristomal cleansing should be taught, using plain water and toi-

Table 17.2 Aspects of appliance and stoma management to include in a teaching plan

Normal stomal function
Type of appliance required: size/measurement, preparation, application, removal
Caring for the stoma and peristomal skin
Obtaining supplies
Storing supplies
Disposal of used appliances at home
Exemption from prescription charges
Recognizing complications
Dealing with problems: leakage, soreness, odour, flatus

let tissue or a disposable cloth, followed by thorough drying before the new appliance is fitted. Some patients may require the use of accessories such as filler pastes and skin barriers to ensure that leakage and skin problems do not arise. However, careful selection of an appliance with a sufficient area of hypoallergenic skin protective and an appropriately sized or cut aperture will ensure that most patients' needs for skin protection can be met.

Sufficient time should be spent exploring individual home circumstances with the patient so that they can make appropriate arrangements for obtaining, storing and disposing of their appliances (see Chapter 18).

It is worth exploring whether written documentation can be improved so that a clear and accurate record of the patient's progress can be maintained. There is a choice between the use of a special chart that details

Some simple steps to going home	
Name .... Stoma type································· Date of surgery .... Discharge: name of appliance .... size of appliance................ Frequency of bag change.......................	
When the patient has achieved all these steps he/she will be, with regard to stoma care, ready to go home	Please tick and date this column when patient has achieved the step and feels confident about it.
11 Whole procedure without supervision	
10 Whole procedure under supervision	
9 Disposal of soiled bag/tissues	
8 Reapply the new bag (identify the name and size of bag)	
7 Cleanses skin, dries skin around stoma	
6 Removes soiled bag	
5 Prepares the new bag	
4 Can identify all equipment needed to take to bathroom for bag change	
3 Has observed stoma	
2 Can empty bag with supervision, and refasten clip	
1 Able to fasten clip on bag	
This must be updated by stoma care nurse specialist and ward staff on a daily basis.	

Fig. 17.1 Stoma care discharge form.

the steps of a complete appliance change (Fig. 17.1) and the use of the nursing care plan; sometimes both systems are used concurrently. Whichever system is adopted, key issues that need to be addressed are the avoidance of duplication, responsibility for completion, and the document's status as a nursing record.

Where care plans exist, these constitute a primary nursing record, and the qualified nurse who directly cares for the patient is responsible for their completion. If 'inability to meet elimination needs due to stoma formation' or a similarly phrased problem is identified, the nurse should record the patient's progress appropriately and the stoma care nurse can also contribute to this record. The problem of duplication of written information sometimes arises when a special chart is introduced to document progression towards self-care; unless time is taken to discuss the importance of completing the chart and ward nurses as well as stoma care nurses are involved in this documentation, some will see this additional charting as the responsibility of the stoma nurse and will not update it. However, the stoma care nurse is not usually present at all appliance changes so there is a risk that the chart also fails to reflect the current abilities of the patient. If the chart is used alone, there is sometimes insufficient space to record relevant information relating to patient progress. The chart can, however, be used for additional purposes, such as enabling the patient to record when he or she feels competent and confident to undertake each step and is ready to progress to the next, or be used as an evaluative written record that the patient has carried out all stages successfully in the presence of the nurse prior to discharge. Whichever documentation is chosen will obviously depend on negotiation between the stoma care nurse and the ward nursing staff, but there should be good communication and agreement about both the responsibility for completion and the minimum detail required within the nursing record. Finally, it should be established that any additional chart will be kept with the nursing care plan when the patient's records are stored following discharge.

PSYCHOLOGICAL AND SOCIAL ADAPTATION

The process of adapting to the presence of a stoma, its daily management and resuming a normal lifestyle takes time. With a general trend towards reduction of the postoperative hospital stay, the true impact of surgery may only become apparent after discharge home. Whilst regaining physical independence and self-care are priorities, patients' psychological needs should not be underestimated.

With physical recovery comes a lessening of the close observation and nursing attention of the early postoperative phase, but this is sometimes interpreted by the patient as a form of rejection (Dudas 1986). Referring to his own experience of ileostomy formation, Kelly (1985) wrote that, 'I thought I was getting less attention from the nurses. I was short tempered and each visiting time would gasp a list of complaints to my wife' (p. 520). Reasons for changes in care and level of support should be discussed with the patient. Negotiation of self-care responsibility as new skills are developed, together with reinforcement that practical stoma care can be achieved should help to maintain self-esteem, decrease fears of rejection and facilitate psychological adaptation. Ongoing assessment within an open, sensitive and trusting nurse–patient relationship will provide nurses with insight into appropriate ways of helping individual patients with a newly formed stoma at a time when emotional strength and readiness to learn are labile.

The presence of a supportive spouse, partner or family member is influential in helping the patient to adjust to a new stoma (Wade 1989). Positive attitudes and the demonstration of loving concern help to resolve fears of rejection, maintain feelings of self-worth and provide patients with a sense of continued acceptance by those who have significance in their lives. The patient's partner and family should be provided with opportunities to obtain information and themselves receive support so that they can understand the implications of surgery, have realistic expectations of progress in the postoperative period and following discharge home and be able to participate in a helpful way with the patient's rehabilitation and re-integration into society.

Plans for discharge need to be made with the patient and close relatives as most support provided in the early days at home is inevitably provided by the family. Many partners express an interest in the practicalities of stoma management and, if the patient is in agreement, it is helpful to teach them the procedure during the hospital stay. Unless, owing to a poor prognosis or disability, a partner or spouse is to assume responsibility for daily stoma care, it is often appropriate to wait to do this until the patient has achieved a sufficient degree of competence and confidence to be able to personally demonstrate the appliance change. Besides providing reassurance for the partner that the stoma can be adequately managed, this approach also decreases the possibility that, in an effort to be supportive, they will promote dependence by performing the procedure for the patient after discharge.

Postoperatively, patients may express doubts that they will ever achieve a return to their previous lifestyle. Being given the opportunity to talk to an established ostomist who has adapted well to life after surgery can allay such apprehensions; subjects in Kelly and Henry's (1992) study evaluated this event very positively. Their perceptions were of somebody who looked normal and was living a normal life; moreover, the information provided by those who had experienced a similar situation and coped successfully was deemed to be more credible than that obtained from other sources. A sense of isolation on returning home can also be reduced by the provision of information about appropriate voluntary associations and the knowledge that advice can be obtained through telephone contact.

Thorough preoperative assessment and insights into the patient's lifestyle obtained through the development of a supportive nurse–patient relationship should permit the nurse to anticipate specific concerns and focus discussion on these in the later postoperative period, including relatives where appropriate so that they are sufficiently prepared to support the patient on returning home. Adaptation can be promoted by making sufficient time available for the patient to consider aspects of daily life and how these may be affected by the presence of a stoma and providing sufficiently detailed

Table 17.3 Resuming a normal lifestyle – issues to explore

Diet
Clothing
Work: returning, coping with the stoma
Specific cultural issues
Social activities: sport, holidays, travel, going out
Personal relationships: partner, spouse, family members, disclosure to others
Sexual relationships, pregnancy
Sources of help: support groups, contact with a fellow ostomist, health care professionals, appliance manufacturers' helplines, information booklets

information to enable him or her to make reasonable adjustments and be prepared to deal with any problems that might arise on returning home. Table 17.3 identifies issues that commonly need to be explored.

Nurses who regularly care for patients with a newly formed stoma will often have sufficient knowledge and experience to support appropriate teaching, and this can be reinforced by making available information booklets that consider particular aspects of living in detail. Information given needs to be consistent and accurate and it is necessary to liaise closely with the stoma care nurse, the key multi-disciplinary team member in preparing the patient for discharge. Through the provision of continuing care the stoma care nurse ensures that issues to which patients assign low priority, or which they are not ready to address in the hospital environment, can be considered at a later time, according to individual needs.

Relatives and others close to the patient may ask how they can assist the patient on returning home. Price (1993) has built on the work of Cohen and McKay (1984) to develop a framework of social support categories that demonstrates the range of ways in which a positive contribution can be made (Table 17.4). Assessment of the stage of recovery and rehabilitation achieved, the patient's unique personal and social circumstances and the readiness and ability of others to help should enable the

Table 17.4 Social support categories

Tangible	Practical help – e.g. assistance with appliance change, obtaining stoma care supplies from chemist, accompanying on outings
Appraisal	Helping the patient to evaluate progress Listening to concerns, achievements; demonstrating empathy
Self esteem	Providing positive regard for the patient Making favourable comments about patients' appearance and abilities
Sense of belonging	Providing introductions back into the social setting Briefing others about body image concerns, patient sensitivities and patient-preferred ways of discussing or dealing with same

Source: Cohen and McKay (1984).

nurse to suggest appropriate options and activities for assistance, using the framework as a source of ideas.

Schover (1986) identified the return to a normal social schedule as one of the important factors in resuming a close and intimate relationship, the others being acceptance of being seen partially or completely unclothed by a partner and sharing the same bed. A private and supportive environment is required for the discussion of personal issues; an opening to explore these can be created by asking the patient, and the partner, if they have anticipated making any modifications to their normal arrangements and the reasons for them. This can provide an opportunity to assess the accuracy of current understanding, give relevant information to allay fears that physical contact may hurt the stoma, and help to confirm that normal life can gradually be resumed. It is usually advisable to do this with each partner separately at first as it cannot be assumed either that they will wish to discuss such issues together or that, in an effort to protect, support or reassure a partner, each will be openly communicative about their own feelings and anxieties.

It is known that patients who return home understanding that their stoma is to be temporary are less happy, experience less enjoyment of life, are less active and also reduce their social activities to a greater extent than those who have had a permanent stoma (Wade 1989). This is not surprising, as many temporary stomas occur as a result of emergency surgery. These patients face the prospect of a major change for which they have been little prepared; some may also live in hope of early reversal and may try to cope in the intervening period by ignoring the presence of the stoma or simply waiting this out (Wood and Watson 1977). Other patients, who have acquired a stoma as part of a palliative operative procedure for carcinoma, will require highly skilled and sensitive care in the postoperative period; they face an unpredictable but apparently hopeless future, living with the knowledge that surgery has not cured them of disease. Such patients may have extreme difficulty in reaching acceptance of the stoma and require the specialist experience and expertise of stoma care nurses, provided for as long as necessary and adapted to their changing individual needs. As plans for discharge are made and the time for returning home approaches, their hospital and community based role is irreplaceable in maintaining the therapeutic relationship, supporting patients and their relatives as they express their emotions and grief, and adapting physical care of the stoma to ensure that comfort and dignity are achieved.

THE ROLE OF THE STOMA CARE NURSE IN DISCHARGE PLANNING

The clinical nurse specialist role was first established to improve the quality of patient care and nursing practice (Georgopolous and Christman 1970). Today it is accepted that the role should remain patient centred and built around the provision of expert clinical care (Hamric and Spross 1989). The way in which individual stoma care nurses interpret their role in practice in relation to the process of discharge planning depends on the knowledge and skills of the ward nursing team, the needs and problems of individual patients and the division of the specialist's time between hospital and the community. Stoma care nurses obtain a considerable amount of job satisfaction from their patient care role and the help and support they provide (Hingley and Marks 1991). However, a heavy caseload and workload is a recognized source of occupational stress. The time available for care of individual patients is a finite resource and consideration has to be given to the most appropriate and effective use of time in the discharge planning role.

Earlier in the chapter the importance to patients of acquiring the ability to manage the stoma independently before discharge was stressed. Major responsibility for leading the effort to co-ordinate continuing care is assumed by the stoma care nurse (Rorden and Taft 1990), and this may be fulfilled in a number of ways. It is not possible or appropriate for all continuing direct care to be undertaken by the nurse specialist but the proportion of time spent on this aspect of the role will vary (Fig. 17.2) according to the competence of the nursing team and the constraints within which they work. Nurses regularly participating in the care of patients with newly formed stomas will have acquired sufficient experience and expertise to enable them to help the majority of patients to develop self-care abilities in a progressive and individualized way. Many are likely to have benefited from the teaching activities of the stoma care nurse or from a course of study such as the ENB 980, both of which will be designed to increase competence for the provision of optimum care.

An established link worker system can enhance patient care by promoting liaison and communication between the stoma nurse and other care team members; link nurses will act as a resource for colleagues to enable them to plan and implement appropriate care for patients with a

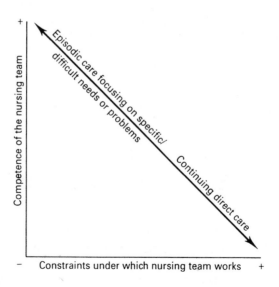

Fig. 17.2 Role of the stoma care nurse in the provision of direct patient care.

stoma in the absence of the specialist nurse, and evaluate its effectiveness. This system also frees the specialist nurse to focus his or her efforts on patients with specific, often complicated needs and problems. However, the context within which the nursing team works and the constraints to which they are subject do need to be taken into consideration. Factors such as skill mix, the organization of care delivery and the changing workload within the clinical area will all influence the stoma care nurse's role and will at times require him or her to exercise flexibility and alter the degree of continuing care provided as an individual to ensure that standards are maintained. One aim of the specialist nurse's intervention should be to develop the knowledge and skills of the nursing team so that their potential to provide effective care increases and, to this end, the ward nurse who has primary responsibility for the care of an individual with a stoma should be involved in all aspects of discharge planning and consulted about the patient's progress towards self-care.

The stoma care nurse can also plan to ensure that the patient's discharge needs are included and met appropriately by devising written protocols that can be discussed with nursing staff and then implemented in practice. Mead (1994) has described the use of a protocol designed to ensure that the practical aspects of stoma care have been covered prior to discharge home (Table 17.5); similar initiatives have been developed by other stoma care nurses.

The specialist nurse also has a good knowledge of the health resources available to the patient on returning home and will normally be responsible for informing the GP and district nurse of the patient's progress and degree of adjustment to the stoma together with details about current stoma management, including the appliance and any accessories used. It may, on occasion, be appropriate for the district and stoma care nurses to visit the newly discharged patient together shortly after returning home; this will be included in discharge planning arrangements either by direct

Table 17.5 Stoma care protocol – acute unit audit – 24 hours prior to discharge

Patient or carer can demonstrate ability to competently change the stoma pouch independently

Patient or carer can describe safe disposal of pouch at home

Patient or carer can identify normal skin, and the action to be taken if problems arise

Patient or carer can identify normal stoma function, and is aware of what action to take if abnormal function should occur

Patient or carer can identify his/her preferred supplier of stoma equipment, has detailed written information, and is given an adequate supply of correct appliances according to agreed policies

Patient or carer is offered a home visit and, if agreed, a date is arranged

Patient or carer has written information on how to contact the stoma nurse

© CliniMed Ltd (1994).

contact or through the discharge planning co-ordinator/community liaison sister.

The quality of care provided for patients with a newly formed stoma should be periodically reviewed and formally evaluated, and this is another facet of discharge planning in which the stoma care nurse participates. The information obtained is valuable, not only to enable informed decisions to be made about service development and improvement but also to permit achievement to be measured against specific defined standards.

In the current political and economic climate within the health service, purchasers are required to obtain an efficient, cost effective and high quality service, so it is imperative that the value of the service provided by the stoma care nurse can be clearly demonstrated. The role of the specialist nurse in stoma care is already being evaluated; Wade (1989) concluded that outcomes for patients with a stoma are better in health districts that employ stoma care nurses – patients are more knowledgeable, more proficient in self-care and more satisfied with the care they receive. Moreover, the presence of the stoma nurse who can provide continuity of care has enabled patients to be discharged earlier from hospital, although the study findings did not directly link a shorter stay to the intervention of a specialist nurse. The majority of stoma care nurses are, or have been, involved in defining the level of care they wish to achieve and the desired outcomes of that care, and in writing standards of care. Through this process it is possible to make explicit the responsibilities of the stoma care nurse in relation to discharge planning and the specialist input required to achieve high quality care.

Auditing the stoma care service can produce valuable evidence that efficient, effective professional care is being provided. The degree of patient satisfaction with the stoma care service was measured by Goodwin (1992) who specifically asked about preparation for discharge in the questionnaire she devised: 86.5% of respondents described themselves as confident on discharge. The patients' perspective is an important one, but additional objective evidence about the quality of the discharge planning process can be obtained by setting a standard for discharge planning and developing a specific audit tool. Audit tools developed for the stoma care nursing service at the Royal Marsden Hospital collected data from three perspectives – patient opinion, professional opinion (the specialist nurse) and documentation (Luthert and Robinson 1993). These demonstrate the approach of one specialist health care organization and are a useful resource to which to refer. However, stoma care nurses need to consider the nature of their individual services within their local health care system and determine in this context for themselves what should be achieved in relation to discharge planning and how this can be measured. Relevant and appropriate evidence will pertain to efficiency, effectiveness and the level, nature and outcomes of care provided but the criteria used for measurement and the way in which information is obtained are variable.

The formation of a stoma is an event that requires significant adjustment by patients if they are to be able to cope positively and return to a normal lifestyle in the future. In the postoperative period, skill and understanding demonstrated by the nursing team will promote the development of self-care abilities and initiate psychological adaptation. The specialist nurse in stoma care has a key function in co-ordinating care in hospital and 'bridging the gap' between hospital and home through the provision of continuity of care. The specialist role encompasses additional activities such as patient advocacy, liaison with and education of staff so that optimum care can be provided, and providing information and teaching for patients and their relatives so that they are confident of their ability to cope at home. In the present climate of the National Health Service, it is imperative that the central role of the stoma care nurse is recognized in the discharge planning process and measures taken to audit this aspect of care, initiate improvements if necessary and inform managers and purchasers of the quality of the service provided to ensure that this unique contribution is recognized.

REFERENCES

Cohen, S. and McKay, G. (1984) Interpersonal relationships as buffers of the impact of psychological stress on health. In: Baum, A., Singer, J. and Taylor, S. (eds) *Handbook of Psychology and Health.* Erlbaum: Hillsdale, NJ.

Collins, R. (1988) Patient teaching and stoma care. *Irish Nursing Forum and Health Services*, **6** (5): 29–31.

Curry, A. (1991) Returning home with confidence. *Professional Nurse*, **6** (9): 536–539.

Donaldson, I. (1989) Communication can help ostomists accept their stoma. *Professional Nurse*, **4** (5): **242**: 244–245.

Dudas, S. (1986) Psychosocial aspects of patient care. In: Smith, D. and Johnson, D. (Eds) *Ostomy Care and the Cancer Patient.* Grune & Stratton: Orlando, pp. 93–102.

Ewing, G. (1989) The nursing preparation of stoma patients for self care. *Journal of Advanced Nursing*, **14**: 411–20.

Georgopoulos, B. and Christman, L. (1970) The clinical nurse specialist: a role model. *American Journal of Nursing*, **70** (5): 1030–9.

Goodwin, K. (1992) An insight into patient satisfaction. *Professional Nurse*, **8** (3): 153, 155–6.

Hamric, A. and Spross, J. (1989) *The Clinical Nurse Specialist in Theory and Practice*, 2nd edn. W.B. Saunders: Philadelphia.

Hingley, P. and Marks, R. (1991) Stoma care: a stressful occupation. *Nursing Times*, **87** (25): 63, 65–6.

Kelly, M. (1985) Loss and grief reactions as responses to surgery. *Journal of Advanced Nursing*, **10**: 517–25.

Kelly, M. and Henry, T. (1992) A thirst for practical knowledge. *Professional Nurse*, **7** (6): 350–1, 354–6.

Luthert, J. and Robinson, M. (Eds) (1993) *Royal Marsden Hospital Manual of Standards of Care.* Blackwell Scientific: Oxford.

Malby, R. (1992) Discharge planning. *Surgical Nurse*, **5** (1): 4, 6–8.

Mead, J. (1994) An emphasis on practical management. *Professional Nurse*, **9** (6): 405–6, 408–10.

Orem, D. (1980) *Nursing: Concepts of Practice.* McGraw-Hill: London.

Price, B. (1993) Profiling the high risk altered body image patient. *Senior Nurse*, **13** (4): 17–21.

Rorden, J. and Taft, E. (1990) *Discharge Planning for Nurses.* W.B. Saunders: Philadelphia.

Schover, M. (1986) Sexual rehabilitation of the ostomy patient. In: Smith, D. and Johnson, D. (Eds) *Ostomy Care and the Cancer Patient.* Grune & Stratton: Orlando, pp. 103–19.

Wade, B. (1989) *A Stoma is for Life.* Scutari: London.

Wilson, E. and Desrisseaux, B. (1983) Stoma care and patient teaching. In: Wilson Barnett, J. (Ed.) *Recent Advances in Nursing*, vol. 6: *Patient Teaching.* Churchill Livingstone: Edinburgh.

Wood, R. and Watson, P. (1977) People with temporary colostomies. *Canadian Nurse*, **73**: 28–30.

18 Continuing care in the community

Theresa Porrett and Jacqueline Joels

Successfully rehabilitating a stoma patient in the community means continuing the care provided in the hospital and preparing the patient for a new phase of life.

Black (1990)

INTRODUCTION

The role of the clinical nurse specialist in stoma care has four well defined areas: clinical practice, education, management/administration and as a resource or consultant. Continuing care of the patient in the community encompasses each of these facets. How these skills may be best employed in identifying problems and helping the individual towards rehabilitation are examined in this chapter.

WHY IS COMMUNITY STOMA CARE NECESSARY?

The stoma care nurse is one of very few health care professionals working within both the hospital and the community setting, often having a remit within each trust. He or she therefore provides a vital link to smooth the transition and aid communication at a point where there is potential for breakdown.

Discharge from the hospital environment, in which there is 24-hour support and help if required, is an extremely stressful and testing time for the new ostomist. 'Even with good preoperative counselling and effective practical teaching of basic stoma care, many patients do not fully realise the true impact of stoma surgery until they have been discharged from hospital' (Bradley 1990).

On returning home patients face the task of adaptation, aiming towards reintegration into society and their previous lifestyle. They require sound practical advice and the ability to put the practical skills learnt in hospital into everyday practice – reinforcement of these with informative literature as a point of reference is often valuable. Stoma care nurses are ideally placed to support patients through this transition as they have had the opportunity to develop a trusting and supportive relationship with them during the period of hospital admission. It is this continuity of care that is beneficial to patients in providing a stable background in which they can regain their confidence and self-esteem.

Once patients are physically feeling stronger and when they have time to reflect, the psychological impact of what has happened descends and patients often grieve for the loss of their former self and body part (Price 1990). Recognizing the stages through which they may pass during the grieving process helps their family to understand behaviour, which at times may be difficult. Wade (1989) identified 10 weeks postoperatively as being a 'low point' for patients psychologically. An appointment to attend the stoma clinic at this time may be worthwhile to ensure that all is well or offering a follow-up home visit, whilst remembering that the proverbial 'would you like a cup of tea, nurse?' may well mean 'I want to talk'.

One cannot prescribe continuing care in the community. There is much debate about the timing and frequency of home visits, but each patient needs to be assessed on an individual basis and care planned accordingly and in liaison with the district nurses. The 1980 DHSS paper on the provision of a stoma care service states that ostomists require continued care and advice after discharge from hospital but that the extent of these needs varies among patients. These variations depend on such factors as age, family circumstances, type of employment, whether the stoma is temporary or permanent and whether there are other associated nursing problems.

In summary, our aim is to assist individuals in their return to a fulfilling life, while maintaining a fine line between their feeling supported but not dependent. 'My confidence is maintained by the knowledge that help and advice is readily available should the need arise' (Jefferies et al. 1992).

CLINICAL PRACTITIONER

Central to the role of clinical nurse specialist in stoma care is the possession of expert knowledge and clinical skills. It is part of the role of clinical practitioner to instruct patients postoperatively to achieve self-care and to monitor their progress following discharge. A home visit provides the perfect opportunity to view patients holistically within their own surroundings to assess their level of stoma management and adaptation and to detect any problems, be they real or potential – making them aware of action to take and when to seek help. The most prevalent of these problems and suggested methods for treatment/future prevention are highlighted below.

Home visits also provide an opportunity to meet other family members or carers, who will often ask questions and express their fears and worries. These can act as indicators as to how the patient is adapting and being accepted.

Poor bathroom facilities

When they get home, many patients find it difficult to adapt the stoma management routine they developed in hospital. Perhaps they no longer have the convenience of a washbasin and toilet in the same room, a strategically placed full-length mirror and privacy.

A home visit allows the nurse to assess the bathroom facilities and perhaps offer practical advice to ease the situation. If necessary it will be possible to liaise with the social services regarding making any necessary changes.

Obtaining supplies

Obtaining regular supplies of appliances can initially be an area of great anxiety for patients. Before discharge patients will have been given a list of their stoma requirements to give to the GP. Patients who have a permanent stoma are exempt from prescription charges: an exemption certificate can be obtained from the GP's surgery. Once their prescription has been received, patients can either take it to the chemist, who will order the products and should have them ready for collection within five days, or they can use one of the many home delivery services available. The advantages of the delivery service are that patients do not have to collect the often bulky appliances from the chemist; appliances can be pre-cut on the receipt of a template from the stoma care nurse; patients also receive free disposable bags and free cleaning wipes. Storage of appliances needs to be discussed; for people with limited space, this can be a problem. Appliances need to be kept cool and out of direct sunlight; often a cupboard under the stairs or a spare room is used.

The first follow-up visit is a good opportunity to ensure that supplies have been received and to reinforce the procedure for reordering, remembering to keep a box in reserve to allow time for delivery. The stoma may need to be remeasured and prescription details altered as shrinkage occurs.

Poor technique

Talking to patients will highlight any practical stoma management problems, but watching patients perform an appliance change in their own home is useful to check their technique and assess their living conditions. 'Life with a stoma demands adaptation and changes in ingrained habits of personal hygiene' (Elcoat 1986). Subtle health education might be appropriate, advice regarding use of appropriate cleansing agents or the frequency of appliance changes.

Disposal

Is the patient disposing of the appliance in a responsible way? During the home visit this can be reinforced and the patient's understanding of the need for safe disposal reinforced.

To date, only one type of appliance is biodegradable and therefore can be flushed down the toilet. All other appliances need to be emptied of faeces and wrapped in a plastic bag or newspaper before being put in the dustbin. For those using a drainable appliance, this just means emptying it before removing the appliance. But for those using a closed type of appliance the bag needs to be cut using scissors and the faecal matter rinsed out either by holding it under the toilet flush or by filling it with water from a jug. This is time consuming and for many patients it is the aspect they find most unpleasant and degrading. We feel sure that a number of patients do not follow this procedure to the letter, but just place the used closed appliance in a sealed plastic bag in the dustbin. Disposal in public conveniences is almost impossible. The situation can be eased by using toilets for the disabled, in which there is a sink and plenty of space. Keys can be obtained – for a small charge – through RADAR (12 City Forum, 250 City Road, London EC1 8AF; tel. 0171-250 3222).

In many districts a soiled dressing collection facility is offered. However, this is not ideal as it means storing used appliances for a week in a yellow bag, and placing this outside the front door on the morning of collections. To many patients it is yet another stigma they can do without. For those living in accommodation without a garden, they have to keep the appliances indoors, which is not hygienic or pleasant. If this is a problem, a unit can be purchased which individually seals each bag and stores them within an odour-proof container until they can be disposed of.

Stoma care nurses should do all they can to ensure that patients are aware of the correct disposal for appliances and the rationale behind it – the fact that the appliances will probably be buried in landfill sites. If some patients choose not to follow these guidelines, there is very little that can be done. Recently, a patient said she did not feel that she should have to undertake what she described as a 'dirty and demeaning task'. She added 'How many mothers do you know who remove the faecal matter from a disposable nappy before they put it in the dustbin?'

POTENTIAL PROBLEMS

Skin soreness

This is without doubt the most commonly encountered physical problem in the community. However, recent years have seen the evolution of superior skin-protecting adhesives that have done much to overcome this, and barrier creams and wipes specifically for use in stoma care are now available. Early referral to the stoma care nurse allows the cause of the soreness to be identified and treated before the skin breaks down, leading to a myriad of problems with adhesion.

Causes

Decrease in stoma size can lead to sore skin and leakage problems. In the weeks following discharge from hospital the stoma may shrink as post-operative oedema resolves, so the size of the stoma requires monitoring as a smaller template or pre-cut appliance may be needed.

Soreness, caused by an *allergic sensitivity* to the appliance adhesive, is usually easily recognizable because it presents as a visible ring in accordance with the wafer's shape; it is not uncommon for this to occur after many years of using one product. Introduction of an alternative adhesive usually resolves the problem, but in cases where there is multi-sensitivity, 'patch testing' to exclude the offending one(s) is worthwhile.

Leakage beneath the appliance adhesive can rapidly lead to skin soreness, particularly if it is of small bowel fluid which contains digestive enzymes. Leakage is also distressing for the patient. Observing an appliance change will help to identify problems of poor technique, or potential channels for leakage such as skin creases, dips or scars.

Granulomas commonly form at the stoma edge; these are areas of over-granulated tissue, often caused as a result of friction from the appliance. Granulomas are harmless but may cause problems either from persistent bleeding or by hindering application of the bag. If so, they are easily treated by means of local cauterization with a silver nitrate pencil obtainable from chemists.

PARASTOMAL HERNIA

The development of a parastomal hernia can be a distressing situation for many patients; fears that a tumour may be recurring can initially cause a great deal of anxiety until the correct diagnosis is confirmed. For many people, the hernia may seem yet another alteration to their body image. If the hernia is small and is presenting no problems regarding stoma management, all that is required is regular monitoring of the hernia to ensure it is not increasing in size.

Parastomal hernias develop at any stage following stoma formation, so they tend to be reported to the stoma care nurse on a follow-up visit. There is a risk, as with all hernias, that the herniated loop of bowel may become strangulated and the blood supply cut off: this can lead to symptoms of acute pain and nausea/vomiting necessitating urgent surgical intervention. For the most part, though, parastomal hernias produce few symptoms and are treated conservatively unless the size of the hernia makes it impossible to apply a stoma pouch securely.

Problems may be caused when applying a pouch owing to the uneven contours of the hernia. The patient might need to be taught how to pleat the appliance to ensure a secure fit. A change to a different appliance with a more flexible flange may help in improving security, as may an appliance with an oval-shaped flange, which may adhere better around hernias than some conventionally shaped appliances.

If the hernia is large, it may cause a muscular dragging sensation around the stoma which can be uncomfortable. A corset/support girdle can be fitted for the patient, which not only supports the hernia, thereby reducing the dragging sensation, but also holds the hernia firmly in place, reducing its size and making it less visible under clothing. A number of companies produce these support girdles or belts, which are available on prescription. The fitting measurements can be taken by the appliance officer at the local hospital or by the stoma nurse; alternatively, a representative from the chosen company can be requested to do the fitting. These products have improved greatly over recent years and now look more like standard undergarments than surgical appliances.

AREAS FOR ADVICE

Discharge from the back passage

This can cause much distress to patients who often believe that something has gone wrong with their operation. Before patients go home it is important to forewarn them that it is not unusual, at times, to pass old faecal matter or mucus from the back passage; it is produced as the bowel's natural lubrication.

Bleeding from the stoma

As the stoma has such a good blood supply, slight bleeding may occur when cleaning. Advice must be sought if blood appears from inside the bowel.

Constipation/diarrhoea

Patients should be told that they can still be affected by constipation or diarrhoea. Certain foods or medications may be the cause, and they can adjust their diet accordingly. If either problem persists they should contact the stoma care nurse or GP for further advice.

Diet

Diet appears to be one of the main areas of confusion and conflicting advice. During the first home visit patients may well have many queries. Questioning them might reveal that they are restricting themselves to a bland and soft diet, often because this was the type of food they were eating in hospital after the surgery.

Many patients restrict their dietary intake in an attempt to reduce stoma output, so diet must be discussed fully with them. It is important to stress the importance of eating regularly to control stoma output and to promote normality by eating a varied and balanced diet whilst identifying and avoiding foods that cause flatus or diarrhoea.

An ileostomist must be aware that certain foods high in roughage may cause discomfort or even obstruction if eaten in large quantities. As long as these foods are chewed well, there is no reason why they should not be eaten in moderation. The key in these early stages must be experimentation. Patients should be encouraged to introduce items back into their diet and not to cut out certain foods because they have read somewhere that it did not agree with someone else. There should be no hard and fast rules regarding diet, but patients should be advised on an individual basis.

RELATIONSHIPS/SEXUAL PROBLEMS

A consultation at 10 weeks after surgery, whether in the patient's home or in the stoma clinic, is an appropriate time to establish whether physical relationships have resumed and if they are experiencing difficulties. Help and advice should be offered. It is often during a home visit that patients express their fears about sexual matters or personal relationships. They may well feel more able to discuss these very intimate matters with the stoma care nurse in the privacy of their own home rather than in hospital.

'Regular visits to the patient's home establishes a rapport with the patient, and the nurse is regarded as a confidante and friend with whom intimate subjects can be discussed' (Black 1990). This view was supported by the findings of Jefferies et al. (1995), whose research revealed that 96% of patients they interviewed felt they had received ample opportunity to discuss their feelings with their stoma care nurse (Fig. 18.1).

By exploring feelings with a person who is non-judgemental patients are often able to come to terms with their feelings. Stoma care nurses must, however, recognize their limitations as few are trained counsellors: if it is felt that a patient has severe emotional or sexual problems that exceed the nurse's area of expertise, the possibility of referral to a specialist should be discussed.

RETURNING TO WORK

There are a number of information leaflets on the subject that are useful for the patient to have as reference. Returning to work is a major achievement in the patient's rehabilitation but is also a time that can be fraught with anxiety. Some patients may be anxious about the reaction of their colleagues and employer, and it may be necessary for the stoma care nurse to liaise with the employer or occupational health department.

If it is not possible for a patient to return to a heavy manual job, advice may be required, in liaison with the disablement resettlement officer, about retraining or changing employment.

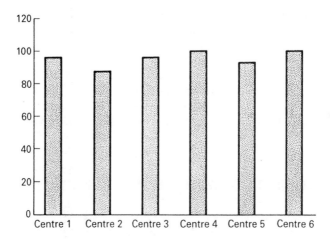

Fig. 18.1 Patient satisfaction with stoma care nurse. Patients were asked 'Do you feel that the stoma care nurse has given you ample opportunities to discuss your feelings?' Of the respondents, 95% knew how to contact their stoma care nurse; of these, only 1% did not feel free to do so.

RETURNING TO SOCIAL ACTIVITIES

Returning to social activities can prove difficult at first as patients may lack confidence and will have to work up to this slowly. For many, the first trip to the corner shop is a major stepping stone on which to build their further rehabilitation.

A study by Rubin and Devlin (1987) on the quality of life with a stoma found that, of the ileostomists and colostomists surveyed, 20% felt their social life to be restricted by fears of problems. A comparison of lifestyles before and after surgery was included in the research of Jefferies et al. (1995): it was pleasing to discover that, after just 3 months, 89% of the sample felt able to attend to their stoma away from home (Fig. 18.2).

Once patients are progressing well in their rehabilitation, it is time to stop regular home visits. Support can be offered in the form of clinic appointments for advice in resuming activities such as sports and travel as necessary. Rather than having formal, regular, clinic appointments, this ability to self-refer gives control back to the patients and allows them to choose how closely their progress is monitored. This informal patient-directed system of follow-up places responsibility with the individual but at the same time gives them the support they need.

RESOURCE/CONSULTANT

As a clinical nurse specialist, the stoma care nurse is considered an expert in his or her field and as such can be used as a resource person to be called on for advice when necessary. In the community, as in hospital, the stoma care nurse is working as part of a team. In the community this team

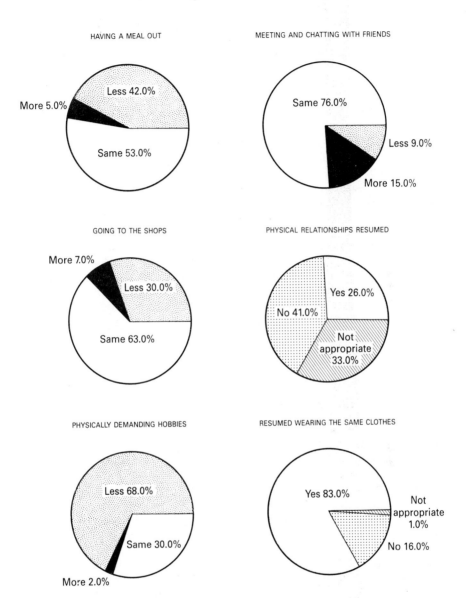

Fig. 18.2 Comparing lifestyles before and after operation. (Note that the questionnaires were answered only three months after the date of surgery.)

may consist of district nurse, GP, social services, voluntary organizations, pharmacy and home delivery service. As part of this team the stoma care nurse is responsible not only for the clinical monitoring of the patient but also for ensuring that all the other team members have the information and support that they require. The stoma care nurse can act as a link between team members, thereby ensuring that patients receive the support they need. It is worth remembering that the average GP practice may only have four or five stoma patients on their lists. They may therefore require a great deal of information regarding correct stock for ostomists, ensuring that the appliances are appropriate for each individual, reducing the incidence of skin problems and leakage, and thereby providing cost effectiveness. They may also need information on suitable medications for ostomists, for example codeine phosphate and loperamide for the treatment of a high output/fluid ileostomy.

It is the stoma care nurse who can help the development of local branches of the national ostomy support groups. These organizations can be called on to visit patients pre- or postoperatively. 'The ideal situation would be to have an integrated approach with the professional and voluntary helpers available for the patient's benefit during rehabilitation' (Black 1990). The visitors from the ostomy support voluntary organizations all have stomas themselves and are specially trained to talk to other patients. They can provide support for the patients and their families, based on their own experience.

Open days can be held in the community, when ostomy product manufacturers exhibit their products. These open days are an opportunity for patients to view and keep up to date on the latest products available but are also useful for hospital and community staff as a means of keeping up to date on current products.

EDUCATOR

The role of educator/teacher extends into the community. Not only are stoma care nurses educators for ostomists and their families, but they are also a teaching support for district nurses.

The teaching support required by district nurses will vary from district to district. In some instances all that will be needed is a joint home visit from the stoma nurse and the district nurse to highlight specific aspects of the patient's management. Often, more formal teaching sessions are requested by district nurses. These formal updates can take the form of full study days where a variety of topics, such as correct choice and fitting of appliances, skin care, fistula management, continence procedures and alternative methods of colostomy management are covered. Alternatively, half-day sessions can be held, looking at one subject in detail. The venue for these sessions can then be alternated among the various health centres, which allows a greater number of nurses the opportunity to attend.

Open days held in a local community venue are ideal opportunities to update patients and staff alike on new product developments. Representatives from the appliance manufacturing companies can be invited to attend, providing an exhibition of new appliances and accessories that patients and staff may not have been aware of. This also provides patients with the opportunity to obtain samples of products they might like to try.

Patients' information booklets and teaching aids are a valuable educational resource. Many of these information booklets have been written by stoma care nurses and have then been published by stoma appliance manufacturers. The booklets can be of great use in the community as a resource for district nurses, and can be obtained via the appliance company's representative. Currently, many study days and conferences are organized and financed by appliance manufacturers. This educational support has done much to further stoma education for nurses.

ADMINISTRATOR

The administrative role of the stoma care nurse is of vital importance if there is to be continuity of care and dissemination of information into the community. Records are kept on all stoma patients and it is essential that this information is up to date and available to district nurses when required. Many stoma care nurses use a written referral letter as a means of communicating patient details and progress on discharge. Although many nurses currently use handwritten patient record cards, there is a gradual move towards computerized record and data keeping which could greatly improve the dissemination of information as districts develop networking systems.

In the current climate of health care reforms and the development of trusts, many stoma care nurses are being called upon to write business plans for their service. These plans highlight the service provided and are of great use to the purchasers when looking at the range of cost-effective services they will buy.

Statistical data regarding the stoma care service are of great importance when it comes to identifying the work that is carried out in the community. A weekly record should be kept of the number of home visits made, the number of patients seen in the outpatient department, the number of patients seen in health centre-based stoma clinics and the number of telephone checks/follow-ups made. If possible, records should also be kept of the amount of time spent travelling to and from home visits. This information can be presented in the form of an annual report, which can be circulated not only to the hospital-based manager and surgeons but also to the district nurse manager.

With the division of many hospital and community services as they become separate trusts, there is a risk that the continuity of care enjoyed by patients and nurse specialists may be lost as the latter become employed by one trust only and their service is not purchased by the local community trust. Accurate statistical data identifying the amount and type of follow-up care carried out in the community will be useful if contracts need to be drawn up regarding the provision of stoma care in the community. These contracts may specify precisely the number and nature of home visits that will be purchased in the course of a year: accurate data from the previous year will be invaluable in the realistic negotiation of contracts.

CONCLUSION

It can be concluded that to prescribe the timing, frequency and level of care for patients in the community would be inappropriate and unrealistic, as each person will have specific needs requiring individual assessment.

Although striving towards a common goal, the delivery of care amongst stoma care nurses is diverse. Nevertheless, the study conducted by Jefferies et al. (1995) found that if patients are assured of a given degree of commitment both in hospital and in the community, and this is carried out, they will feel supported.

We have examined how the many facets of the stoma care nurse's role are a vital link for the multi-disciplinary team and in smoothing the transition for patients in their return to the community. It would be a great shame, therefore, if the advent of GP fundholders and separate trusts purchasing and providing services meant that this continuity of care became no longer available.

REFERENCES

Black, P. (1990) Community stoma care. *Nursing Standard*, **4** (43): 54–5.

Bradley, C. (1990) The role of the stoma care nurse. *Nursing*, **4** (18): 9–11.

Elcoat, C. (1986) *Stoma Care Nursing*. Baillière Tindall: London.

Harlow, J. (1988) Waste disposal. *Nursing Times*, **84** (8): 72, 75.

Jefferies, E., Butler, M., Cullum, R., et al. (1995) A service evaluation of stoma care nurses' practice. *Journal of Clinical Nursing*, **4** (4): 235–42.

Macdonald, L.D. (1984) Stigma in patients with rectal cancer: a community study. *Journal of Epidemiology and Community Health*, **38**: 284–90.

Price, B. (1990) *Body Image: Nursing Concepts and Care*. Prentice Hall: pp. 108–24.

Rubin, G.P. and Devlin, H.B. (1987) The quality of life with a stoma. *British Journal of Hospital Medicine*, **38** (4): 300–6.

Sadler, C. (1992) Working together. *Nursing Times*, **88** (22): 61–2, 64, 66.

Wade, B. (1989) *A Stoma is for Life*. Scutari Press: London.

Index